# CRITICAL CARE IN PATIENT TRANSPORT

Evidence-Based Textbook Covering Hemodynamic Support, Ventilator Strategies, and Multisystem Trauma for Flight Nurses



**Ramon C. Henson, MD**

This textbook is intended solely for educational and informational purposes and is designed to support the continuing professional development of licensed healthcare providers. The clinical content presented herein reflects information believed to be accurate and current at the time of publication; however, medicine evolves rapidly, and readers are advised that new research findings, updated clinical practice guidelines, and revised regulatory approvals may alter or supersede information contained in this work after its publication date.

Nothing in this publication constitutes medical advice, clinical guidance specific to any individual patient, or a substitute for the independent professional judgment of a licensed and qualified healthcare provider. No clinician-patient relationship is established, implied, or intended by the use of this textbook or any portion thereof. All clinical decisions, including but not limited to diagnosis, therapeutic selection, drug dosing, and patient monitoring, must be individualized based on thorough and direct assessment of the patient, the totality of current published evidence, applicable clinical practice guidelines, institutional protocols, and the informed professional judgment of the responsible clinician.

Drug information, dosages, treatment protocols, and therapeutic recommendations presented in this publication are offered for educational reference only and must be independently verified against current prescribing information, pharmacopeial references, and applicable regulatory approvals prior to clinical application. The author and publisher have made every reasonable effort to ensure the accuracy and completeness of the information presented; nevertheless, they expressly disclaim all liability for any adverse outcomes, clinical errors, patient harm, loss, or injury alleged to arise, directly or indirectly, from the use, misuse, or application of any information, recommendation, protocol, or clinical guidance contained in this publication.

# TABLE OF CONTENTS

# PREFACE

A critically ill patient does not become more stable by virtue of being moved. The ventilator settings, the vasoactive drips, the injured brain's fragile pressure balance, the coagulopathy still declaring itself—all of it travels with the patient into a vehicle or an aircraft, where the resources of the sending intensive care unit no longer exist and the resources of the receiving one have not yet arrived. The clinician managing that patient during transit is not practicing a lesser version of critical care medicine. They are practicing the same discipline under a narrower margin, with fewer hands, less monitoring redundancy, and a physiologic environment—altitude, vibration, acceleration, cabin pressure—that acts on an already unstable patient in ways a bedside ICU never has to consider.

This text exists because the clinical knowledge required to manage that patient safely is not simply critical care medicine plus a set of transport logistics bolted on. It is a distinct clinical competency: the ability to anticipate how a specific disease process, a specific device, or a specific injury will behave when altitude drops a ventricular assist device's flow, when a thirty-minute climb changes the volume of gas in an endotracheal cuff, when forty-five minutes of vibration and unmonitored positioning obscures the earliest signs of a bleed reaccumulating. The evidence is unambiguous that critical events during interfacility transport cluster predictably—around baseline instability, around mechanical ventilation, around specific windows of time in transit—and yet the clinician's training has rarely been organized around that predictability. This book is organized around it.

Every chapter in this text carries **The In-Transit Deterioration Signature System**, a structured pattern-recognition framework built directly into the clinical content. Each Signature names a specific, anticipatable deterioration pattern; identifies the Movement Trigger—the specific altitude, positional, or motion-related stress that provokes or unmasks it; names the Early Tell—the earliest deviation a clinician can catch before overt decompensation; walks through the Trap Logic that separates it from benign look-alikes; and closes with a Signature Anchor, the decisive threshold or intervention that resolves the clinical question. These Signatures are not an add-on. They are built into the same clinical narrative that teaches the underlying pathophysiology, so that recognizing the pattern and understanding why it occurs happen in the same breath.

At the back of the book, **The In-Transit Deterioration Master Signature Atlas** consolidates every Signature introduced across the text into a single indexed reference, organized by organ system and cross-referenced to its chapter of origin—built to be scanned in the seconds before wheels-up, not studied at leisure.

This is a clinical reference, not an examination preparation product. It contains no practice questions, no board-style items, and no self-assessment drills of any kind. Its purpose is to teach the reasoning a flight or ground critical care clinician uses to keep a patient the same—or better—for the whole of the transport, not merely at its start and its end.

# CHAPTER 1: PHYSIOLOGIC PRINCIPLES OF CRITICAL CARE TRANSPORT

**Learning Objectives**

1. Apply the gas laws governing pressure, volume, and partial-pressure behavior to predict how altitude will affect a specific patient's physiology and equipment.
2. Anticipate the hemodynamic and monitoring consequences of acceleration, vibration, and deceleration during air and ground transport.
3. Recognize the thermoregulatory and sensory stressors unique to the transport environment and their effect on clinical assessment and equipment performance.
4. Calculate oxygen reserve requirements and anticipate cuff-volume and pleural-space behavior under cabin pressurization changes.
5. Distinguish the cumulative physiologic burden of prolonged ground transport from the acute stressors of flight.
6. Adapt altitude and motion physiology principles to pediatric, geriatric, and other physiologically vulnerable transport populations.

**Chapter Outline**

This chapter establishes the physiologic vocabulary that recurs throughout the remainder of the text: the gas laws that govern altitude's effect on the body and its equipment, the mechanical stresses of acceleration and vibration, the thermal and sensory environment of the vehicle or aircraft, and the specific behavior of gas-filled and cuffed structures under pressurization change. Later chapters assume fluency with these principles and apply them to specific disease processes.

The physiology of critical illness does not change when a patient leaves the intensive care unit. What changes is the environment acting on that physiology, and the resources available to respond to it. A patient with a marginal cardiac output tolerates a bedside position change poorly enough; the same patient tolerates a rotor-wing ascent, a stretcher tilt during loading, and forty minutes of engine vibration according to physiologic rules that a purely bedside training never addresses. This chapter builds the foundation for recognizing, before it happens, how the transport environment itself becomes a variable in the patient's clinical course.

Throughout this text, **The In-Transit Deterioration Signature System** identifies the specific, recurring patterns by which transport-environment stress converts a stable-appearing patient into a deteriorating one. This chapter introduces the first two Signatures, both rooted directly in the physiology developed below.

## Gas Laws and Altitude Physiology in Flight

### Boyle's Law and Gas-Filled Space Expansion

Boyle's law states that at a constant temperature, the volume of a gas is inversely proportional to the pressure acting on it. As an aircraft climbs, ambient pressure falls, and any gas-filled space in or around the patient expands accordingly. This is not a trivial consideration confined to esoteric flight physiology; it is a direct predictor of clinical deterioration in structures the clinician may not be actively monitoring at the moment ascent begins. An endotracheal tube cuff inflated to an appropriate seal at sea level will expand as cabin altitude increases, because the cuff itself is a closed gas-filled space subject to the same pressure-volume relationship as the lungs. An occult pneumothorax too small to produce clinical signs on the ground can expand sufficiently during ascent to convert into a tension physiology within minutes, because the same law that expands the endotracheal cuff expands trapped pleural air. Gastric distention, pneumocephalus following recent neurosurgery, and air in central venous catheters or intravenous tubing are all subject to the identical relationship, and all represent silent liabilities that declare themselves only once altitude has already been gained.

The magnitude of this expansion is predictable and worth internalizing as a working rule rather than an abstraction: ascent from sea level to a typical unpressurized rotor-wing cruising altitude of eight to ten thousand feet increases gas volume by roughly thirty to forty percent, a figure large enough that a cuff or pleural pocket that was clinically silent on the ground can become clinically decisive in flight. Because most rotor-wing platforms are unpressurized, this expansion is not a hypothetical to be managed only on fixed-wing missions; it applies to the majority of scene and interfacility helicopter transports as well, and crews who treat gas-law effects as a fixed-wing-only concern are missing the more common exposure.

### Dalton's Law and Alveolar Oxygen Tension at Altitude

Dalton's law establishes that the total pressure of a gas mixture equals the sum of the partial pressures of its constituent gases. Because atmospheric pressure falls with altitude while the fractional composition of air remains constant, the partial pressure of inspired oxygen falls proportionally even though the percentage of oxygen in ambient air does not change. A patient whose oxygenation is already marginal at sea level--tolerating a saturation in the low nineties on a fixed fraction of inspired oxygen--may cross into clinically significant hypoxemia purely as a function of cabin altitude, independent of any change in the underlying pulmonary pathology. This relationship is the physiologic basis for cabin altitude restriction policies used by fixed-wing programs, and it is the reason a patient's oxygenation reserve must be assessed not only for the ground-level moment of transport but for the specific cabin altitude the aircraft will reach.

### Cabin Altitude Restriction and Supplemental Oxygen Strategy

Most fixed-wing critical care transport aircraft are capable of cabin pressurization to an altitude substantially lower than the aircraft's cruising altitude, and the degree of pressurization selected for a given flight is itself a clinical decision, not merely an operational one. A patient with borderline oxygenation, elevated intracranial pressure, or recent thoracic or ophthalmologic surgery may require the crew to request a lower cabin altitude than the aircraft would otherwise use, at the cost of fuel efficiency and range.

The clinician's role in this decision is to translate the patient's specific physiologic tolerance into a concrete cabin altitude request, rather than assuming that standard pressurization is adequate for every patient. Rotor-wing and ground transport lack cabin pressurization control entirely, which shifts the entire burden of altitude tolerance onto route and altitude selection, oxygen supplementation, and, where the terrain allows, the choice of a lower-altitude flight path.

### Pediatric and Geriatric Vulnerability to Altitude and Motion Stress

The gas laws described above act with particular force on physiologically vulnerable populations at both extremes of age. Neonates and young infants have a proportionally higher metabolic rate and oxygen consumption relative to their functional residual capacity, which narrows their margin for the alveolar oxygen tension decline described by Dalton's law and makes even modest cabin altitude increases more consequential than in an adult with greater reserve. A neonate's eustachian tube anatomy and incompletely developed middle-ear ventilation also predispose to disproportionate discomfort and vagally mediated bradycardia during pressure changes, which can be misread as a primary cardiac event if the transport crew does not recognize the pressure-change context. Older adults, particularly those with emphysematous lung disease, fixed cardiac output from valvular or ischemic disease, or reduced thermoregulatory reserve, tolerate the combined stresses of hypoxemia, gas expansion, and temperature swings less well than younger adults with equivalent baseline organ function, and deserve the same proactive cabin-altitude and oxygen-reserve planning applied to any patient with marginal pulmonary or cardiac reserve, regardless of the absence of a specific diagnosis that would otherwise flag them as high risk.

| Physical Principle | Clinical Structure Affected | Anticipated Change With Ascent | Transport Action |
|---|---|---|---|
| Boyle's Law | Endotracheal or tracheostomy cuff | Cuff volume increases; overinflation risk | Use saline-filled or pressure-monitored cuff; recheck cuff pressure at altitude |
| Boyle's Law | Pleural air (occult pneumothorax) | Expansion toward tension physiology | Consider prophylactic chest tube or heightened surveillance before ascent |
| Boyle's Law | Gastric or bowel gas | Distention; aspiration and ventilatory compromise risk | Nasogastric decompression before ascent in at-risk patients |
| Dalton's Law | Alveolar-arterial oxygen gradient | Falling PaO2 at fixed FiO2 | Recalculate oxygen reserve for planned cabin altitude; request lower cabin altitude if marginal |

| | | | |
|---|---|---|---|
| Charles's Law | Ambient and equipment temperature | Gas volume shifts with temperature; device performance drift | Anticipate infusion pump and ventilator behavior changes in extreme cold |

**Figure 1.1: Gas-Filled Space Expansion With Altitude**

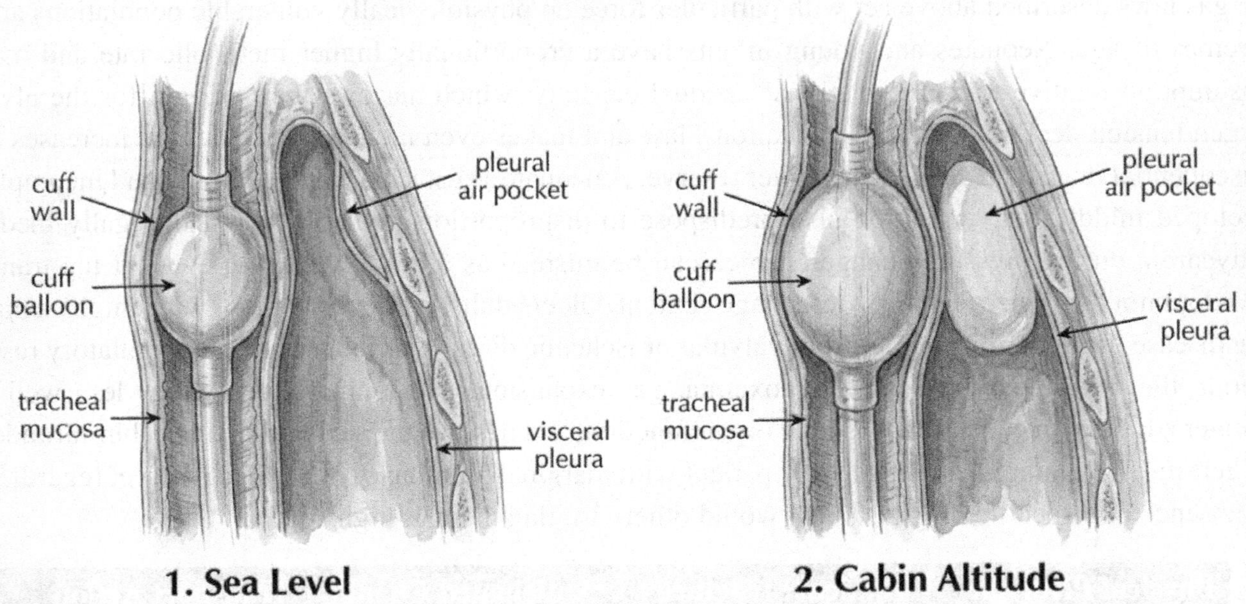


**Pre-Transport Physiologic Risk Assessment and Mission Planning**

The gas-law principles developed above are only clinically useful if they are applied systematically before departure rather than recalled reactively once a problem has already declared itself in flight. A structured pre-transport physiologic risk assessment walks through each gas-filled or pressure-sensitive structure in the patient in turn--airway cuff, pleural space, gastrointestinal tract, cranial vault in the post-neurosurgical patient, any indwelling catheter balloon--and asks explicitly whether that structure carries meaningful expansion risk at the planned cabin altitude. This is not a theoretical exercise performed once during initial training; it is a mission-specific checklist applied to every patient, because the same diagnosis carries different risk depending on the specific altitude profile of the specific mission, the specific aircraft's pressurization capability, and the specific patient's baseline reserve.

This risk assessment should also explicitly incorporate the mission's planned cabin altitude as a negotiable variable rather than a fixed constraint. A crew that identifies a borderline oxygenation or occult-pneumothorax risk during pre-transport assessment has genuine options: request a lower cabin altitude from the flight crew at the cost of range or fuel efficiency, place a prophylactic chest tube before departure, upsize the oxygen supply carried, or, in the least time-sensitive cases, delay departure until a decompensating trend has been further characterized. Treating the cabin altitude and the pre-departure interventions as jointly adjustable, rather than treating altitude as fixed and the patient's physiology as the only variable available to manage, is the conceptual shift that separates anticipatory transport medicine from reactive transport medicine, and it is the organizing idea behind every Signature introduced in this text.

| Structure Assessed | Key Question Before Departure | Action If Risk Identified |
|---|---|---|
| Airway cuff | Air-filled or saline-filled? Pressure-monitored? | Convert to saline fill or establish pressure monitoring before ascent |
| Pleural space | Any current or recent pneumothorax, or plausible mechanism? | Consider prophylactic chest tube; heighten surveillance threshold |
| Gastrointestinal tract | Ileus, bowel obstruction, or recent abdominal surgery? | Nasogastric decompression before ascent |
| Cranial vault | Recent neurosurgery with potential pneumocephalus? | Confirm with neurosurgical team whether altitude restriction is required |
| Oxygenation reserve | Saturation and FiO2 margin at planned cabin altitude? | Recalculate for cabin altitude; request lower cabin altitude if marginal |

## Effects of Acceleration, Vibration, and Deceleration on Critical Illness

### Hemodynamic Effects of G-Forces During Ascent and Descent

Acceleration and deceleration forces during takeoff, climb, descent, and landing produce transient but clinically meaningful shifts in venous return and afterload. During acceleration and climb, gravitational and inertial forces acting along the body's long axis reduce venous return from the lower extremities, decreasing preload in a patient who may already be volume-depleted or vasoplegic. In a patient dependent on a mechanical circulatory support device, this preload reduction is not merely a transient nuisance; because device flow in most continuous-flow ventricular assist devices is preload-dependent, a reduction in venous return during ascent can produce a measurable drop in device flow that the crew must anticipate rather than discover on the flow display after the fact. Positioning maneuvers that improve venous return--leg elevation, sequential compression devices, or, in an awake patient, active calf contraction--are effective countermeasures when applied proactively before or at the onset of ascent rather than reactively once flow has already fallen.

Deceleration on descent and landing produces the reverse hemodynamic pattern: a transient increase in venous return that is generally well tolerated in patients with preserved cardiac reserve but can precipitate acute pulmonary edema or right heart strain in a patient already operating near the top of the Frank-Starling curve, such as one with decompensated heart failure or severe pulmonary hypertension. Anticipating this transition--rather than being surprised by a new oxygen requirement or crackles on descent in a patient who was stable throughout cruise--allows the crew to have diuretic or afterload-reduction strategies ready rather than improvised.

### Vibration-Induced Monitoring Artifact and Signal Loss

Continuous engine and airframe vibration, particularly in rotor-wing and fixed-wing turboprop platforms, degrades the signal quality of noninvasive monitoring modalities more severely than most clinicians anticipate from ground-based experience. Pulse oximetry waveforms become intermittently unreadable, noninvasive blood pressure cycling becomes unreliable during periods of turbulence, and capnography sampling lines are prone to mechanical disruption. This is the physiologic argument for early conversion to invasive arterial pressure monitoring in any patient whose hemodynamic trajectory is uncertain: an arterial waveform, once established, degrades far less under vibration than a noninvasive cuff cycle, and it provides continuous rather than intermittent data at exactly the moments when intermittent data is least trustworthy.

Practically, this means the threshold for invasive line placement should be lower before a transport begins than it would be for an equivalent patient remaining in a stationary intensive care unit bed, because the cost of establishing access after vibration has already degraded the crew's ability to trend the patient's status is considerably higher than the cost of establishing it proactively during the calmer pre-departure window.

### Patient Positioning and Restraint Considerations

Stretcher positioning during loading and unloading imposes brief but real postural stress, and patients with intracranial hypertension, unstable spinal injury, or precarious airway control are disproportionately vulnerable to the head-down or head-up transients that occur during litter loading onto an aircraft or ambulance cot. A deliberate loading sequence--head-of-bed position confirmed and locked before movement begins, airway and lines secured against the direction of anticipated tilt, and verbal confirmation of the loading angle with the transport team--converts an uncontrolled positional stress into a controlled and anticipated one.

### THE IN-TRANSIT DETERIORATION SIGNATURE SYSTEM — Ascent-Triggered Device Flow Compromise

---

**The Signature:** A progressive, unexplained fall in ventricular assist device flow or continuous cardiac output monitor readings that begins within minutes of takeoff or the start of climb, in the absence of any change in device settings, medication administration, or overt hemodynamic event.

**Movement Trigger:** Acceleration and sustained climb reduce venous return from the lower extremities via gravitational pooling, decreasing right-sided preload delivered to the device or native heart at the exact moment device flow depends on it most.

**Early Tell:** A flow decrement of even ten to fifteen percent from the pre-ascent baseline, appearing within the first five minutes of climb, before any accompanying change in blood pressure or heart rate becomes apparent.

**Trap Logic:** This pattern is frequently misread as device malfunction or thrombus, prompting alarm troubleshooting that delays the correct response. The discriminating feature is timing: a flow drop that begins precisely at the onset of climb and stabilizes once level flight is reached points to a preload phenomenon, not a device or clotting problem.

**Signature Anchor:** Confirm euvolemia before ascent whenever feasible, apply leg elevation or sequential compression at the first sign of flow decline, and treat a climb-onset flow drop as a preload event to be corrected with positioning and volume assessment before escalating to device-focused troubleshooting.

**CLINICAL PEARL:** A flow alarm that resolves spontaneously once level flight is reached, without any intervention, retrospectively confirms a preload-mediated mechanism rather than a device fault--but the crew should not wait for level flight to intervene if the flow decline is significant.

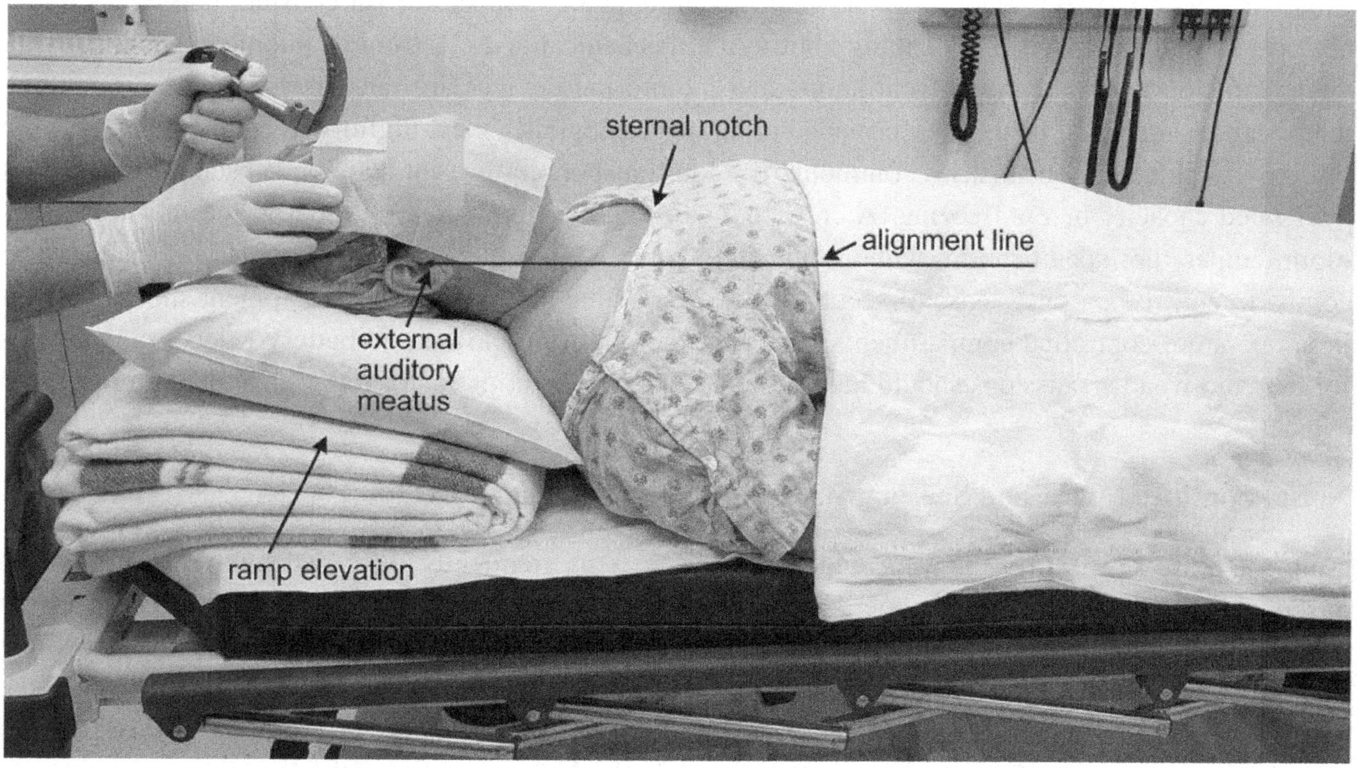

## Thermoregulation and Environmental Stressors in Transit

### Hypothermia Risk in Prolonged Transport

The transport environment predisposes critically ill patients to unintentional hypothermia through several converging mechanisms: exposure during extrication or loading, the cooling effect of unwarmed intravenous fluids, radiant heat loss in an unheated or poorly insulated cabin, and the impaired thermoregulatory capacity of sedated, paralyzed, or hemodynamically unstable patients. Hypothermia below thirty-five degrees Celsius has measurable consequences for coagulation, cardiac rhythm stability, and drug metabolism, and in the trauma population specifically, hypothermia is one leg of the lethal triad alongside acidosis and coagulopathy. Active warming--forced-air warming blankets, warmed intravenous fluids, and passive insulation--should be initiated proactively at the start of transport rather than reactively once a temperature drop has already been recorded, because the confined, difficult-to-access environment of a moving vehicle makes rewarming considerably harder to achieve than prevention.

### Equipment Performance and Battery Behavior in Temperature Extremes

Charles's law--the direct relationship between gas volume and temperature at constant pressure--applies not only to the patient's own physiology but to the mechanical and electronic equipment accompanying them. Infusion pumps, portable ventilators, and monitoring devices are rated for a specified operating temperature range, and battery performance in particular degrades meaningfully in cold conditions, with lithium-based battery chemistries commonly used in transport equipment losing a substantial fraction of their rated capacity below freezing. A crew that calculates battery reserve based on the manufacturer's room-temperature specification, without adjusting for a winter tarmac exposure or an unheated cargo compartment, risks a false sense of security about remaining device runtime. Equipment should be kept in temperature-controlled compartments whenever the platform allows, and battery reserve calculations for extreme-weather missions should include a conservative derating factor rather than the nominal rated capacity.

### Noise, Confined Space, and Sensory Stress Effects on Assessment

Ambient noise levels in rotor-wing and fixed-wing cabins frequently exceed the threshold at which auscultation, verbal patient assessment, and even alarm recognition become unreliable, requiring the clinician to rely more heavily on visual monitor trends, waveform capnography, and tactile assessment than would be necessary at the bedside. The confined working space around the patient limits the clinician's ability to reposition for a difficult airway attempt, obtain additional vascular access, or perform chest compressions with full mechanical efficiency, all of which argues for anticipating these limitations--securing additional access, confirming airway backup plans, and pre-positioning equipment--before departure rather than during an in-flight crisis.

**CAUTION:** A subjective patient report of pain or dyspnea may be entirely inaudible over cabin noise; a clinician who relies on verbal cues alone in a high-noise environment risks missing early deterioration that objective monitoring would have flagged.

## Cabin Pressurization and Oxygenation Considerations

### Endotracheal and Other Cuff Volume Changes With Altitude

Building directly on the gas-law principles established earlier in this chapter, every air-filled cuff on the patient--endotracheal, tracheostomy, or urinary catheter balloon--is subject to expansion during ascent. The clinical standard for critical care transport is to either replace air in the endotracheal cuff with saline, which is essentially incompressible and does not expand with altitude, or to use a cuff pressure monitor that allows the crew to actively deflate the cuff incrementally as altitude increases and reinflate during descent. Failure to manage cuff volume across a flight profile risks either an underinflated cuff at altitude, with an air leak and loss of ventilation, or tracheal mucosal injury from overinflation if the cuff was filled with air and not adjusted.

### Chest Tube and Pneumothorax Considerations at Altitude

A chest tube connected to a one-way valve or underwater seal drainage system generally continues to function appropriately across altitude changes, provided the system remains upright and the valve mechanism is intact; the concern is not the functioning tube but the undrained or occult pneumothorax. Any patient with a recent pneumothorax, even one that appears radiographically resolved, or any patient with multiple rib fractures and a plausible mechanism for occult pleural air, should be assessed for prophylactic chest tube placement before a flight that will reach a cabin altitude sufficient to expand a small, currently asymptomatic pocket of pleural air into a clinically significant one.

### Oxygen Supply Calculation and Reserve Planning

Every transport requires an explicit calculation of oxygen consumption against oxygen supply carried, accounting for the patient's minute ventilation, fraction of inspired oxygen, any supplemental high-flow or nebulized therapy in use, and a safety margin for unanticipated delay. This calculation must be performed for the specific flight profile and cabin altitude planned, not simply for ground-level consumption, since oxygen demand at a given saturation target may rise as cabin altitude increases and the alveolar-arterial gradient in Dalton's law reduces the oxygen tension delivered per liter of flow.

### Oxygen Delivery Device Selection and Altitude Interaction

The choice of oxygen delivery interface carries altitude-specific implications beyond simple flow-rate math. High-flow nasal cannula systems and noninvasive positive pressure devices depend on blender and flow-generator performance that can drift at altitude if the device is not specifically rated for aeromedical use, and a device that performs predictably at sea level may deliver a different effective fraction of inspired oxygen or driving pressure at a reduced cabin pressure. Portable ventilators intended for ground-based use only, without aeromedical certification, may likewise miscalculate delivered tidal volume or trigger sensitivity at altitude because their internal flow sensors are calibrated against sea-level barometric pressure. Selecting equipment explicitly rated and tested for the altitude range of the planned mission, rather than assuming ground-hospital equipment will perform identically, is a a foundational safety decision that precedes any disease-specific management choice made later in transport.

| Oxygen Source | Typical Capacity | Flow-Dependent Duration Consideration |
|---|---|---|
| D cylinder | ~425 L usable | At 15 L/min continuous flow, approximately 28 minutes |
| E cylinder | ~625 L usable | At 15 L/min continuous flow, approximately 41 minutes |
| Portable liquid oxygen unit | Program-dependent, typically several hours | Verify unit-specific duration chart against planned flow rate before departure |

**THE IN-TRANSIT DETERIORATION SIGNATURE SYSTEM — Occult Pneumothorax Expansion at Altitude**

**The Signature:** Progressive desaturation, rising peak airway pressures, and new hemodynamic instability that develops during or shortly after ascent in a patient with any plausible mechanism for undrained pleural air, in the absence of any other identified cause.

**Movement Trigger:** Boyle's law expansion of trapped pleural air as cabin altitude increases and ambient pressure falls, converting a subclinical pocket of air into a space-occupying, and ultimately tension-physiology, process.

**Early Tell:** A subtle but sustained rise in ventilator peak inspiratory pressure or a fall in dynamic compliance beginning within the first ten to fifteen minutes of climb, often preceding any change in oxygen saturation.

**Trap Logic:** This pattern is easily mistaken for a primary ventilator or airway problem--tube migration, mucus plugging, or bronchospasm--particularly because the desaturation and pressure changes can resemble any of those processes. The discriminating feature is the temporal relationship to ascent and any trauma or thoracic history, however remote, that makes occult pleural air plausible.

**Signature Anchor:** In any patient with a plausible mechanism for occult pneumothorax, treat a new pressure or saturation change occurring during or immediately after ascent as pleural in origin until excluded, and proceed to needle or finger decompression without delay if tension physiology develops, rather than exhausting airway troubleshooting first.

## Physiologic Effects of Prolonged Ground Transport

### Cumulative Stress of Extended Transport Time

Ground critical care transport, particularly over rural or long interfacility distances, exposes the patient to a different physiologic burden than the acute altitude and acceleration stresses of flight: sustained low-amplitude vibration, prolonged fixed positioning, and an extended window during which any slow-developing process--evolving compartment syndrome, gradually accumulating hemothorax, or progressive intracranial pressure elevation--has more time to declare itself before arrival. The absence of altitude-related gas expansion does not make ground transport physiologically neutral; it substitutes an acute stressor profile for a cumulative one.

**Rural and Long-Distance Transport Considerations**

Transport times exceeding thirty to forty-five minutes have been independently associated with a measurably higher rate of clinical deterioration in interfacility transport cohorts, which argues for a structured reassessment interval--vital signs, neurologic status, ventilator parameters, and line and tube security--performed on a fixed schedule throughout a long transport rather than only at the beginning and end. A crew that reassesses only when something seems wrong will, by definition, miss the earliest and most treatable phase of a slowly evolving deterioration.

Extended ground transport also carries logistical consequences distinct from flight: the crew cannot request a change in cabin altitude or divert to a closer facility with the same flexibility as an aircraft, medication and fluid supplies must be calculated for a longer worst-case duration including potential traffic or weather delay, and the physical fatigue of sustained manual monitoring and reassessment over two or more hours is itself a patient-safety variable, since clinician vigilance measurably declines over a sufficiently long unbroken task. Programs that routinely perform long rural ground transports benefit from building in a structured crew rotation or deliberate re-engagement checkpoint--not only a patient reassessment interval but a moment for the crew itself to pause, re-orient to the working diagnosis, and confirm equipment and line status--precisely because fatigue-driven inattention is a more realistic threat on a two-hour ground transport than on a forty-minute flight.

**Structured Communication and Documentation During Extended Transport**

A long ground transport also multiplies the number of discrete clinical moments that must be reliably captured and communicated to the receiving team, and a crew relying on memory alone across ninety minutes or more of continuous patient management will reliably lose fidelity in the retelling. Structured, time-stamped documentation performed at each scheduled reassessment interval--rather than reconstructed from memory after arrival--preserves the specific sequence of any deterioration, which vital sign or examination finding changed first, and what intervention was given in response, all of which materially affects the receiving team's ability to understand the trajectory rather than only the endpoint. For transports crossing between emergency medical services regions or between institutions with different electronic documentation systems, a standardized verbal handoff structure--covering mechanism or diagnosis, interventions performed, trend since departure, and any anticipated needs on arrival--should be rehearsed as deliberately as any procedural skill, since the handoff is the single point at which the entire transport's clinical value can be lost if the receiving team does not receive an accurate and complete picture of what occurred en route.

Consider a forty-eight-year-old man transported by ground critical care ambulance following a motor vehicle collision, with a known small subdural hematoma managed nonoperatively and stable vital signs at the time of departure from the referring facility. The transport distance is ninety minutes over rural highway. At the midpoint reassessment, the crew notes a two-point decline in Glasgow Coma Scale score and a new asymmetric pupillary response, neither of which was present at departure. Because the crew had established a fixed twenty-minute reassessment interval rather than relying on the patient's initial stability, the change is caught at the midpoint rather than at arrival, allowing early notification of the receiving neurosurgical team and a change in transport priority to the nearest appropriate facility rather than the originally planned destination.

A second illustrative case involves a sixty-one-year-old woman with a continuous-flow left ventricular assist device transported by fixed-wing aircraft for a device-related complication evaluation, clinically euvolemic and hemodynamically stable at departure. Approximately four minutes into climb, the flow display shows a decline from 4.8 to 4.1 liters per minute with no change in pump speed or power, and the crew, recognizing the Ascent-Triggered Device Flow Compromise Signature introduced earlier in this chapter, elevates the patient's legs and confirms euvolemic status rather than initiating device-fault troubleshooting. Flow recovers to 4.6 liters per minute within ninety seconds and remains stable for the remainder of the cruise phase. Had the crew instead interpreted the flow decline as a primary device problem, the resulting alarm-focused workup would have consumed critical early minutes without addressing the actual, preload-mediated cause--an outcome the Signature framework is specifically designed to prevent by naming the pattern and its correct first response in advance of ever encountering it in flight.

These two cases, one ground-based and one airborne, illustrate the same underlying principle from opposite directions: the ground case shows that time itself is a risk factor requiring structured vigilance, while the flight case shows that a specific, brief physiologic event requires immediate pattern recognition rather than a generic troubleshooting sequence. Both outcomes depended not on more advanced equipment or a different level of clinician training, but on the crew's advance familiarity with the specific way the transport environment was going to act on this specific patient's physiology--which is precisely the anticipatory framework this text is built to provide.

## Henry's Law and Dissolved Gas Behavior in Transit

### Nitrogen Narcosis and Decompression Considerations

Henry's law states that the amount of gas dissolved in a liquid is proportional to the partial pressure of that gas above the liquid, and while this principle is most commonly associated with diving medicine, it has direct relevance to certain transport populations. A patient who has recently completed a scuba dive and subsequently requires aeromedical evacuation carries a residual nitrogen load dissolved in blood and tissues that, under the reduced ambient pressure of altitude, can come out of solution and form bubbles--producing decompression sickness during what would otherwise be a routine flight. Current recommendations specify altitude restrictions following diving that the flight crew must be aware of, and the transport clinician should specifically screen for recent diving history in any patient requiring aeromedical transport, since the combination of a recent dive and altitude exposure can produce neurologic, pulmonary, and musculoskeletal symptoms that mimic other acute conditions and may not be attributed to their true cause unless the diving history is elicited.

### Dissolved Oxygen and Carbon Dioxide Kinetics at Altitude

The behavior of dissolved oxygen and carbon dioxide in the bloodstream at altitude follows the same Henry's law relationship: as the partial pressure of oxygen in inspired air falls with altitude, the amount of oxygen dissolved in plasma (as distinct from hemoglobin-bound oxygen) decreases proportionally, reducing the oxygen dissolved fraction that contributes to tissue oxygen delivery. While hemoglobin-bound oxygen constitutes the majority of blood oxygen content, the dissolved fraction is the component that is immediately available to cross into tissue, and its reduction at altitude can become clinically relevant in patients with already-marginal oxygen delivery--specifically, patients with severe anemia, in whom the hemoglobin-bound component is reduced, and patients with carbon monoxide poisoning, in whom hemoglobin is functionally occupied by carbon monoxide and the dissolved fraction becomes proportionally more important. The transport clinician managing either of these populations at altitude should recognize that supplemental oxygen at altitude is not merely replacing inspired oxygen but is specifically defending the dissolved fraction that these patients depend on disproportionately.

## Humidity and Fluid Balance at Altitude

### Insensible Losses and Dehydration During Prolonged Flight

The ambient humidity inside aircraft cabins--particularly fixed-wing cabins at cruising altitude--can fall below fifteen percent, dramatically lower than the thirty to sixty percent range found in most indoor environments, producing an accelerated rate of insensible water loss through the respiratory tract and exposed skin surfaces. In a healthy passenger this dehydration is a minor inconvenience; in a critically ill patient who is already volume-depleted, receiving diuretic therapy, or dependent on precise fluid balance for hemodynamic management, the additional insensible losses from low cabin humidity can produce a clinically significant volume deficit over a multi-hour flight that is easy to overlook because it is invisible--no measurable drainage, no hemorrhage, simply an accelerated evaporative loss that accumulates quietly. The transport clinician should account for these insensible losses in the fluid balance calculation for any transport exceeding two hours, particularly in intubated patients breathing dry gas and in patients with extensive burn surface area.

### Humidification of Inspired Gas During Extended Transport

Mechanical ventilation with inadequately humidified gas produces progressive drying of airway secretions, increasing the viscosity of mucus, promoting mucus plugging that can obstruct the endotracheal tube or produce atelectasis, and damaging the ciliated airway epithelium that is the respiratory tract's primary defense against infection. The heat-and-moisture exchange filters discussed earlier in this chapter provide adequate humidification for transports of moderate duration, but their capacity is finite and their effectiveness diminishes over time as the filter saturates, making them less reliable for extended transports exceeding several hours. Transport programs that routinely perform long-duration fixed-wing missions should consider carrying active heated humidification capability, or at minimum should plan for filter replacement at defined intervals during extended transports, rather than relying on a single filter for the entire mission duration.

## Gravitational Effects on Intravascular Lines and Monitoring Equipment

### Transducer Leveling and Pressure Artifact During Flight

Invasive pressure monitoring--arterial, central venous, and intracranial pressure transducers--requires leveling to a consistent anatomic reference point, and any change in the patient's position or the transducer's position relative to the patient during transport introduces a hydrostatic pressure artifact that can be mistaken for a genuine physiologic change if the transducer is not re-leveled. The magnitude of this artifact is approximately 0.7 millimeters of mercury per centimeter of vertical displacement, which means that a transducer that has shifted even five centimeters from its reference point during loading or repositioning can produce a three-to-four-millimeter-of-mercury error in the displayed pressure--small in the context of arterial pressure monitoring but potentially significant for intracranial or central venous pressure monitoring, where the clinical decision thresholds are narrow and absolute.

The practical implication is that pressure transducers should be re-leveled and re-zeroed after every position change during transport, and the crew should develop the habit of performing this re-leveling as an automatic component of any repositioning sequence rather than as a troubleshooting step performed only when the displayed pressure looks unexpectedly different. In aircraft, the additional consideration of cabin pressurization changes during climb and descent means that transducer readings may drift even without any change in patient position, since the transducer's atmospheric pressure reference changes as cabin altitude changes, and a brief re-zeroing at the start of cruise provides a corrected baseline for the level-flight phase of the transport.

### Intravenous Infusion Rate Effects of Altitude and Position

Gravity-dependent intravenous infusions--those not driven by an infusion pump but relying on hydrostatic head pressure for flow--are susceptible to flow rate changes during the position and altitude changes of transport. A fluid bag hung at a given height above the patient at sea level develops a specific hydrostatic driving pressure; at altitude, the reduced atmospheric pressure against which the infusion flows produces a relative increase in driving pressure that can increase the flow rate, while a change in the height of the bag relative to the patient during a stretcher tilt or aircraft maneuver can dramatically alter or stop flow entirely. This is the physiologic argument for running all critical infusions through calibrated infusion pumps rather than gravity-dependent lines during transport, since a pump maintains a set flow rate independent of bag height, patient position, and ambient pressure, eliminating an entire category of infusion variability that gravity-dependent administration introduces.

## Fatigue Physiology and the Transport Clinician's Performance Envelope

### Circadian Rhythm Disruption and Its Clinical Consequences

Transport clinicians frequently work shifts that span circadian low points--the early morning hours between two and six o'clock, when cognitive performance, reaction time, and situational awareness are at their physiologic nadir--and the transport environment's sensory demands do not compensate for this circadian trough in the way that a busy, well-lit emergency department might. A darkened aircraft cabin, a steady engine vibration, and a monotonous monitoring task during a stable cruise phase combine to produce conditions that maximize the circadian performance decrement, and a clinician who is unaware of this effect may not recognize that their assessment quality and decision-making speed are objectively impaired during these hours despite their subjective sense of alertness. Transport programs that schedule crews through the early morning circadian low point should build in structured alertness strategies--brief physical activity, caffeine timed appropriately, and deliberate, forced-pace reassessment intervals--rather than relying on passive vigilance to carry the crew through the performance trough.

### Altitude Hypoxia Effects on Crew Performance

The same Dalton's law reduction in alveolar oxygen tension that affects the patient also affects the transport clinician, and at cabin altitudes above approximately eight thousand feet, clinician cognitive performance begins to measurably decline even in healthy individuals--reduced working memory, impaired judgment, and slower reaction times that are particularly dangerous because the clinician experiencing them typically does not recognize the impairment. Pressurized fixed-wing aircraft maintain cabin altitudes well below this threshold under normal operations, but rotor-wing aircraft and unpressurized fixed-wing platforms can expose the crew to cabin altitudes in the range where performance effects are measurable, and a crew member who notices progressive headache, difficulty concentrating, or a sense of euphoria during a flight at meaningful altitude should consider supplemental oxygen for themselves as a patient safety intervention, not merely a personal comfort measure.

## Radiation Exposure Considerations for Frequent Flyers

### Cosmic Radiation and the Transport Clinician's Cumulative Exposure

Transport clinicians who fly frequently--particularly those operating on fixed-wing platforms at high cruising altitudes--accumulate cosmic radiation exposure at rates that exceed ground-level background radiation and, over a career, can approach the annual occupational exposure limits recommended by radiation protection agencies. The exposure rate increases with altitude and with proximity to the magnetic poles, and a clinician who logs several hundred flight hours per year at typical aeromedical cruising altitudes accumulates a radiation dose that is comparable to several chest radiographs per year. While the individual-flight dose is trivially small, the cumulative career dose is non-trivial, and transport programs should inform their flight crews of this occupational exposure, maintain flight-hour logs that allow individual dose estimation, and provide guidance for crews who are pregnant or planning pregnancy, since the developing fetus is more sensitive to radiation exposure than the adult.

### Pregnancy and Radiation Considerations for Transport Crew

A pregnant transport clinician faces the dual consideration of cosmic radiation exposure to the developing fetus and the physical demands and environmental exposures of transport duty, and most transport programs offer modified duty assignments that reduce or eliminate flight exposure during pregnancy while maintaining the clinician's ground-based clinical role. The decision to modify duty should be made in consultation with the clinician's obstetrician and the program's occupational health advisor, using the estimated cumulative radiation dose for the remaining pregnancy based on the clinician's typical flight profile, and should be treated as a routine occupational health accommodation rather than a career-limiting event.

## Integration of Transport Physiology Into Clinical Decision-Making

### Building the Pre-Mission Physiologic Risk Profile

The gas-law, hemodynamic, thermoregulatory, humidity, and gravitational principles described in this chapter converge into a single practical output: a pre-mission physiologic risk profile that the transport clinician should construct mentally or explicitly for every patient before departure. This profile identifies the specific physiologic vulnerabilities that the specific transport environment will impose on the specific patient: which gas-filled spaces are at risk for expansion, how much oxygenation reserve exists at the planned cabin altitude, what positional hemodynamic effects to anticipate, what temperature and humidity management is needed, and what monitoring adjustments are required for the specific flight profile and duration. Building this profile before departure, rather than discovering these vulnerabilities reactively during flight, is the foundational application of the anticipatory transport medicine framework that the rest of this text is built on.

The pre-mission physiologic risk profile is not a form to be filled out or a checklist to be completed; it is a cognitive process that integrates the patient's specific disease process, the specific transport platform's environmental characteristics, and the specific mission profile's altitude, duration, and route into a unified assessment of where the transport environment is most likely to threaten this particular patient. A patient with ARDS and marginal oxygenation on a two-hour fixed-wing flight at altitude has a fundamentally different physiologic risk profile from the same patient on a thirty-minute ground transport at sea level, even though the disease and its management are identical in every other respect. The ability to construct this profile accurately and act on it proactively is the clinical skill that this chapter is designed to develop, and it is the skill that every subsequent chapter in this text assumes the clinician already possesses.

**CLINICAL PEARL:** The pre-mission physiologic risk profile asks one question about every gas-filled space, every marginal physiologic parameter, and every environmental vulnerability in the patient: what will happen to this specific finding at the specific altitude, duration, and route of this specific mission? Building this profile before wheels-up is the single most valuable cognitive act the transport clinician performs.

## Barometric Pressure Effects on Medical Devices and Implants

### Implanted Device Behavior at Altitude

Beyond the gas-filled physiologic spaces discussed earlier, the transport environment affects a range of implanted and external medical devices through the same barometric pressure mechanisms. Programmable ventriculoperitoneal shunt valves may exhibit flow rate changes at altitude as the pressure differential across the valve changes with cabin pressurization, potentially producing either overdrainage (with risk of subdural hematoma) or underdrainage (with rising intracranial pressure) depending on the specific valve design and the direction of the pressure change. Tissue expanders, breast implants containing saline, and surgically placed wound VAC devices all contain gas or fluid volumes that respond to Boyle's law expansion, and the transport clinician should specifically inquire about these devices during the pre-transport assessment and anticipate their behavior at the planned cabin altitude.

### Air Splint and Pneumatic Device Behavior

Pneumatic anti-shock garments, air splints for extremity fracture immobilization, and air-filled cervical collars are external devices that expand with altitude and constrict during descent, and their pressure must be monitored and adjusted throughout the flight profile to maintain therapeutic effectiveness without producing the tissue ischemia that over-inflation causes or the loss of immobilization that under-inflation permits. The practical approach is to inflate these devices to the minimum effective pressure at ground level, monitor for tightness during ascent (releasing air as needed to prevent over-compression), and re-inflate during descent to maintain effectiveness as the contained air contracts with increasing ambient pressure.

### Medication Delivery Device Behavior at Altitude

Metered-dose inhalers, which deliver medication by releasing a propellant-drug mixture from a pressurized canister, may produce variable dose delivery at altitude as the pressure differential between the canister and the ambient environment changes with cabin pressurization, though this effect is generally small enough to be clinically negligible for most patients. More consequentially, air bubbles in intravenous tubing and medication syringes expand at altitude just as any other gas-filled space does, and the transport clinician should de-air all infusion lines and syringes before ascent with particular care, since a bubble that was too small to notice at sea level may expand to a size that produces a clinically relevant air embolus at altitude or that interrupts infusion pump flow detection and triggers a false air-in-line alarm.

### Contact Lens and Ophthalmic Considerations

Patients wearing gas-permeable contact lenses may experience corneal bubble formation at altitude as dissolved nitrogen comes out of solution in the tear film, producing pain, visual disturbance, and corneal abrasion. While this is a minor consideration in most transport patients, it becomes clinically relevant in the conscious patient with facial trauma or neurologic injury whose visual assessment is part of the ongoing monitoring plan, since a new visual complaint attributed to a contact lens issue should not be confused with a neurologic deterioration requiring urgent intervention. The transport clinician should document the presence of contact lenses during the initial assessment and consider removing them before flight if the patient's cooperation and clinical status allow.

### Hyperbaric Considerations Following Altitude Exposure

Patients who have undergone recent altitude exposure--whether from a prior transport flight, a mountain rescue, or recreational high-altitude activity--and who subsequently require hyperbaric oxygen therapy for decompression sickness, carbon monoxide poisoning, or other hyperbaric indications present a specific transport challenge: the residual nitrogen load from the altitude exposure may worsen upon re-ascent if the patient requires a second flight to reach a hyperbaric facility, producing a decompression syndrome during a transport intended to treat a condition that was itself caused or worsened by altitude. The transport clinician should screen for prior altitude exposure history in any patient being transported for hyperbaric therapy and should coordinate with the hyperbaric facility and the flight crew to establish the lowest feasible cabin altitude for the transport, with ground transport considered as a safer alternative when the distance and patient condition allow.

### Spatial Disorientation and Motion Sickness in the Conscious Patient

Conscious patients, particularly those with vestibular injuries, recent head trauma, or ongoing vertigo from any cause, may experience worsening symptoms or acute motion sickness during the acceleration, banking, and vibration phases of transport that can produce vomiting with aspiration risk, autonomic instability, and severe distress that degrades the patient's cooperation with their own care. Prophylactic antiemetic therapy before departure, positioning the patient to minimize vestibular stimulation (head stabilized in the midline, visual fixation on a stable point if the patient is able), and forewarning the patient about the expected motion sensations all reduce the incidence and severity of transport-induced motion sickness and should be part of the routine preparation for any conscious patient being transported by air.

### Third-Spacing and Altitude-Enhanced Capillary Leak

Patients with systemic inflammatory states--sepsis, major burns, pancreatitis, post-surgical systemic inflammatory response--exhibit increased capillary permeability that produces third-spacing of fluid into the interstitial and extravascular compartments. The reduced atmospheric pressure at altitude can theoretically enhance this third-spacing effect by reducing the external hydrostatic pressure that partially opposes transcapillary fluid movement, though the clinical magnitude of this effect at typical cabin altitudes is debated. The practical implication for the transport clinician is that a patient who is already third-spacing at sea level may third-space more rapidly at altitude, producing an accelerated intravascular volume depletion that requires more aggressive resuscitation during flight than the same patient would need during a ground transport at sea level. Monitoring urine output, hemodynamic trends, and serial hematocrit (which rises as plasma volume is lost to third-spacing) provides the trend data needed to detect this accelerated volume loss.

## THE IN-TRANSIT DETERIORATION SIGNATURE SYSTEM — Foundational Movement-Triggered Patterns

**Signatures Introduced This Chapter:** Ascent-Triggered Device Flow Compromise (preload-mediated flow decline with climb) and Occult Pneumothorax Expansion at Altitude (Boyle's law expansion of trapped pleural air).

**Shared Movement Trigger Logic:** Both Signatures in this chapter are driven by predictable physical laws--gravitational preload shift and gas-volume expansion--rather than by primary disease progression, which is why anticipatory action taken before or at the onset of ascent is more effective than reactive troubleshooting after a flow or pressure change has already occurred.

**Cross-Reference Forward:** Chapter 7 (Mechanical Circulatory Support Devices in Transit) extends the Ascent-Triggered Device Flow Compromise Signature to intra-aortic balloon pumps and extracorporeal circuits; Chapter 12 (Pneumothorax, Chest Trauma, and Thoracic Emergencies in Transit) extends the Occult Pneumothorax Expansion Signature to acute traumatic presentations.

## Summary and Key Concepts

Boyle's, Dalton's, and Charles's laws predictably govern how altitude affects gas-filled structures, oxygen tension, and equipment performance, and should be applied proactively to specific patients and specific flight profiles rather than treated as background physiology.

Acceleration and vibration produce preload and monitoring-signal effects that are frequently misattributed to primary device or airway problems unless their timing relative to ascent is recognized.

Pediatric, geriatric, and other physiologically vulnerable patients tolerate the combined stresses of altitude, temperature, and gas expansion less well than patients with equivalent baseline organ function, and warrant proactive planning regardless of a specific flagging diagnosis.

Thermoregulatory and sensory stressors in the transport environment degrade both the patient's physiologic reserve and the clinician's assessment tools, and should be mitigated proactively; equipment performance itself is temperature-sensitive and must be planned for accordingly.

Cuff management, oxygen reserve calculation, oxygen delivery device selection, and pneumothorax risk assessment must be performed against the specific planned cabin altitude, not against ground-level assumptions.

Prolonged ground transport substitutes a cumulative physiologic burden and clinician fatigue risk for the acute stressors of flight, and warrants a fixed reassessment interval and deliberate crew re-engagement to catch slowly evolving deterioration.

# CHAPTER 2: THE CRITICALLY ILL PATIENT IN TRANSIT: ASSESSMENT, MONITORING, AND HANDOFF

**Learning Objectives**

1. Apply a rapid, problem-based physiologic framework to assess a critically ill patient inherited mid-course from a sending facility.
2. Select and interpret invasive and noninvasive hemodynamic monitoring modalities appropriate to the transport environment.
3. Extract the clinically decisive elements of a sending facility's workup within a time-limited bedside interaction.
4. Distinguish trend-based deterioration recognition from fixed-threshold vital sign interpretation in patients whose baseline is already abnormal.
5. Deliver a structured, complete handoff that preserves clinical trajectory information for the receiving team.
6. Communicate effectively with family members and non-clinical stakeholders present during interfacility transport.

**Chapter Outline**

This chapter addresses the cognitive and procedural work that precedes and accompanies every transport: rapidly building an accurate physiologic picture of a patient the clinician has known for minutes rather than days, choosing monitoring appropriate to that picture, and communicating it faithfully at both ends of the transport. These skills are foundational to every disease-specific chapter that follows.

The defining feature of critical care transport, as distinct from bedside intensive care, is that the clinician is not the first to formulate a diagnosis or begin treatment. They are inheriting a patient mid-course: a working diagnosis already established, interventions already initiated, and a trajectory already in motion, all of which must be rapidly absorbed, verified where possible, and then actively managed for the specific window of the transport before responsibility passes to a third team at the receiving facility. This chapter builds the assessment and communication framework that makes that mid-course inheritance safe.

## Rapid Assessment and Problem-Based Physiologic Framework

### The Problem List as an Organizing Structure

Rather than attempting to reconstruct a complete diagnostic narrative at the bedside of a sending facility, the transport clinician is better served by rapidly constructing a physiologic problem list: airway status, ventilation adequacy, oxygenation adequacy, hemodynamic stability, neurologic status, and any active bleeding or metabolic derangement, each assessed independently and each assigned a working plan for the transport window. This structure is deliberately diagnosis-agnostic at the outset, because it generates an actionable plan even before the underlying diagnosis is fully understood, and because a patient's physiologic problems--not their diagnosis--are what will actually threaten them during transit.

Constructing this problem list is not a one-time event performed at the bedside and then set aside; it is a living document, revisited explicitly at each scheduled reassessment interval during transport, with each item re-graded as improving, stable, or worsening. A problem list that is built once at departure and never revisited functionally degrades into the same kind of stale snapshot that Chapter 1 warned against for vital sign trending, and the discipline of active re-grading is what keeps the framework useful throughout a transport of any meaningful duration.

### Physiologic Reserve Estimation Under Time Pressure

Beyond simply cataloguing current status, the rapid assessment should generate an explicit estimate of physiologic reserve--how much additional physiologic insult, whether from the transport environment itself or from an evolving disease process, this specific patient can tolerate before decompensation becomes likely. A patient maintaining an adequate blood pressure only through an already near-maximal vasopressor dose has essentially no reserve, even though the displayed number looks acceptable, whereas a patient with an identical blood pressure achieved on a low, easily titratable dose has considerably more room to absorb an unexpected stressor. This reserve estimate, made explicitly rather than left implicit, directly informs decisions made throughout the remainder of this chapter and the disease-specific chapters that follow: how aggressively to invest in invasive monitoring, how low the threshold should be for early intervention rather than watchful waiting, and how the crew should prioritize their limited attention across a patient with multiple simultaneous physiologic problems.

### Time-Limited Primary and Secondary Survey

A structured primary survey--airway, breathing, circulation, disability, exposure--performed within the first minutes at the bedside, regardless of how much sending-facility documentation is available, establishes an independent baseline that the transport crew can trust as their own rather than one inherited secondhand. This is not redundant with the sending team's assessment; it is the transport crew's own point of reference against which every subsequent change during transit will be measured, and it frequently identifies findings--a subtly diminished breath sound, a new petechial rash, a pupillary asymmetry--that were not the focus of the sending team's more diagnosis-specific evaluation.

A secondary survey, performed once the primary survey confirms no immediately life-threatening finding, should systematically examine each body region and each indwelling line, tube, and drain for security, position, and function, since a dislodged or malpositioned device discovered mid-transport is considerably harder to correct than one identified and secured before departure. This survey should also explicitly note baseline skin integrity and pressure points, particularly for transports anticipated to exceed thirty minutes, since prolonged immobility on a transport stretcher carries its own, distinct risk of pressure injury that is easy to overlook amid higher-acuity concerns.

**KEY POINT:** The transport crew's own hands-on primary survey, however brief, becomes the true baseline for the transport--not the sending facility's last documented vital signs, which may already be minutes to hours old by the time of departure.

### Team Role Allocation During Initial Assessment

A two- or three-person transport crew arriving at a sending bedside benefits substantially from an explicit, pre-briefed division of labor during the initial assessment window rather than allowing each member to independently and redundantly examine the same findings while other elements go unassessed. A common and effective allocation assigns one clinician to the hands-on primary survey and equipment verification, a second to extracting the decisive elements of the sending documentation and speaking directly with the sending team, and, where a third crew member is present, a dedicated role confirming line, tube, and medication security in preparation for movement. This division should be established as a standing team convention before ever arriving at a specific bedside, since negotiating roles in real time at an unfamiliar sending facility consumes exactly the time the framework is designed to conserve. Cross-training every crew member in every role remains essential, since patient acuity or staffing on a given mission may require any individual to assume any role without notice.

## Invasive and Noninvasive Hemodynamic Monitoring in Transit

### Matching Monitoring Modality to Physiologic Uncertainty

The decision to establish invasive arterial or central venous monitoring before departure should be driven by the degree of physiologic uncertainty and instability anticipated during transit, not solely by whether the sending facility had already placed such lines. A patient on even a low-dose vasopressor infusion, or one whose hemodynamic trajectory over the preceding hour has been anything other than flat and reassuring, benefits from arterial line placement before departure, both because it provides continuous rather than intermittent pressure data and because, as established in Chapter 1, noninvasive cuff cycling is disproportionately unreliable under transport vibration.

### Continuous Waveform Interpretation as a Monitoring Discipline

Once invasive monitoring is established, the transport clinician should treat continuous waveform review--arterial pressure tracing, capnography waveform, and, where present, central venous or pulmonary artery pressure tracing--as an active surveillance task rather than a passive number on a screen. Waveform morphology frequently signals a developing problem before the corresponding numeric value crosses an alarm threshold: a narrowing pulse pressure on the arterial tracing, a rising capnography baseline suggesting rebreathing or hypoventilation, or a new respiratory variation in the arterial waveform suggesting volume responsiveness, are all findings visible in the waveform well before they would be reflected in an intermittent vital sign reading.

### Point-of-Care Ultrasound as a Transport-Adapted Monitoring Extension

Portable point-of-care ultrasound, where crew training and equipment allow, extends the monitoring picture beyond what waveforms and numeric trends alone can provide, particularly for rapid reassessment of a new hemodynamic change: a focused cardiac view can distinguish a volume-responsive picture from a new pericardial effusion or right heart strain pattern within moments, information that would otherwise require a return to a fixed diagnostic imaging suite unavailable during transit. A brief, protocolized examination--assessing cardiac contractility, inferior vena cava size and collapsibility, and the presence or absence of lung sliding--can be performed within the confines of a moving vehicle or aircraft cabin with practice, and its principal transport-specific limitation is image quality degradation under vibration, which argues for pausing or bracing against a stable surface during image acquisition rather than attempting to scan through active turbulence.

Figure 2.1: Arterial Waveform Morphology and Early Deterioration Signals

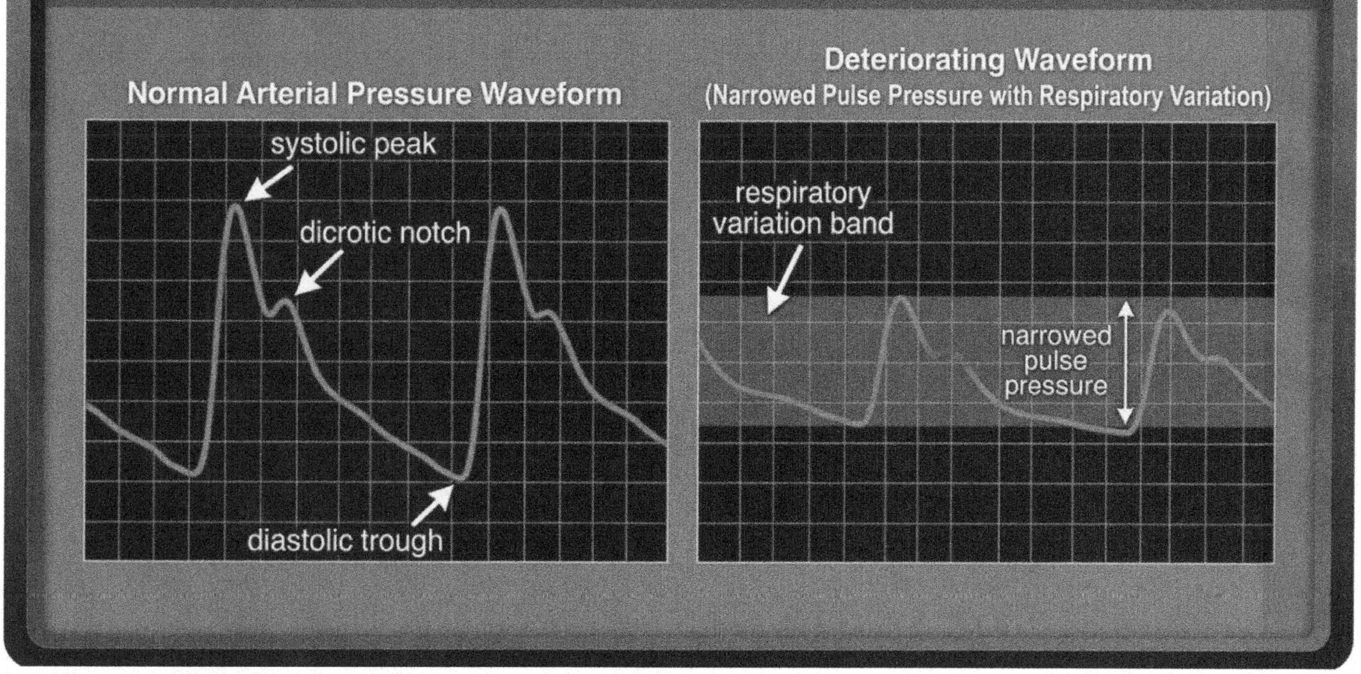


### Vasoactive Infusion Management and Line Security

Continuous vasoactive infusions require particular attention to line security and pump function during transport, since an interrupted or dislodged infusion in a patient dependent on it for hemodynamic support can produce a rapid and severe deterioration that is entirely preventable with adequate preparation. Before departure, the crew should confirm that all vasoactive infusion lines are clearly labeled, secured against inadvertent traction at the connection points most likely to be jostled during loading and movement, and connected to a pump with sufficient battery reserve independently verified for the full anticipated transport duration plus a safety margin, following the same derating logic for cold-weather battery performance introduced in Chapter 1. Wherever multiple vasoactive infusions run simultaneously, a clear, crew-wide understanding of which line delivers which medication, confirmed verbally before departure, prevents a dangerous mix-up if a line requires troubleshooting mid-transport.

| Monitoring Modality | Primary Transport Advantage | Key Limitation in Transit |
|---|---|---|
| Invasive arterial line | Continuous, vibration-resistant pressure data; waveform morphology visible | Requires procedural time and skill before departure |
| Noninvasive blood pressure cuff | No procedure required | Unreliable during vibration and turbulence; intermittent only |
| Continuous capnography | Continuous ventilation adequacy and rebreathing surveillance | Sampling line prone to mechanical disruption |
| Point-of-care ultrasound | Rapid structural and functional reassessment without imaging suite | Image quality degrades under vibration; operator-dependent |
| Central venous pressure monitoring | Trend data for volume status and right heart function | Absolute values less reliable than trend; requires central access |

**Figure 2.2: Point-of-Care Ultrasound Probe Positioning for Focused Cardiac and Lung Views**

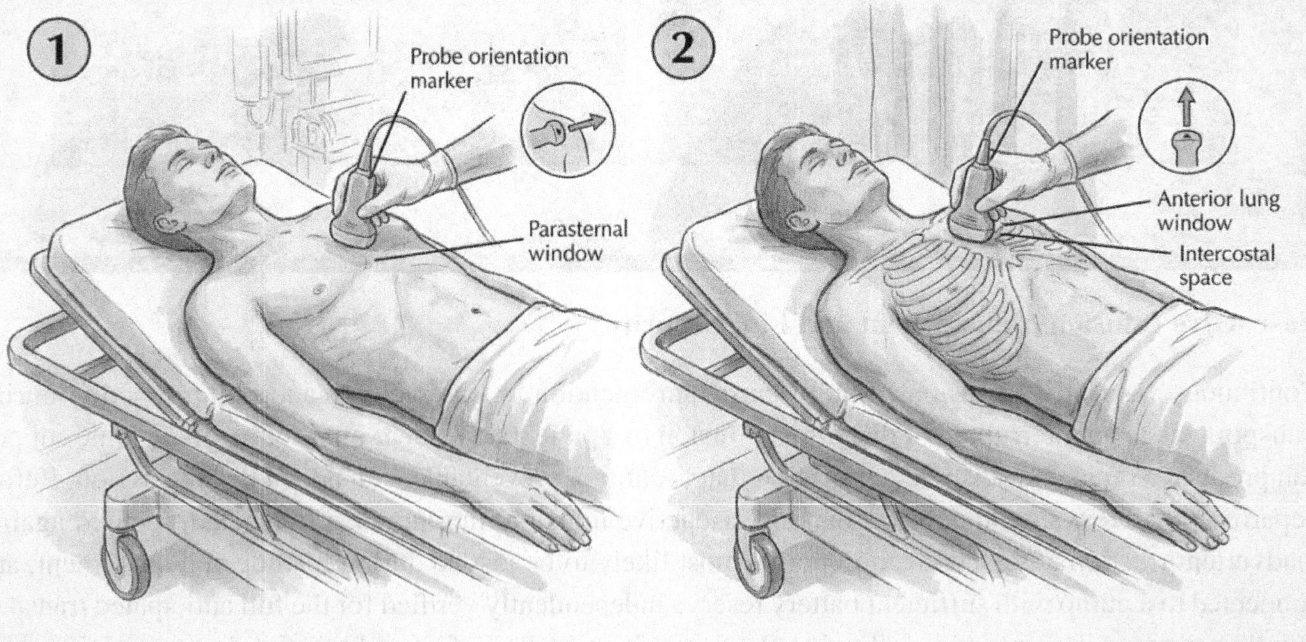

### Transitioning Monitoring Modalities Mid-Transport

Occasionally a patient's monitoring needs escalate mid-transport--a previously borderline patient develops a clear indication for invasive arterial monitoring after departure, or a peripheral intravenous line providing vasoactive infusion access becomes compromised and central access must be considered under transit conditions. Establishing new invasive monitoring or access mid-transport is procedurally more difficult than at a stationary bedside, given confined space, vibration, and lighting limitations, and the decision to attempt it in transit versus request an unscheduled stop or diversion should weigh the specific urgency of the need against the specific procedural difficulty the environment imposes. As a general principle, any procedure that is not time-critical should be deferred to the next planned stop or to arrival rather than attempted under suboptimal transit conditions purely for the sake of avoiding a brief delay, since a failed or complicated procedural attempt in transit carries greater risk than the delay itself.

## Interpreting the Inherited ICU Workup

### Extracting the Decisive Elements Under Time Pressure

A sending facility's chart may contain hours of laboratory trends, multiple imaging studies, and a detailed narrative note, none of which can be fully absorbed within the time available at a bedside handoff. The transport clinician's task is to extract the specific elements that will change management during transit: the most recent arterial blood gas and its trend direction, the current ventilator settings and how recently they were adjusted, the trajectory of any vasoactive infusion over the preceding hour, and any critical imaging finding that establishes a structural diagnosis relevant to in-flight risk, such as an aortic dissection flap location or a pneumothorax size. Everything else is useful context but not decision-critical within the transport window.

### Verifying Rather Than Assuming Sending-Facility Data

Wherever feasible within the time available, the transport clinician should independently verify at least the most consequential elements of the inherited workup rather than accepting them uncritically: confirming tube or line position by direct assessment rather than relying solely on a chart note, confirming the current infusion rate at the pump rather than the rate documented an hour earlier, and confirming allergy and code status information verbally with the sending team or family when time allows, since documentation errors and stale data are more common in a rapid interfacility handoff than in routine inpatient care.

### Communicating With the Sending Team Under Time Constraints

The sending team is frequently managing multiple competing demands at the moment of transport handoff, and the transport clinician's ability to extract decisive information efficiently depends heavily on asking targeted, closed-ended questions rather than open-ended ones that invite a lengthy narrative response. Questions structured around the physiologic problem list developed earlier in this chapter--"has the vasopressor requirement changed in the last two hours," "what was the most recent blood gas and when was it drawn," "is there any reason to expect this airway to be difficult"--yield decision-relevant answers efficiently, whereas an open request to "walk me through the case" often consumes disproportionate time relative to the clinically actionable information it returns. This targeted questioning style should be practiced deliberately, since it runs counter to the more narrative handoff style common in routine inpatient nursing report.

### THE IN-TRANSIT DETERIORATION SIGNATURE SYSTEM — Undisclosed Trajectory Mismatch

**The Signature:** A patient who appears stable at the moment of transport departure but whose sending-facility trend data, if reviewed carefully, actually shows a worsening trajectory over the preceding one to two hours that was not verbally emphasized during handoff.

**Movement Trigger:** The handoff moment itself, in which a busy sending team communicates a snapshot rather than a trend, and the receiving transport crew, working from that snapshot, departs without recognizing that the patient is already moving in an unfavorable direction before any transport-specific stress has even been applied.

**Early Tell:** A vasopressor or ventilator support requirement that has been escalating, even gradually, over the hour or two preceding transport, rather than one that has been flat or improving.

**Trap Logic:** This pattern is easily missed because the single most recent vital sign set, viewed in isolation, may still fall within an acceptable range; the discriminating feature is not the most recent value but the slope of the trend leading up to it, which requires actively requesting and reviewing trend data rather than a single snapshot.

**Signature Anchor:** Before every departure, explicitly request the trend of support requirements--vasopressor dose, ventilator settings, oxygen requirement--over the preceding two hours, not merely the current value, and treat a worsening trend as grounds for a lower threshold to escalate monitoring and intervention readiness during transit, even if the single most recent value looks acceptable.

**CLINICAL PEARL:** Asking a sending nurse or physician the specific question, "has this patient's support requirement gone up, down, or stayed flat over the last two hours," often surfaces trend information that a chart review under time pressure would miss entirely.

### Medication Reconciliation and Allergy Verification

A focused medication reconciliation, distinct from a complete review of the sending facility's medication administration record, should confirm the identity, concentration, and current rate of every active infusion, the timing and dose of the most recent analgesic, sedative, or paralytic administration, and any recently administered medication with a delayed or ongoing effect relevant to transport--a loading dose of an antiarrhythmic, a bolus of a reversal agent, or a recently administered thrombolytic. Allergy status, verified verbally rather than assumed from a chart field that may not have been updated, is a small but consequential check, since a transport crew that discovers a documented allergy only after administering a medication has lost the entire value of a verification step that would have taken seconds to perform proactively.

## Trending Versus Threshold-Based Vital Sign Interpretation

### Why Fixed Normal Ranges Fail the Already-Abnormal Patient

Standard vital sign reference ranges are calibrated to a physiologically normal population, and applying them unmodified to a patient who is, by definition, already critically ill produces a monitoring strategy that is both insensitive to real deterioration and prone to false reassurance. A patient whose baseline mean arterial pressure has been sixty-two millimeters of mercury for the preceding several hours on a stable vasopressor dose is not necessarily deteriorating at that same pressure an hour into transport; conversely, a fall from a baseline of ninety to seventy, even though seventy might appear acceptable on a generic reference range, represents a meaningful deviation that deserves the same clinical attention as an objectively abnormal number in a healthier patient.

### Establishing and Using a Patient-Specific Baseline

The practical application of this principle is straightforward: at the start of every transport, the crew should explicitly record the patient's own baseline across each monitored parameter, and every subsequent reassessment should be interpreted primarily as a deviation from that specific baseline rather than as a comparison against a population reference range. This is particularly consequential in patients with chronic hypertension, chronic hypoxemia from underlying lung disease, or a neurologically abnormal baseline mental status, all of whom would generate false alarms under threshold-based monitoring and false reassurance under a purely snapshot-based assessment that never establishes what normal looks like for this specific patient.

### Special Considerations in Chronic Disease Populations

Patients with chronic obstructive pulmonary disease frequently maintain a baseline oxygen saturation in the high eighties to low nineties that would prompt aggressive intervention in a patient without underlying lung disease, and applying a universal saturation target risks either unnecessary intervention or, through excessive supplemental oxygen, precipitation of hypercapnic respiratory failure in a patient dependent on a degree of hypoxic respiratory drive. Similarly, a patient with longstanding, poorly controlled hypertension may tolerate--and in fact require--a higher mean arterial pressure to maintain adequate cerebral and renal perfusion than a normotensive patient, a consideration directly relevant to blood pressure management targets discussed further in the neurologic and cardiovascular chapters that follow. Establishing each patient's chronic baseline explicitly, rather than defaulting to a universal target, is not a refinement of monitoring practice but a precondition for interpreting any subsequent change correctly.

### Documenting and Displaying Trend Data for Rapid Reference

A patient-specific baseline is only useful if it remains readily visible to the entire crew throughout transport rather than existing only in one clinician's memory or buried in a written note. Writing the established baseline values in a fixed, visible location--a dedicated line on the transport monitoring sheet, or a grease-pencil notation on the monitor bezel itself where institutional practice allows--ensures that any crew member glancing at the current display can immediately compare it against the patient-specific reference rather than a generic range, and this small documentation habit is what actually operationalizes the trending principle described above under the time pressure of an active transport rather than leaving it as an abstract best practice.

## Structured Handoff and Interfacility Communication

### A Standardized Handoff Structure at Both Ends of Transport

A structured handoff format--covering the working diagnosis, the physiologic problem list established at the start of this chapter, interventions performed and their timing, the trend observed during transit, and specific anticipated needs on arrival--should be used consistently both when receiving the patient from the sending facility and when delivering the patient to the receiving facility. Consistency in structure, rather than a free-form narrative that varies by clinician, reduces the likelihood that a decisive piece of information is omitted under the time pressure and cognitive load of a bedside-to-bedside transfer.

### Communicating Trajectory, Not Only Status

The single most valuable piece of information a transport crew can deliver to a receiving team, beyond the patient's current status, is the trajectory observed during transit: whether the patient trended better, worse, or unchanged, and what specific event or intervention, if any, corresponded to a change in that trajectory. A receiving team that hears only "the patient is currently stable" without any trajectory context has lost the clinical narrative that the transport crew alone was positioned to observe, and that narrative frequently changes the receiving team's index of suspicion and initial management priorities.

### Handling Discrepancies Between Sending and Transport Assessment

When the transport crew's independent assessment meaningfully diverges from the sending facility's characterization--a physical examination finding not previously documented, a trend the sending team had not emphasized, or a monitoring value that differs from what was reported--this discrepancy should be communicated directly and specifically to the receiving team rather than smoothed over or omitted to avoid the appearance of contradicting the sending facility. The goal of this disclosure is not to assign fault but to ensure the receiving team has the most complete and accurate picture available, since a receiving team that is never told about a discrepancy cannot factor it into their own initial assessment and may anchor on an outdated or incomplete characterization. Framing this communication factually and without editorializing--"on our exam we noted X, which was not mentioned in the sending report"--preserves collegial working relationships across facilities while still ensuring the clinically relevant information is transmitted.

### Family Communication During Transport

Family members present at the sending facility, and occasionally accompanying the patient during ground transport, require a distinct communication approach from the clinical handoff described above: brief, honest, jargon-free language describing what is happening and what to expect next, delivered with attention to the family's evident level of distress and comprehension rather than as a condensed version of the clinical report. Providing a family member with a specific point of contact and an estimated arrival time, even when the clinical picture remains uncertain, meaningfully reduces family distress without requiring the crew to overstate their confidence in the outcome, and this brief communication should be treated as a genuine element of the transport clinician's role rather than an optional courtesy fit in only if time allows.

Consider a thirty-four-year-old woman transferred by ground critical care ambulance for a suspected pulmonary embolism, hemodynamically borderline at the sending facility with a heart rate in the low one hundreds and a systolic pressure in the low nineties, characterized by the sending team as "stable for transport." The transport clinician's independent primary survey confirms these findings but also notes, on direct examination, a subtly cool and mottled distal extremity exam not commented on in the sending documentation. Rather than accepting the "stable for transport" characterization uncritically, the crew establishes their own baseline, places an arterial line given the borderline pressure and physiologic uncertainty, and monitors closely through a forty-minute transport during which the pressure trends gradually downward from ninety-two to eighty-one systolic despite an unchanged clinical appearance otherwise.

Because the crew had established their own baseline and was tracking trend rather than reassessing against the sending facility's threshold of "stable," this gradual change is recognized and communicated proactively to the receiving team before arrival, allowing the emergency department to have escalation resources--including consideration of thrombolytic therapy--ready immediately on arrival rather than reassessing from a colder start. The patient's husband, riding in the front of the ambulance, is given a brief, honest update at the midpoint of transport--that the patient's blood pressure has trended down somewhat and that the team is actively monitoring and has already alerted the receiving hospital--rather than being left uninformed until arrival, which the crew later notes measurably eased his visible anxiety without requiring any overstatement of certainty about the outcome. This case illustrates the chapter's central argument: the transport clinician's value lies not in repeating the sending facility's assessment, but in independently establishing a baseline, tracking deviation from it with discipline, and communicating that trajectory faithfully to whoever--clinical team or family--receives the patient's story next.

## Advanced Assessment Techniques for the Transport Environment

### Integrating Physical Examination With Continuous Monitoring Data

The transport clinician's assessment integrates two fundamentally different information streams that must be reconciled continuously: the continuous, automated data from monitors (heart rate, blood pressure, oxygen saturation, capnography, and where present, invasive pressures) and the intermittent, manually obtained data from physical examination (mentation, skin perfusion, breath sounds, abdominal examination, and neurologic findings). Neither stream alone provides a complete picture. A monitor can display a normal heart rate and blood pressure while the patient's skin is mottled and cool, indicating compensated shock that the monitor alone would miss. Conversely, a patient who appears clinically unchanged may be developing a subtle but sustained arterial waveform change that indicates a hemodynamic shift detectable only on the continuous monitor. The transport clinician who relies exclusively on one information stream and neglects the other will systematically miss one category of deterioration, and the discipline of actively integrating both streams at each reassessment interval is what separates expert transport assessment from adequate monitoring.

### Developing a Mental Model of the Patient's Expected Trajectory

Beyond establishing a baseline and monitoring for deviation, the expert transport clinician develops a mental model of the patient's expected trajectory for the transport window: what should this patient look like in twenty minutes, in forty minutes, at arrival? This trajectory projection is based on the known natural history of the patient's condition, the expected response to therapies already initiated, and the specific transport-environment stressors that will be imposed during the mission. A patient with septic shock who received a fluid bolus and vasopressor initiation fifteen minutes before departure should show some hemodynamic improvement by twenty minutes into the transport; if they do not, the absence of the expected improvement is itself a finding, signaling either inadequate resuscitation, an additional hemodynamic insult, or a more severe shock state than initially appreciated. This expected-trajectory mental model is the cognitive tool that allows the clinician to detect deterioration before the numbers cross an alarm threshold, because the clinician is comparing the current state not against a population normal but against what this specific patient should be doing right now if the working assessment is correct.

## Pre-Departure Decision Framework: To Transport or Not

### Assessing Whether the Patient Is Safe to Move

The transport clinician arriving at the sending facility faces a decision that is sometimes overlooked in the urgency to move: is this patient actually safe to transport right now, or would a brief stabilization period at the sending bedside produce a meaningfully safer transport? The sending facility has already decided to transfer--that decision is made--but the transport crew retains the clinical authority to delay departure for stabilization if the patient's current condition represents an unacceptable risk for the specific transport environment. Situations that may warrant a brief stabilization delay include: an unsecured airway in a patient with predicted difficulty (intubate before departure rather than in transit), hemodynamic instability that has not yet responded to initial resuscitation (stabilize before loading), an uncontrolled seizure (terminate before movement), or an equipment readiness problem (resolve before departure). The general principle is that a ten-to-fifteen-minute delay at the sending bedside to convert an unstable patient into a stabilized one almost always produces a safer and ultimately faster transport than departing immediately with an actively deteriorating patient whose in-transit management will be more difficult and more dangerous.

### Communicating the Stabilization Decision to the Sending Team

The decision to delay departure for stabilization can create tension with a sending facility that has been waiting for transport and expects immediate departure, and the transport clinician must communicate this decision clearly and professionally: "We need to stabilize X before we can safely transport. This will take approximately Y minutes. Here is what we need to do." This communication should be framed as a patient safety decision, not as a criticism of the sending facility's management, and the specific stabilization tasks should be identified and assigned to avoid ambiguity about what needs to happen before departure can proceed. A sending team that understands the specific clinical reasoning behind the delay is generally supportive, while a sending team that perceives an unexplained delay may become frustrated in ways that degrade the collaborative relationship between facilities.

## Continuous Reassessment Architecture During Transport

### Structured Versus Opportunistic Reassessment

Transport reassessment can be either structured (performed at defined time intervals regardless of the patient's apparent clinical status) or opportunistic (performed when something triggers the clinician's attention, such as an alarm, a visible change, or an internal sense that something is different). Expert transport clinicians use both, but the structured component is the more important of the two, because opportunistic reassessment depends on the clinician noticing a change, which in turn depends on attention, vigilance, and the signal-to-noise ratio of the transport environment--all of which degrade over time, with fatigue, and under cognitive load. A structured reassessment interval ensures that every monitored parameter and every relevant physical finding is systematically reviewed at a frequency that matches the patient's acuity, regardless of whether anything has triggered the clinician's attention in the interval.

### Determining the Appropriate Reassessment Interval

The reassessment interval should be matched to the patient's acuity and the expected rate of change of their clinical condition: a hemodynamically unstable patient on multiple vasoactive infusions may warrant reassessment every five minutes, a stable patient on a single low-dose vasopressor every ten to fifteen minutes, and a fully stable, monitored patient being transferred for an elective procedure every fifteen to twenty minutes. These intervals should be explicitly decided and communicated to the crew before departure rather than left to each clinician's individual judgment, since an undefined reassessment interval in practice means that the interval stretches progressively longer as the transport continues without incident and the clinician's vigilance fades--exactly the scenario in which a slowly developing deterioration is most likely to be missed.

### The Reassessment Bundle: What to Check Every Time

Each structured reassessment should follow a consistent, complete sequence rather than a selective survey of whichever parameters the clinician happens to think of: airway security and ventilator parameters (tube depth, circuit integrity, delivered tidal volume, peak and plateau pressures, capnography waveform), hemodynamic status (arterial pressure trend, heart rate, rhythm, vasopressor dose and trajectory, urine output since last check), neurologic status (level of consciousness, pupil size and reactivity, motor response), and equipment status (infusion rates and remaining volumes, battery reserves, line and tube security, monitoring lead integrity). This bundle should take no more than sixty to ninety seconds for a stable patient and produces the comprehensive, multi-system trend data that the receiving team depends on for trajectory assessment, data that a selective, parameter-by-parameter check reliably misses through inconsistency.

## Documentation Standards for Transport Medicine

### Real-Time Versus Retrospective Documentation

Documentation performed in real time--at the moment of the assessment, intervention, or clinical change--is categorically more accurate than documentation reconstructed from memory after arrival, particularly for the specific timing and sequence of events that the receiving team needs to understand the patient's trajectory. A vital sign recorded at the moment it was obtained carries the correct timestamp; the same vital sign reconstructed from memory ten minutes later may carry an estimated timestamp that is minutes off, and in a time-critical condition like acute stroke or STEMI, those minutes materially affect the receiving team's management decisions. The practical challenge is that real-time documentation competes with clinical care for the clinician's attention, and the solution is a documentation system--whether electronic, paper-based, or a combination--that allows rapid capture with minimal distraction: tick-boxes for structured data, pre-formatted time entries, and free-text fields only for narrative that cannot be captured in a structured format.

### What the Receiving Team Needs From the Transport Record

The transport record serves two purposes: a medicolegal document of the care provided during transport, and a clinical communication tool that transfers information from the transport crew to the receiving team. For the second purpose, the receiving team needs specific, actionable information: the patient's baseline at departure, every intervention performed and its timing, every significant vital sign change and its temporal relationship to an intervention or transport event, the current status of all infusions and devices, and the specific trajectory observed during transport (improving, stable, or worsening, with details). A receiving team that reads the transport record should be able to reconstruct the entire transport narrative--what happened, when, what was done about it, and what the response was--without needing to interview the transport crew, since the crew may have already departed for another mission by the time the receiving team needs the information.

### Verbal Handoff Structure: SBAR and Its Limitations

The Situation-Background-Assessment-Recommendation framework provides a structured format for verbal handoff that reduces omission of critical information, and most transport programs use either SBAR or a program-specific variant as their standard handoff format. The transport-specific limitation of SBAR is that the standard format does not include an explicit trajectory component--the trend observed during transport--which, as argued throughout this chapter, is the single most valuable piece of information the transport crew can provide. A modified format that adds a Trajectory element between Assessment and

Recommendation (SBATR) ensures that the receiving team hears not only what the patient looks like now but what direction they were heading during the transport, a distinction that frequently changes the receiving team's initial management posture. The verbal handoff should be delivered to the specific clinician who will be assuming the patient's care, not to a triage nurse or registration clerk, and the transport clinician should confirm that the receiving clinician has no further questions before departing the receiving facility.

## Legal and Regulatory Considerations in Transport Assessment

### EMTALA Obligations and the Transport Crew's Role

The Emergency Medical Treatment and Labor Act requires that the sending facility provide an appropriate transfer when the patient requires a level of care beyond the facility's capability, and the transport clinician should understand their role within this legal framework: the sending facility is responsible for stabilizing the patient within its capability before transfer, the transport crew is responsible for maintaining that stabilization during transport, and the receiving facility is obligated to accept the transfer and provide the needed care. The transport clinician's assessment at the sending bedside serves a secondary legal function: it documents the patient's condition at the moment of transfer and becomes part of the legal record should the appropriateness of the transfer be questioned. Thorough, real-time documentation of the patient's condition, stability, and the transport crew's independent assessment protects all parties in the transfer chain.

### Scope of Practice and Protocol Authority During Transport

Transport clinicians operate under medical control authority that defines standing orders, protocol-based interventions, and the circumstances requiring real-time physician consultation. The scope of practice for transport nurses, paramedics, and respiratory therapists varies by state, by program, and by medical director preference, and the transport clinician must know their specific scope of practice boundaries, particularly for interventions that exceed standard EMS or hospital-floor nursing scope--blood product administration, vasoactive infusion titration, chest tube management, and advanced airway procedures--that are routine in critical care transport but may not be within the clinician's base scope without specific transport protocols or medical control authorization. When a clinical situation arises that exceeds the crew's standing protocols, contacting medical control should be the first step rather than the last resort, and the communication should use the same structured format (SBAR or equivalent) used for receiving-facility handoff to ensure complete information transfer.

## Telemedicine Integration in Transport Assessment

### Real-Time Video Consultation During Transport

Telemedicine technology increasingly allows real-time video consultation between the transport crew and a remote physician specialist during transit, enabling expert guidance for clinical decisions that exceed the crew's scope of practice or comfort level. The transport clinician should understand the specific telemedicine capabilities available on their platform--cellular-based video, satellite communication, or dedicated telemedicine hardware--and the connectivity limitations of each during different phases of transport. A telemedicine consultation that drops mid-sentence during a mountain pass or a communication dead zone is worse than no consultation at all if the crew has already begun an intervention based on partial guidance, and the crew should confirm communication reliability before initiating a telemedicine consultation for a complex clinical decision.

### Transmitting Clinical Data to the Receiving Facility

Beyond voice and video communication, some transport programs have the capability to transmit clinical data--12-lead ECGs, monitor waveform snapshots, and even point-of-care imaging--directly to the receiving facility during transport. This data transmission capability transforms the receiving team's preparation from one based on a verbal description to one based on their own review of the objective clinical data, and for time-critical conditions such as STEMI and large vessel occlusion stroke, the ability to transmit the ECG or CT angiography images directly to the receiving specialist can save minutes in the activation sequence. The transport clinician should know which data types can be transmitted from their specific platform, how to initiate the transmission, and who at the receiving facility should receive it.

### Remote Medical Control: When to Call and What to Communicate

Medical control consultation during transport serves two purposes: clinical guidance for decisions that exceed standing protocols, and medicolegal authorization for interventions that require physician order. The transport clinician should contact medical control proactively--before a clinical situation has become critical--rather than reactively after a deterioration has already progressed beyond easy management. The communication format should follow the same SBAR structure used for facility handoff, with the addition of a specific request: "I am calling for guidance on X" or "I need authorization for Y," so that the medical control physician can provide a focused, actionable response rather than a lengthy differential diagnosis. The crew should document the medical control conversation, including the physician's name, the guidance provided, and the time of the call, as part of the transport record.

### GPS and Geolocation in Transport Decision-Making

Modern transport platforms integrate GPS and geolocation data that provide the crew with real-time information about their position relative to potential receiving facilities, diversion airports, and ground EMS staging areas, information that directly affects clinical decisions about diversion, destination selection, and estimated time of arrival communication. When a patient deteriorates during transport and the crew must decide between continuing to the originally planned receiving facility or diverting to a closer facility, the GPS-derived time-to-each-destination calculation provides the objective data needed for a rational decision rather than a guess. The transport clinician should know how to access this information on their specific platform and should incorporate destination-time data into every diversion decision.

## Cognitive Load Management During Complex Transports

The cognitive load imposed on the transport clinician during a complex transport--a patient on multiple vasoactive infusions, a mechanical circulatory support device, and a challenging airway, being transported during turbulence with intermittent communication capability--can exceed the working memory capacity of even experienced clinicians, producing errors of omission (forgetting to perform a scheduled reassessment), commission (administering a medication at the wrong dose or through the wrong line), and fixation (becoming cognitively locked on one clinical problem while others evolve unmonitored). Effective cognitive load management uses external memory aids--checklists, written medication logs, alarm-based reassessment reminders--to offload tasks from working memory onto reliable external systems, freeing the clinician's cognitive resources for the clinical judgment and decision-making that cannot be externalized.

## Shared Mental Models Between Crew Members

A shared mental model between crew members--a common understanding of the patient's condition, the current plan, the anticipated trajectory, and the contingency responses--reduces the communication overhead required to coordinate care during a crisis, since each crew member can anticipate the other's actions without explicit direction. Building a shared mental model requires a deliberate pre-departure briefing that covers not only the patient's current status but the expected trajectory, the planned monitoring and intervention schedule, the most likely deterioration scenario, and the specific role each crew member will play if that scenario occurs. This briefing takes two to three minutes and produces a team whose crisis response is coordinated by shared expectation rather than real-time direction, a distinction that saves critical seconds during a time-sensitive emergency.

## Patient and Family Expectations Management

The patient and family's understanding of what the transport involves--the duration, the expected sensations (noise, vibration, temperature changes), what they can and cannot bring, who will accompany the patient, and what will happen on arrival--significantly affects the smoothness of the transport and the patient's psychological state during transit. A brief, proactive explanation before departure, delivered at a pace and level appropriate to the family's distress and comprehension, prevents the anxiety-driven questions and requests that consume crew attention during the transport and that can be misinterpreted as clinical changes when an anxious patient's heart rate and blood pressure rise from psychological rather than physiologic stress.

**THE IN-TRANSIT DETERIORATION SIGNATURE SYSTEM — Assessment and Handoff Patterns**

**Signature Introduced This Chapter:** Undisclosed Trajectory Mismatch (a worsening pre-transport trend obscured by a reassuring single snapshot at handoff).

**Shared Assessment Logic:** This Signature is fundamentally a data-interpretation pattern rather than a physiologic-mechanism pattern, and it underlies every disease-specific Signature introduced in later chapters: a snapshot vital sign, however reassuring, is never a substitute for an actively solicited trend.

**Cross-Reference Forward:** Every subsequent chapter assumes the trend-based, patient-specific-baseline framework established here; disease-specific Signatures in Chapters 4 through 19 build on this chapter's assessment discipline rather than repeating it.

## Summary and Key Concepts

A diagnosis-agnostic physiologic problem list--airway, breathing, circulation, disability, exposure--generates an actionable transport plan even before the underlying diagnosis is fully understood, and should be actively re-graded, not set once and forgotten.

An explicit physiologic reserve estimate, not just current status, should drive decisions about monitoring intensity and intervention threshold throughout transport.

Invasive monitoring should be established proactively based on anticipated physiologic uncertainty, not merely matched to what the sending facility had already placed.

Extracting the decisive elements of an inherited workup through targeted, closed-ended questioning matters more under time pressure than absorbing the complete chart or a narrative handoff.

Vital signs must be interpreted against the patient's own established baseline, not a population reference range, particularly in patients with chronic abnormal baselines such as COPD or chronic hypertension.

A structured handoff that communicates trajectory, not merely current status, preserves the clinical value the transport crew alone was positioned to observe, and honest, brief family communication is a genuine part of that same discipline.

# CHAPTER 3: AIRWAY AND VENTILATOR MANAGEMENT IN TRANSIT

**Learning Objectives**

1. Perform a structured difficult airway assessment and select an appropriate rapid sequence intubation strategy adapted to the field or transport environment.
2. Select portable ventilator modes and settings appropriate to specific disease processes encountered in transport.
3. Apply lung-protective ventilation principles consistently across the transport window, including during equipment transitions.
4. Interpret ventilator waveforms to identify and troubleshoot common in-transit problems.
5. Recognize and manage airway emergencies, including loss of airway and difficult rescue ventilation, in a moving vehicle or aircraft.

**Chapter Outline**

This chapter addresses airway and ventilator management as a continuous discipline spanning pre-departure decision-making, in-transit maintenance, and emergency rescue, building directly on the altitude and gas-law physiology introduced in Chapter 1 and the monitoring and assessment framework established in Chapter 2.

Airway and ventilator management carry disproportionate weight in critical care transport practice, and for good reason: a secure airway and adequate ventilation are prerequisites for the safe application of nearly every other intervention discussed elsewhere in this text, and the confined, resource-limited transport environment converts an airway problem that would be readily manageable at the bedside into a genuine emergency with fewer hands, less light, and less room to work. This chapter builds the anticipatory framework that keeps airway and ventilator management proactive rather than reactive.

## Difficult Airway Assessment and Rapid Sequence Intubation in the Field

### Structured Difficult Airway Prediction Before Departure

Every patient being transported with an unsecured airway, or with an airway that may require re-securing during transit due to accidental extubation risk, should undergo a structured difficult airway assessment before departure, evaluating mouth opening, thyromental distance, neck mobility, and any anatomic distortion from trauma, edema, or prior surgery. This assessment differs in one crucial respect from its bedside counterpart: the transport clinician must also assess difficulty specific to the transport environment itself--patient positioning constraints within the vehicle or aircraft, available lighting, and the physical space available for a rescue approach if the first attempt fails--none of which factor into a standard hospital-based airway assessment.

### Adapting Rapid Sequence Intubation to the Transport Environment

Rapid sequence intubation performed in the field or at a sending facility immediately before transport follows the same pharmacologic and procedural principles as an in-hospital intubation, with several transport-specific modifications: induction and paralytic agent selection should account for the hemodynamic fragility common in transport patients, favoring agents with a more favorable hemodynamic profile where the clinical picture allows; a fully prepared rescue airway plan, including a supraglottic device and surgical airway kit immediately accessible, should be confirmed before any paralytic is administered, since the transport environment offers less immediate backup than a hospital operating room or emergency department; and the decision to intubate before departure versus during transit should default strongly toward securing the airway before movement begins whenever the clinical trajectory suggests intubation will likely become necessary during the transport window regardless, since airway management in a moving vehicle is categorically more difficult than at a stationary bedside.

### Confirming and Securing the Airway for Movement

Following successful intubation, tube position must be confirmed by waveform capnography, not color-change detection alone, and the tube must be secured using a method resistant to the traction forces anticipated during loading, movement, and any planned patient repositioning, since a tube that migrates even one to two centimeters during transit can result in mainstem intubation or inadvertent extubation. Depth at the lip or teeth should be explicitly documented and re-verified at each scheduled reassessment interval established in Chapter 2, using the same trend-based discipline applied to every other monitored parameter.

**CAUTION:** Color-change capnometry alone is insufficient confirmation for a transport intubation; continuous waveform capnography must be established and maintained for the duration of transport, since a colorimetric device provides only a single point-in-time confirmation and cannot detect subsequent tube migration.

### Pre-Oxygenation and Apneic Oxygenation Strategies in the Field

Thorough pre-oxygenation before any rapid sequence intubation attempt is particularly consequential in the transport setting, where a failed first attempt has fewer readily available rescue resources than a hospital operating room. High-flow nasal oxygen continued through the apneic period, where equipment allows, extends the safe apnea window and reduces the urgency-driven pressure to complete laryngoscopy quickly, converting a rushed attempt into a more controlled one. Positioning for optimal laryngoscopic view--ramped positioning in the obese or short-necked patient, and careful attention to external auditory meatus alignment with the sternal notch--should be actively arranged rather than accepted as whatever position the patient happens to be found in on the stretcher, since a suboptimal starting position measurably increases first-attempt failure rates.

## Cricoid Pressure and Manual In-Line Stabilization Considerations

In trauma patients with a plausible cervical spine injury, manual in-line stabilization must be maintained throughout laryngoscopy, and the crew should anticipate that this stabilization will meaningfully worsen the laryngoscopic view compared to a patient whose neck can be freely positioned, which argues for having a video laryngoscope, where available, as the primary rather than backup device in this population, since video laryngoscopy has been shown to improve first-attempt success specifically when cervical motion is restricted. The evidence base for routine cricoid pressure application has grown more equivocal over time, and many transport programs have moved toward selective rather than routine application; regardless of local protocol, if cricoid pressure is applied and is judged to be worsening the laryngoscopic view, it should be released or adjusted rather than maintained reflexively at the cost of a successful first attempt.

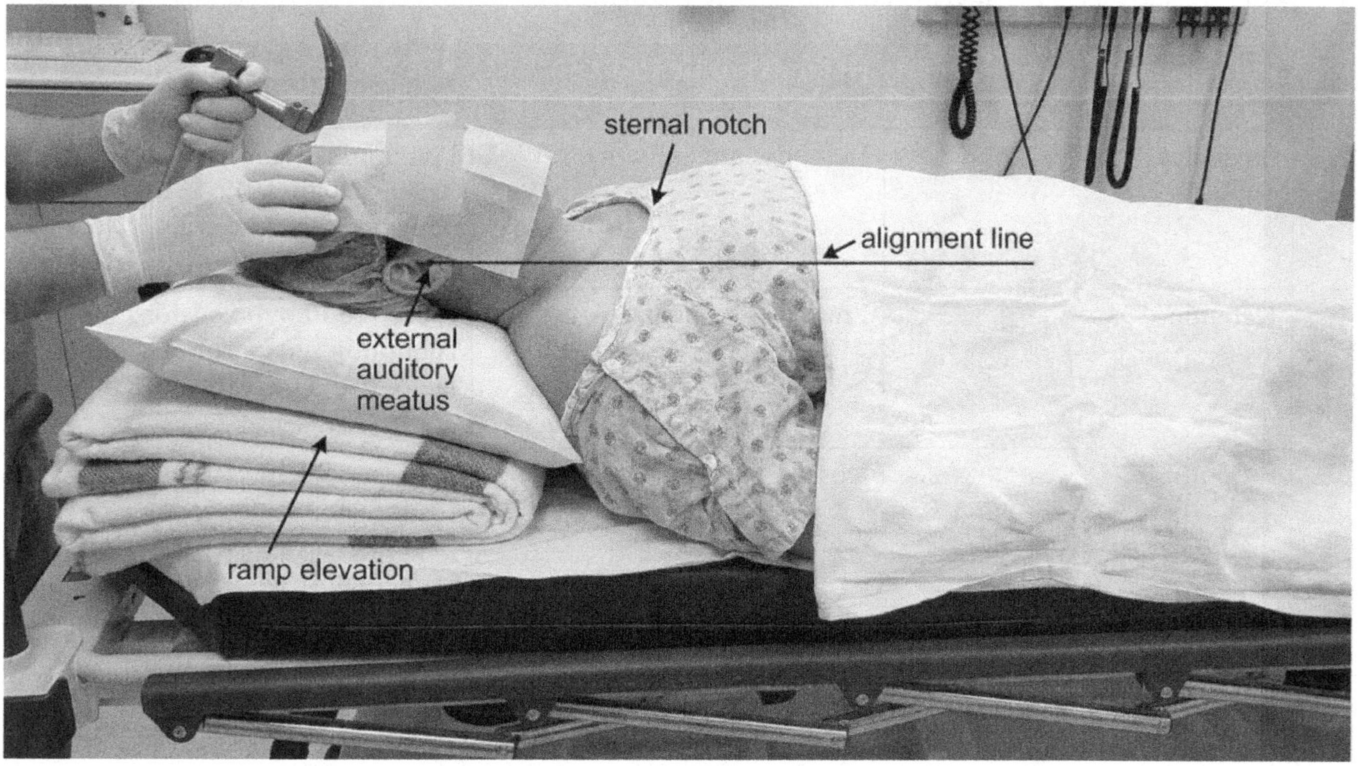


## Pharmacologic Considerations for Transport Rapid Sequence Intubation

Induction agent selection for rapid sequence intubation in the transport population must account for the hemodynamic fragility that distinguishes most transport patients from the general emergency department intubation population. Etomidate, while hemodynamically neutral relative to most alternatives, carries a recognized risk of adrenal suppression that may be clinically consequential in a patient already in or approaching septic shock. Ketamine preserves sympathetic tone and is increasingly favored for the hemodynamically tenuous patient, though it carries its own considerations in patients with uncontrolled tachycardia or a psychiatric history that may complicate emergence. Propofol, while offering a rapid and predictable induction, produces dose-dependent hypotension that can convert a borderline hemodynamic profile into frank cardiovascular collapse in a volume-depleted or vasoplegic patient if not dose-reduced and paired with an immediate vasopressor readiness plan.

Paralytic selection--succinylcholine versus rocuronium--depends on the specific clinical scenario: succinylcholine's rapid onset and short duration make it attractive when a brief paralytic window is desired, but its contraindications (hyperkalemia risk in burns, crush injury, denervation states, and prolonged immobilization) must be actively screened for rather than assumed absent, since the transport population frequently includes patients with exactly these conditions. Rocuronium at a full intubating dose provides comparable onset time but a considerably longer duration of action, a trade-off that is acceptable when a supraglottic rescue device is immediately available as a backup, since the longer paralysis window allows multiple laryngoscopy attempts if needed without the time pressure of an imminent return of tone. Every transport program should have a standardized, weight-based dosing reference for both induction and paralytic agents immediately accessible, not requiring calculation from memory under time pressure.

| Induction Agent | Hemodynamic Profile | Key Transport-Specific Consideration |
|---|---|---|
| Etomidate | Hemodynamically neutral | Potential adrenal suppression in sepsis; single-dose risk debated but relevant in already-stressed patients |
| Ketamine | Preserves sympathetic tone | Preferred in hypotension; caution in uncontrolled tachycardia or severe coronary disease |
| Propofol | Dose-dependent hypotension | Dose-reduce in hemodynamically fragile patients; have vasopressor immediately available |
| Midazolam | Moderate hypotension; variable onset | Slower, less predictable onset; generally not first-line for RSI in transport |

## Portable Mechanical Ventilation: Modes and Settings

### Selecting a Ventilator Mode for the Transport Environment

Portable transport ventilators offer a narrower range of modes than a full-featured intensive care unit ventilator, and the transport clinician's task is to translate the patient's bedside ventilator settings into the closest clinically equivalent mode available on the transport device, rather than assuming a direct one-to-one translation exists for every parameter. Volume-controlled or pressure-regulated volume-controlled modes are generally preferred for transport given their relative predictability and ease of troubleshooting under the monitoring constraints described in Chapter 1, though a patient with significant spontaneous respiratory effort may be better served by a mode that accommodates patient-triggered breaths rather than one that suppresses them entirely.

### Translating Bedside Settings to the Transport Ventilator

When transitioning a patient from a bedside ventilator to a transport ventilator, the crew should verify, rather than assume, that tidal volume, respiratory rate, positive end-expiratory pressure, and fraction of inspired oxygen have transferred correctly to the new device, and should perform a brief period of side-by-side monitoring--comparing exhaled tidal volume, peak pressure, and oxygen saturation on the new device against the values observed on the bedside ventilator immediately before the switch--to confirm equivalence before fully committing to the transport device and disconnecting the original. This equivalence check is a discrete, deliberate step, not an assumption to be made on the basis of matching displayed settings alone, since delivered tidal volume can differ from displayed tidal volume due to differences in circuit compliance and compensation algorithms between devices.

### Sedation and Analgesia Alignment With Ventilator Strategy

Ventilator mode selection and sedation strategy are interdependent decisions rather than sequential ones: a mode that assumes minimal spontaneous effort requires a sedation depth sufficient to prevent patient-ventilator dyssynchrony, while a mode designed to accommodate spontaneous breathing requires a lighter sedation target that preserves adequate respiratory drive. The transport clinician should explicitly confirm that the sedation plan inherited from the sending facility matches the ventilator mode selected for transport, adjusting one or the other as needed rather than allowing a mismatch to produce dyssynchrony that then gets misattributed to a ventilator malfunction rather than correctly identified as a sedation-mode mismatch.

| Ventilator Mode | Best-Suited Clinical Scenario | Key Transport Consideration |
|---|---|---|
| Volume-controlled (assist-control) | Minimal spontaneous effort; predictable delivered volume needed | Most straightforward to troubleshoot under transport monitoring constraints |
| Pressure-regulated volume control | Variable compliance; need for volume guarantee with pressure limitation | Requires accurate compliance data to set correctly |
| Synchronized intermittent mandatory ventilation with pressure support | Preserved spontaneous effort with partial support | Sedation must be titrated to preserve adequate spontaneous drive |
| Pressure support only (noninvasive or via tracheostomy) | Spontaneously breathing patient requiring augmentation | Requires reliable patient effort; not appropriate for heavily sedated patients |

### Circuit and Humidification Considerations for Extended Transport

Ventilator circuit configuration for transport differs from a bedside intensive care unit setup in several respects that carry clinical consequence over extended mission durations: heat-and-moisture exchange filters, commonly used in transport in place of active heated humidification for reasons of weight and power consumption, provide adequate humidification for shorter transports but may become progressively less effective over several hours, particularly in a patient with thick or copious secretions, and the crew should have a low threshold for suctioning and for monitoring rising airway resistance as a sign of filter-related obstruction on longer missions. Circuit integrity should be visually confirmed at every reassessment interval, checking for condensation pooling, tubing kinks introduced by patient repositioning, and secure connection at every junction, since a circuit leak or occlusion is more likely to develop unnoticed in a moving vehicle than at a stationary bedside whcrc ambient conditions and connections remain undisturbed.

## Lung-Protective Ventilation Strategies During Transport

### Maintaining Lung-Protective Targets Across Equipment Transitions

Lung-protective ventilation--low tidal volume calculated against predicted body weight, plateau pressure limitation, and appropriately titrated positive end-expiratory pressure--is a standard of care that must be maintained continuously across the transport window, not merely at the bedside before departure. The equipment transition described above is a specific point of vulnerability for lung-protective ventilation to lapse, since a transport ventilator's default settings, if not deliberately adjusted, may not reflect the predicted-body-weight calculation performed for the patient's actual settings, and a crew that transfers a numeric tidal volume without re-verifying it against predicted body weight risks inadvertently abandoning lung protection at exactly the transition point most likely to be overlooked.

### Permissive Hypercapnia and Driving Pressure Considerations in Transit

Patients managed with permissive hypercapnia as part of a lung-protective strategy require particular attention during transport, since the altered mental status, agitation, or increased respiratory drive that can accompany a rising carbon dioxide tension may be misattributed to inadequate sedation or primary neurologic change rather than correctly recognized as an expected consequence of the ventilation strategy itself, particularly in a patient the crew has known for only a short time and lacks a full baseline for. Driving pressure--the difference between plateau pressure and positive end-expiratory pressure--should be monitored as an additional lung-protective target where the transport ventilator allows its calculation, since driving pressure has been associated with outcome independent of tidal volume alone in patients with acute respiratory distress syndrome, a topic developed further in Chapter 11.

**THE IN-TRANSIT DETERIORATION SIGNATURE SYSTEM — Silent Lung-Protection Lapse at Equipment Transition**

---

**The Signature:** A patient who was appropriately lung-protectively ventilated at the sending facility but is inadvertently ventilated with a higher tidal volume or plateau pressure after transitioning to the transport ventilator, without any alarm or overt sign at the moment of transition.

**Movement Trigger:** The ventilator equipment transition itself, in which displayed numeric settings are copied across devices without re-verifying delivered tidal volume against the patient's predicted body weight and without accounting for differences in circuit compliance between the bedside and transport devices.

**Early Tell:** A delivered tidal volume or plateau pressure on the transport ventilator that, when explicitly recalculated against predicted body weight, exceeds the lung-protective target that was documented as the goal at the sending facility, detectable only by deliberately performing that recalculation rather than assuming settings transferred correctly.

**Trap Logic:** This pattern generates no ventilator alarm, because the transport device is functioning exactly as set; the failure is not mechanical but cognitive, occurring when the crew accepts numeric equivalence between two different devices without verifying that the actual delivered volume and pressure remain within lung-protective range.

**Signature Anchor:** At every ventilator transition, explicitly recalculate and document tidal volume against the patient's predicted body weight on the new device, rather than assuming the numeric setting transferred correctly, and treat this recalculation as a mandatory step of the transition checklist, not an optional refinement.

**KEY POINT:** Predicted body weight, not actual body weight, drives lung-protective tidal volume calculation; a transport ventilator that defaults to actual-weight calculation on setup can silently produce a clinically excessive tidal volume in an obese or edematous patient.

### Recruitment Maneuvers and Their Transport-Specific Risks

Recruitment maneuvers, intended to re-expand collapsed alveolar units in severe hypoxemic respiratory failure, carry a transport-specific risk profile that argues for particular caution: the transient elevation in intrathoracic pressure that a recruitment maneuver produces can precipitate or worsen hypotension in an already volume-depleted or vasoplegic patient, and if performed in a patient with occult pleural air of the kind discussed in Chapter 1, a recruitment maneuver can accelerate the conversion of a small pneumothorax into a tension physiology. Recruitment maneuvers should generally be reserved for patients with a clearly established indication and performed only with hemodynamic monitoring immediately available and the crew prepared to intervene promptly if blood pressure falls significantly during the maneuver, rather than applied routinely or reflexively during a period of borderline oxygenation.

## Ventilator Waveform Interpretation and Troubleshooting in Transit

### Recognizing Common Waveform Abnormalities

Building on the waveform-interpretation discipline established in Chapter 2 for hemodynamic monitoring, ventilator waveforms--pressure-time, flow-time, and volume-time curves where the transport device displays them--provide early warning of developing problems before they manifest as an alarm or an overt change in oxygenation. A rising peak pressure with a stable plateau pressure suggests an airway resistance problem, such as bronchospasm or a partially obstructed tube, while a rising plateau pressure alongside the peak suggests a compliance problem, such as a developing pneumothorax, worsening pulmonary edema, or breath stacking from inadequate expiratory time, a distinction directly relevant to the Occult Pneumothorax Expansion Signature introduced in Chapter 1.

### A Systematic Approach to In-Transit Ventilator Troubleshooting

When a ventilator alarm sounds or a concerning waveform change is noted during transport, a systematic troubleshooting sequence--rapidly assessing the patient directly rather than the machine first, confirming tube position and patency, auscultating for bilateral breath sounds and new asymmetry, and only then interrogating the ventilator's displayed parameters and waveforms--prevents the common error of extensively troubleshooting equipment while a genuine patient-level emergency, such as a tension pneumothorax or mainstem migration, goes unaddressed. This sequence should be rehearsed as a standing team protocol rather than improvised in the moment, since a confined and noisy cabin is a poor environment for developing a novel troubleshooting approach under time pressure.

**Figure 3.1: Ventilator Waveform Patterns and Their Clinical Correlates**

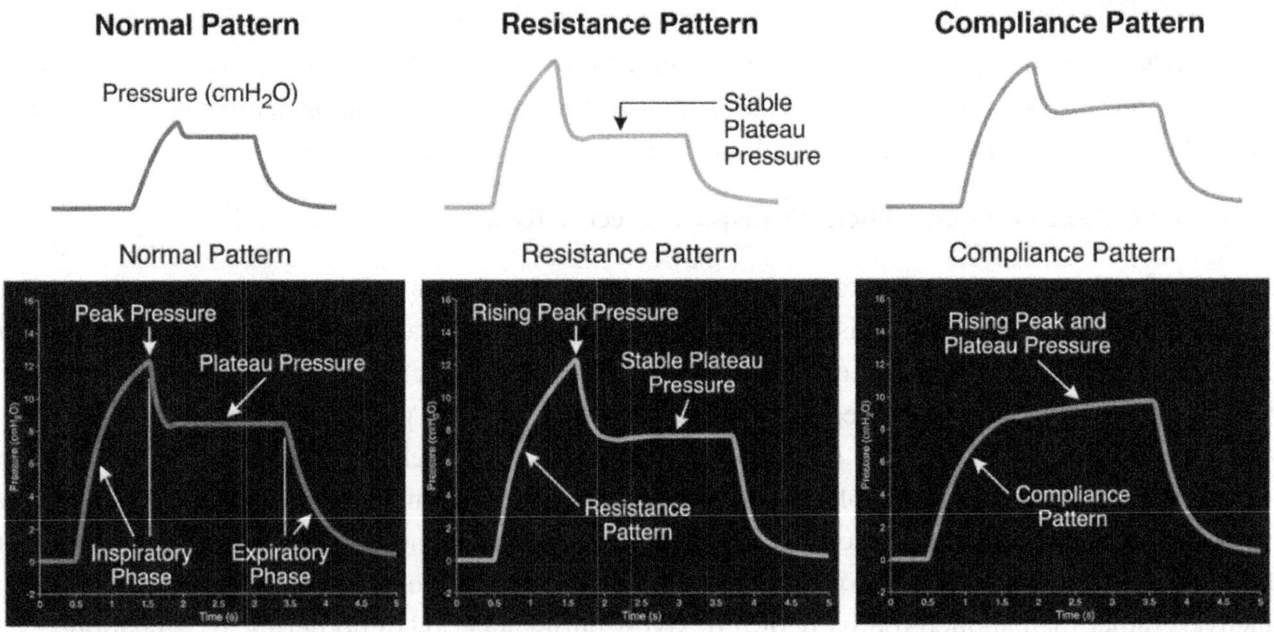

### Alarm Management and Nuisance Alarm Discrimination

Transport ventilators generate alarms for a range of conditions spanning genuine emergencies to nuisance triggers related to circuit motion or brief patient coughing, and a crew that responds to every alarm with equal urgency will experience alarm fatigue that ultimately degrades their response to the alarms that matter most. A structured approach to alarm response--glancing first at the patient's overall appearance and the capnography waveform, which together distinguish a genuine physiologic event from a transient artifact within a second or two, before turning attention to the specific alarm message and underlying parameter--allows the crew to triage alarm urgency efficiently rather than treating every alarm as a full troubleshooting event. Persistent or recurring alarms, even if each individual instance resolves quickly, should prompt a more thorough circuit and patient check rather than repeated dismissal, since a recurring nuisance alarm sometimes represents an early, intermittent signal of a developing problem rather than a truly benign artifact.

## Airway Emergencies and Rescue Techniques En Route

### Recognizing and Responding to Loss of Airway in Transit

Loss of a secured airway during transport--whether from accidental extubation, tube obstruction, or catastrophic equipment failure--requires an immediate, rehearsed response sequence rather than improvisation, given the confined space and reduced immediate backup available compared to a hospital setting. The first response to any sudden desaturation or loss of capnography waveform in an intubated patient should be a rapid assessment for accidental extubation or mainstem migration before assuming a primary pulmonary event, since these mechanical causes are both common and rapidly correctable if identified promptly, whereas time spent escalating oxygen delivery or ventilator settings in response to what is actually a displaced tube delays the correct intervention.

### Rescue Ventilation and Surgical Airway Considerations

A supraglottic rescue airway device should be immediately available and pre-sized for every intubated transport patient, positioned for rapid access rather than packed away in a bag that must be searched during an emergency, and every crew member should be independently capable of placing it without requiring instruction from another team member in the moment. A surgical airway kit, similarly pre-staged and accessible, represents the final rescue option in a cannot-intubate, cannot-ventilate scenario, and while the confined space of a moving vehicle or aircraft makes this procedure more difficult than in a hospital operating room, the decision to proceed should not be delayed by that difficulty once the clinical scenario meets the threshold for surgical airway, since a further delay in a true cannot-ventilate scenario carries greater risk than the procedural difficulty of the confined space.

### Post-Intubation Sedation and Ventilation Optimization

The minutes immediately following a successful intubation in the field represent a critical optimization window that is frequently compressed or overlooked under the pressure to begin movement. Establishing adequate post-intubation sedation and analgesia before the paralytic wears off prevents the dangerous combination of an awake, distressed patient on a ventilator in a moving vehicle, where patient-ventilator dyssynchrony, self-extubation attempts, and acute hypertension or tachycardia from inadequately controlled pain or anxiety can cascade into a genuine emergency. Post-intubation ventilator settings should be verified against the patient's clinical indication and body habitus, not left on default, and the initial post-intubation arterial blood gas or capnography reading should be actively checked and acted upon rather than deferred to arrival, since a ventilation or oxygenation problem identified and corrected in the first ten minutes after intubation is considerably easier to manage than the same problem discovered thirty minutes into a transport when its downstream consequences have already accumulated.

**Crew Rehearsal and Team Preparedness for Airway Failure**

The reliability of an airway rescue response under the stress and constraint of a transport emergency depends more heavily on prior rehearsal than on individual procedural skill, because the confined space, noise, and time pressure of an in-flight airway crisis degrade the cognitive performance of even experienced clinicians, and a pre-rehearsed, role-assigned sequence degrades less under stress than an improvised one. Transport programs that incorporate regular, scenario-based airway failure drills--performed in the actual vehicle or aircraft cabin rather than a simulation center, and including the full equipment access, space limitation, and communication challenges of the real environment--produce crews whose performance under genuine emergency conditions more closely resembles their trained performance than crews whose rehearsal occurs only in classroom settings. This investment in rehearsal is not a training luxury but a direct patient-safety intervention, since the first time a crew attempts a surgical airway in a moving aircraft should not be the first time they have attempted it in any aircraft at all.

Consider a fifty-six-year-old man intubated at a sending facility for airway protection following a large ischemic stroke, transported by fixed-wing aircraft with a stated flight time of ninety minutes. Approximately twenty minutes into cruise, the crew notes a sudden loss of the capnography waveform accompanied by a falling oxygen saturation. Rather than initiating ventilator troubleshooting first, the crew immediately reassesses the airway directly: auscultation reveals absent breath sounds on the left with preserved sounds on the right, and direct visualization confirms the endotracheal tube has migrated to a depth several centimeters beyond what was documented at departure, consistent with mainstem intubation, likely related to the neck flexion that occurred during a routine repositioning several minutes earlier. The tube is withdrawn to the previously documented depth, breath sounds are confirmed bilaterally, and the capnography waveform and oxygen saturation both normalize within moments. Because the crew's troubleshooting sequence prioritized direct patient and airway reassessment over ventilator-focused troubleshooting, the correct diagnosis was reached and corrected within under a minute of the initial alarm, illustrating the chapter's central argument: airway and ventilator problems in transit are usually mechanical and patient-level in origin, and a troubleshooting sequence that checks the patient before the machine will consistently outperform one that does the reverse.

A second illustrative scenario involves a thirty-nine-year-old woman with severe angioedema requiring intubation at a rural sending facility before ground transport to a tertiary center, in whom the sending team's single laryngoscopy attempt was unsuccessful due to severely distorted airway anatomy and the patient was being manually bag-mask ventilated with difficulty at the time of the transport crew's arrival. Recognizing a predicted difficult airway with an already-failed attempt and a deteriorating window for further tries, the transport crew elects to proceed directly to a supraglottic rescue device rather than attempting a second direct or video laryngoscopy attempt with anatomy already known to be unfavorable, successfully establishing ventilation and oxygenation, and transports the patient to the receiving facility with a definitive airway plan--awake tracheostomy versus fiberoptic intubation under controlled conditions--deferred to the receiving team's more resource-rich environment rather than pursued in the field. This decision, prioritizing a reliably functioning rescue airway over a repeated attempt at definitive intubation against known difficult anatomy, reflects the chapter's broader principle that the transport environment's resource constraints should actively inform not just how an airway is managed but what the goal of airway management should be for that specific transport window: adequate oxygenation and ventilation delivered safely, not necessarily a definitive airway achieved by the crew in the field.

## Advanced Airway Decision-Making for Transport

### The Failed Airway Algorithm Adapted to Transport Constraints

The failed airway algorithm in transport medicine follows the same escalation sequence as the hospital-based algorithm--oral attempt, supraglottic rescue device, surgical airway--but the transport environment compresses the decision timeline and narrows the options at each step. A second oral attempt after a failed first attempt should use a different technique, different blade, or different operator if available, since repeating the same approach that failed the first time has a low probability of success and consumes time that could be spent on a rescue approach. The supraglottic airway device should be the immediate fallback rather than a grudging last resort before surgery, since modern supraglottic devices provide adequate oxygenation and ventilation in the majority of cannot-intubate scenarios and can bridge the patient to a controlled surgical airway at the next available stop or at the receiving facility.

### Video Laryngoscopy as the Primary Intubation Approach in Transport

Video laryngoscopy has emerged as the preferred primary intubation approach for transport medicine, displacing direct laryngoscopy as the first-attempt tool, because video laryngoscopy produces a higher first-attempt success rate across the range of airway anatomies and operator experience levels encountered in transport, and because the indirect glottic view it provides is less degraded by the suboptimal positioning and lighting conditions of the transport environment than the line-of-sight view required for direct laryngoscopy. Programs transitioning to video laryngoscopy as their primary approach should ensure that every crew member is proficient with at least one backup technique--direct laryngoscopy, supraglottic device placement, or surgical airway--that does not depend on the video device, since a dead battery, a blood-obscured camera, or a fogged lens can render the video laryngoscope unusable at exactly the moment it is needed most.

### The Bougie as a First-Pass Adjunct in Difficult Transport Airways

The endotracheal tube introducer (bougie) has demonstrated improved first-pass intubation success in both prehospital and emergency department settings, and its use as a routine first-pass adjunct--rather than a rescue device deployed only after a failed attempt--is increasingly adopted by transport programs. The bougie provides tactile feedback of tracheal ring clicks that confirms tracheal placement independent of visual confirmation, which is particularly valuable in the transport environment where blood, secretions, or suboptimal positioning may obscure the glottic view even with video laryngoscopy. The technique involves advancing the bougie through the glottic opening under laryngoscopic guidance, confirming tracheal clicks, and then railroading the endotracheal tube over the bougie, and should be practiced regularly so that the mechanical coordination of bougie advancement, laryngoscope stabilization, and tube threading is fluid rather than clumsy under the stress of a real airway emergency.

### Awake Intubation Techniques and Their Transport Feasibility

Awake fiberoptic or awake video laryngoscopic intubation, the gold standard for the known difficult airway in the hospital setting, is feasible in the transport environment but requires specific preparation: topical anesthesia of the airway with lidocaine (nebulized, atomized, or applied directly to the base of the tongue and posterior pharynx), gentle sedation with a short-acting agent that preserves respiratory drive and protective reflexes, and a patient who is cooperative enough to tolerate the procedure. The transport clinician should consider an awake approach when the airway assessment predicts high difficulty and the patient is currently maintaining their own airway and oxygenation, since the alternative--paralyzing a patient with a predicted difficult airway and then discovering that intubation is indeed difficult--produces a cannot-intubate, cannot-ventilate scenario that is far more dangerous than the controlled discomfort of an awake approach.

## Ventilator Management for Specific Disease Processes

### Ventilation Strategies for Obstructive Airway Disease

Patients with severe asthma or acute exacerbations of chronic obstructive pulmonary disease who require mechanical ventilation during transport present a specific ventilatory challenge: the expiratory airflow limitation that characterizes obstructive disease produces air trapping (auto-PEEP) when the respiratory rate or inspiratory time is set too high, and this trapped gas progressively increases intrathoracic pressure, reduces venous return, and can produce hemodynamic collapse that is easily mistaken for a primary cardiac event if the auto-PEEP is not recognized. The ventilation strategy for obstructive disease prioritizes adequate expiratory time over minute ventilation: a lower respiratory rate, a longer expiratory time (achieved by reducing the inspiratory-to-expiratory ratio), and acceptance of a higher $PaCO_2$ (permissive hypercapnia) to allow the trapped gas to escape before the next breath is delivered.

The transport clinician should monitor for auto-PEEP using the flow-time waveform on the transport ventilator: if expiratory flow has not returned to zero before the next breath begins, auto-PEEP is present and the respiratory rate or tidal volume should be reduced until the expiratory flow reaches zero at end-expiration. In the event of acute hemodynamic collapse in a ventilated patient with obstructive disease, the immediate intervention is to disconnect the patient from the ventilator for several seconds, allowing complete exhalation of trapped gas, which will produce an immediate improvement in venous return and blood pressure if auto-PEEP was the cause--a diagnostic and therapeutic maneuver that takes seconds and can be life-saving.

### Ventilation Strategies for Morbid Obesity

The morbidly obese patient requiring mechanical ventilation during transport presents a compounding set of challenges: the weight of the chest wall and abdominal contents increases the work of breathing and reduces functional residual capacity, the supine position exacerbates these effects by allowing abdominal contents to compress the diaphragm, and the reduced chest wall compliance increases peak airway pressures even with appropriate tidal volume settings, which can trigger high-pressure alarms that are falsely interpreted as an airway or pulmonary problem rather than a chest wall compliance issue. Positioning the morbidly obese patient in a reverse Trendelenburg (head-up) position improves respiratory mechanics by using gravity to displace abdominal contents caudally, and higher PEEP settings than would be used in a normal-weight patient are typically required to maintain alveolar recruitment against the compressive forces of the chest wall and abdomen.

### Managing the Patient on Non-Standard Ventilatory Support

Patients transferred from facilities with advanced ventilatory capabilities may be receiving modes or settings that the transport ventilator cannot replicate: airway pressure release ventilation, high-frequency oscillatory ventilation, or neurally adjusted ventilatory assist are modes available on some ICU ventilators that have no equivalent on most transport platforms. The transport clinician must translate these non-standard modes into the closest achievable equivalent on the transport device, recognizing that the translation is necessarily imperfect and that the patient's gas exchange may change--for better or worse--during the transition. Communication with the sending intensivist about the specific physiologic goals of the non-standard mode (what is it achieving that a conventional mode would not?) allows the transport clinician to target those same goals with the tools available rather than attempting a mechanical replication of mode-specific settings that have no direct equivalent.

## Post-Intubation Complications and Their Transport Management

### Endotracheal Tube Complications During Transport

The three most common endotracheal tube complications during transport are accidental extubation, mainstem bronchus intubation from tube migration, and tube obstruction from secretions or blood, and the transport clinician should monitor for all three at each reassessment interval. Accidental extubation is prevented by secure tube fixation verified before departure and rechecked after every position change; mainstem migration is prevented by documenting tube depth and verifying bilateral breath sounds at each reassessment; and tube obstruction is managed by maintaining adequate humidification, performing suction at defined intervals or when indicated by rising airway pressures, and having a replacement tube immediately available if the current tube becomes irreversibly obstructed. A suction catheter that passes easily to the expected tube length confirms patency; one that meets resistance at a point shorter than the tube length suggests obstruction that may require tube exchange.

### Ventilator-Associated Events During Transport

Ventilator-associated events--including pneumonia, barotrauma, and oxygen toxicity--are primarily concerns of prolonged mechanical ventilation in the ICU rather than the transport window, but certain transport-specific practices can contribute to their risk if not managed carefully. Aspiration during intubation or during tube manipulation in transit introduces oropharyngeal organisms into the lower airway; barotrauma risk is increased if high plateau pressures are not monitored during altitude-related compliance changes; and excessive FiO2 maintained reflexively throughout a transport that started with marginal oxygenation but has since improved exposes the patient to unnecessary oxidative stress. The transport clinician should titrate FiO2 downward as oxygenation allows rather than maintaining maximum oxygen delivery throughout the transport purely as a safety margin, since the margin between adequate oxygenation and unnecessary hyperoxia is itself a clinically relevant management decision.

## Extubation During Transport and Planned Airway Transitions

### When Extubation During Transport Is Appropriate

While the general principle established earlier in this chapter is to maintain the current airway status throughout transport and defer elective changes to the receiving facility, rare circumstances may justify extubation during transport: a patient who was intubated for a self-limited condition (brief seizure, procedural sedation) and has fully recovered airway protective reflexes and respiratory drive, or a patient who is self-extubating repeatedly despite adequate sedation and whose clinical picture suggests that the endotracheal tube is no longer needed. The decision to extubate during transport should be made with the same conservative threshold applied to every other elective procedure in transit: if the patient can safely tolerate remaining intubated for the duration of the transport, they should remain intubated; extubation during transport should be reserved for situations where the intubated state itself is producing a clinical problem (self-extubation attempts producing airway trauma, tube-related agitation worsening intracranial pressure) that outweighs the risks of a planned extubation in a moving vehicle.

### Tracheostomy Patients in Transport

Patients with tracheostomies present specific transport airway management considerations: the tracheostomy tube must be secured against the mechanical forces of transport movement, the tube type (cuffed versus uncuffed, fenestrated versus non-fenestrated) must be confirmed and its implications for ventilation understood, a replacement tracheostomy tube of the same size and a tube one size smaller must be immediately available in case of accidental decannulation, and the crew must understand the specific reinsertion technique for the patient's tracheostomy maturity (a mature tract can usually be re-cannulated directly, while a fresh tracheostomy less than seven to ten days old may close rapidly after decannulation and may require oral intubation as the rescue airway rather than attempted reinsertion through a closing stoma). The transport clinician should also carry an endotracheal tube that can be advanced through the stoma if the tracheostomy tube cannot be reinserted, recognizing that this is a temporizing measure rather than a definitive airway.

### Supraglottic Airway as a Definitive Transport Airway

In certain clinical scenarios--a patient with a known difficult airway in whom intubation has failed but a supraglottic device provides adequate oxygenation and ventilation, or a patient whose clinical condition does not warrant the hemodynamic risks of RSI but who requires a secured airway for safe transport--a supraglottic airway device may serve as the definitive airway for the duration of the transport rather than as a temporary rescue bridge to intubation. The transport clinician using a supraglottic device as a definitive transport airway should confirm adequate ventilation and oxygenation through the device, should monitor continuously for device displacement or loss of seal, should have a plan for conversion to a definitive airway if the supraglottic device fails, and should communicate to the receiving team that the patient is arriving with a supraglottic airway so that definitive airway management resources are available on arrival.

### Laryngeal Mask Airway Versus Second-Generation Supraglottic Devices

Second-generation supraglottic airway devices, which incorporate a gastric drainage channel in addition to the ventilatory channel, offer several advantages over the classic laryngeal mask airway for transport use: the gastric channel allows passage of a nasogastric tube for gastric decompression (reducing aspiration risk), the higher seal pressures achievable with second-generation devices allow positive pressure ventilation at pressures that would leak around a classic LMA, and many second-generation designs can serve as a conduit for intubation if the clinical situation subsequently requires endotracheal tube placement. Transport programs should stock second-generation devices as their standard supraglottic airway rather than classic LMAs, and should ensure that the crew is trained and current in their insertion, since the techniques differ in meaningful ways from classic LMA placement.

### Airway Management in Specific Transport Populations

Certain patient populations encountered in transport present airway management challenges that differ from the general adult airway: the morbidly obese patient, whose redundant pharyngeal tissue, short neck, and chest wall weight produce a fundamentally different airway geometry than the standard-build patient, requiring ramped positioning, potentially larger blade selection, and awareness that desaturation during apnea occurs much more rapidly due to reduced functional residual capacity; the patient with cervical spine trauma, whose neck cannot be extended for laryngoscopy and who requires manual in-line stabilization throughout the intubation attempt, degrading the laryngoscopic view and arguing for video laryngoscopy as the primary approach; the patient with facial trauma, whose disrupted anatomy, blood, and edema can make even video laryngoscopy difficult and who may require a surgical airway as the primary rather than rescue approach; and the pregnant patient, whose airway edema, reduced functional residual capacity, and aspiration risk from a full stomach create a combination of difficult anatomy, rapid desaturation, and high-consequence complications that makes pregnancy-specific airway preparation mandatory before any intubation attempt.

### Awake Versus Asleep Decision Framework for Transport Intubation

The decision between an awake intubation technique and a rapid sequence intubation with paralysis is one of the most consequential airway decisions in transport medicine, and it should be made deliberately based on a structured risk assessment rather than defaulted to RSI out of habit or comfort. The key variables are: the predicted difficulty of laryngoscopy (how likely is it that the glottic view will be adequate?), the patient's current ability to maintain oxygenation and protect their airway (how urgently does the airway need to be secured?), the availability of rescue options if the primary attempt fails (how many backup plans can be deployed in this specific transport environment?), and the patient's cooperation (can they tolerate an awake technique, or is their mental status or agitation level incompatible with an awake approach?). When the predicted difficulty is high but the urgency is moderate, an awake technique preserves the patient's own airway protective mechanisms as a safety net; when the urgency is extreme (active aspiration, complete obstruction), RSI with paralysis provides the best first-attempt success despite the loss of the patient's protective mechanisms.

### The Post-Intubation Checklist: A Mandatory Step Before Movement

After every intubation in the transport setting, a structured post-intubation checklist should be completed before the patient is moved from the bedside to the stretcher or from the stretcher to the vehicle: tube depth confirmed and documented, bilateral breath sounds verified, continuous capnography waveform confirmed, tube secured with a method resistant to transport movement forces, ventilator settings verified against clinical indication and body weight, sedation and analgesia confirmed adequate for the planned ventilator mode, and a rescue airway device pre-sized and immediately accessible. This checklist converts a series of individual clinical actions into a verified, complete, documented preparation for movement, and it is the mechanism by which the transport clinician confirms that the airway is genuinely secured--not just intubated, but secured, confirmed, and ready for the additional challenges of transit.

### THE IN-TRANSIT DETERIORATION SIGNATURE SYSTEM — Airway and Ventilation Transition Patterns

---

**Signature Introduced This Chapter:** Silent Lung-Protection Lapse at Equipment Transition (unverified tidal volume or plateau pressure drift after switching from bedside to transport ventilator).

**Cross-Chapter Pattern Recognition:** This chapter's mainstem-migration case demonstrates the same movement-triggered logic as the Occult Pneumothorax Expansion Signature from Chapter 1: a new pressure, saturation, or waveform change occurring around a positional or equipment-transition event should prompt direct patient reassessment before machine-focused troubleshooting.

**Cross-Reference Forward:** Chapter 11 (Acute Respiratory Failure and ARDS Management in Transit) extends lung-protective ventilation and driving-pressure monitoring in greater depth for the specific population most dependent on strict adherence to these targets.

## Summary and Key Concepts

Difficult airway assessment before transport must account for both anatomic factors and the specific constraints of the transport environment itself.

Ventilator mode and setting translation from bedside to transport equipment requires deliberate verification, not assumption of numeric equivalence, particularly for lung-protective tidal volume targets.

Sedation strategy and ventilator mode are interdependent and must be explicitly reconciled rather than allowed to drift out of alignment.

Ventilator waveform interpretation distinguishes resistance from compliance problems and provides earlier warning than waiting for an alarm threshold to be crossed.

Airway emergencies in transit should be approached by reassessing the patient and airway directly before troubleshooting the ventilator, since most in-transit airway and ventilation problems are mechanical and patient-level in origin.

Rescue airway equipment must be pre-staged, pre-sized, and immediately accessible, and every crew member should be independently capable of using it without in-the-moment instruction.

# CHAPTER 4: PHARMACOLOGY AND INFUSION MANAGEMENT IN TRANSIT

**Learning Objectives**

1. Select, dose, and titrate vasoactive infusions for hemodynamic support under the monitoring constraints of the transport environment.
2. Apply weight-based sedation, analgesia, and neuromuscular blockade protocols adapted to transport duration and patient acuity.
3. Anticipate drug-environment interactions introduced by altitude, temperature, and vibration.
4. Manage multi-infusion logistics, including line labeling, pump programming, and battery reserve verification, before departure.
5. Recognize and respond to pharmacologically mediated deterioration patterns during transport.

**Chapter Outline**

This chapter addresses the pharmacologic dimension of critical care transport as a distinct clinical discipline rather than a subset of bedside intensive care pharmacology. The same medications used in a hospital ICU behave differently when administered through a portable infusion pump operating on battery power, in a vehicle subject to vibration-induced flow irregularities, at an altitude that alters drug metabolism and distribution, and by a clinician who lacks immediate access to a pharmacist, a laboratory, or a resupply chain. Every pharmacologic decision made in transit is simultaneously a logistics decision.

## Vasoactive Agents in Critical Care Transport

### Norepinephrine, Vasopressin, and Phenylephrine: Selection and Titration

Norepinephrine remains the first-line vasopressor for most forms of distributive and septic shock encountered in transport, and its titratability--the ability to adjust dose incrementally in response to continuous arterial pressure monitoring--is one of its principal advantages in the transport environment, where hemodynamic conditions may shift rapidly with altitude, positioning, and the patient's evolving physiology. Vasopressin, typically administered as a fixed-dose adjunct rather than titrated, serves a complementary role in patients whose norepinephrine requirement is escalating, and its catecholamine-independent mechanism provides hemodynamic support through a distinct receptor pathway that is particularly useful in vasoplegia refractory to adrenergic agents alone.

Phenylephrine, a pure alpha-agonist, has a narrower clinical role but is specifically useful in transport scenarios involving hypotension associated with neuraxial anesthesia or spinal cord injury, where the predominant mechanism is loss of peripheral vascular tone without intrinsic cardiac dysfunction, and where the reflex bradycardia that phenylephrine can produce in a patient with intact vagal tone is either absent or desirable. The transport clinician should be aware that phenylephrine can worsen cardiac output in a patient with impaired contractility, and its use in undifferentiated shock without confirmation of preserved ventricular function carries a risk of hemodynamic worsening that is harder to recover from in transit than at the bedside.

### Inotropic Support: Dobutamine, Milrinone, and Epinephrine

When hemodynamic instability is driven by impaired cardiac contractility rather than vasodilation, inotropic support with dobutamine or milrinone may be required, each carrying transport-specific considerations. Dobutamine increases contractility and heart rate through beta-1 stimulation but can produce hypotension through its beta-2 vasodilatory effect, a combination that is poorly tolerated in a patient already requiring vasopressor support and may necessitate concurrent norepinephrine titration. Milrinone, a phosphodiesterase inhibitor with combined inotropic and vasodilatory properties, has a long half-life that makes it difficult to titrate rapidly in response to changing hemodynamic conditions, a characteristic that argues for establishing a stable milrinone infusion rate before departure rather than initiating or significantly adjusting it mid-transport.

Epinephrine, with its combined alpha and beta effects, serves as both a vasopressor and an inotrope and is frequently the agent of choice when a patient requires simultaneous hemodynamic and chronotropic support, particularly in post-cardiac arrest care or anaphylaxis. Its potent chronotropic and arrhythmogenic properties require continuous rhythm monitoring, which should already be in place for any transport patient receiving vasoactive support.

### Push-Dose Pressors for Acute Hemodynamic Rescue

Push-dose epinephrine and phenylephrine, prepared from standard concentration ampules and diluted to a predictable per-milliliter dose, provide a rapid hemodynamic bridge in scenarios where a continuous infusion has not yet been established, has been interrupted by a line malfunction, or is titrating too slowly against an acute decompensation. The preparation of push-dose pressors requires deliberate, rehearsed dilution steps to avoid the well-documented risk of concentration errors that can produce a ten- or hundred-fold overdose from an undiluted or incompletely diluted ampule. Transport programs should maintain pre-diluted push-dose syringes or, failing that, a standardized preparation protocol printed on the syringe storage location itself, so that the dilution can be performed accurately under stress without relying on memory or mental arithmetic.

### Vasoactive Infusion Transition at the Sending Facility

Transitioning a patient from the sending facility's vasoactive infusion setup to the transport team's own pumps and concentrations is a moment of genuine hemodynamic vulnerability that should be performed as a controlled, stepwise process rather than a simultaneous swap. The standard practice is to hang the transport team's infusion alongside the existing one, initiate the transport infusion at the current rate, confirm hemodynamic equivalence over a brief monitoring period, and then discontinue the sending facility's infusion and line in a controlled fashion. Switching both pumps simultaneously, even briefly, risks either a complete loss of vasopressor delivery during the changeover or an inadvertent double-dosing if the timing is imprecise, either of which can produce a clinically significant hemodynamic event that is entirely avoidable with a sequential approach. The transport clinician should also verify that the drug concentration prepared by the sending facility's pharmacy matches the concentration the transport team's pump is programmed for, since a concentration mismatch during a rate-equivalent transition will produce an actual dose change that is invisible on the pump display.

**Figure 4.0: Hemodynamic Waveform Changes During Vasoactive Titration**

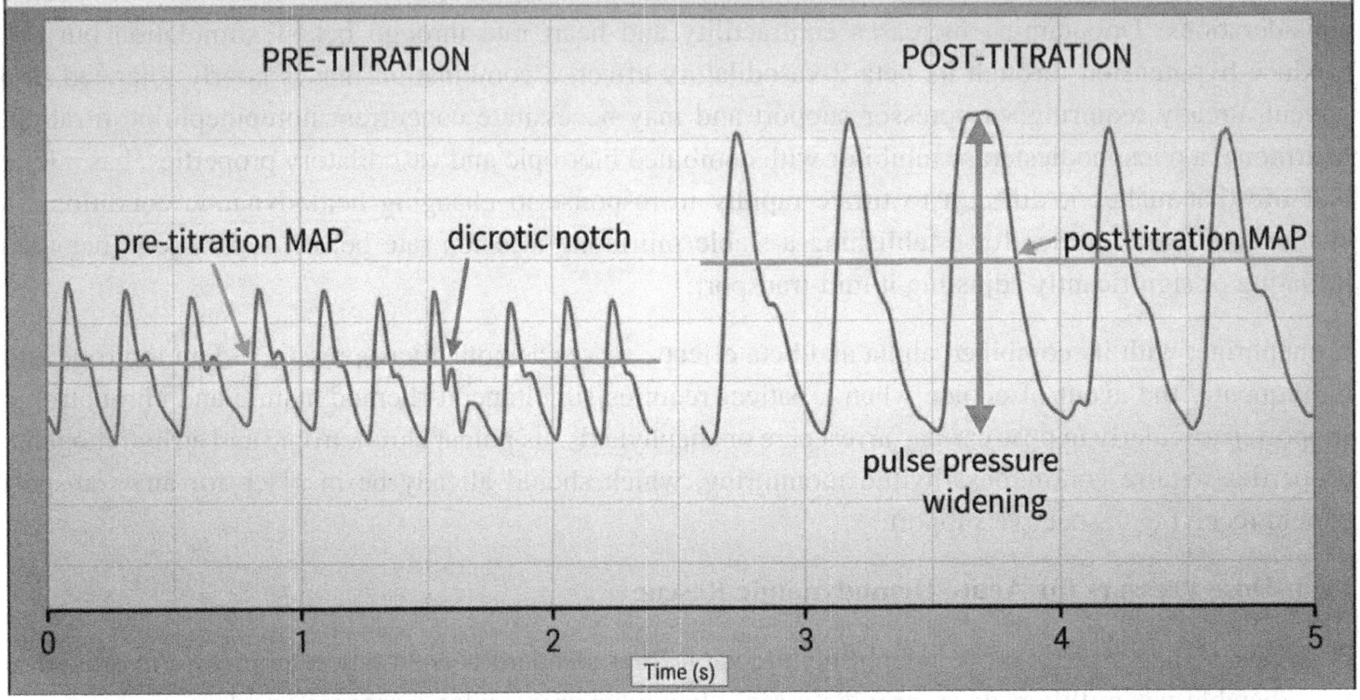


| Agent | Primary Receptor | Hemodynamic Effect | Key Transport Consideration |
|---|---|---|---|
| Norepinephrine | Alpha-1 > Beta-1 | Vasoconstriction with mild inotropy | First-line for most transport shock; highly titratable |
| Vasopressin | V1 | Non-catecholamine vasoconstriction | Fixed dose; catecholamine-sparing; useful in refractory vasoplegia |
| Phenylephrine | Pure Alpha-1 | Vasoconstriction only | Useful in neurogenic shock; avoid in impaired contractility |
| Dobutamine | Beta-1 > Beta-2 | Inotropy with vasodilation | May worsen hypotension; often needs concurrent vasopressor |

| | | | |
|---|---|---|---|
| Milrinone | PDE-3 inhibitor | Inotropy and vasodilation | Long half-life limits rapid titration in transit |
| Epinephrine | Alpha and Beta | Vasoconstriction, inotropy, chronotropy | Arrhythmogenic; requires continuous rhythm monitoring |

## Sedation, Analgesia, and Neuromuscular Blockade in Transit

### Sedation Depth Targets and Assessment During Transport

Establishing and maintaining an appropriate sedation depth is more challenging in the transport environment than at the bedside, because many of the clinical cues that inform sedation assessment--verbal responsiveness, subtle facial expressions, purposeful versus non-purposeful movement--are obscured by ambient noise, restraint, and limited visual access to the patient. A standardized sedation scale, applied at fixed intervals matching the reassessment schedule established in Chapter 2, provides a structured framework for sedation assessment that is less vulnerable to environmental degradation than an unstructured clinical impression, and it generates the trend data the receiving team needs to continue sedation management without interruption.

### Analgesic Selection and Multimodal Pain Management

Pain management in the transport patient serves both a humanitarian purpose and a physiologic one: untreated pain drives sympathetic activation, tachycardia, hypertension, and increased oxygen consumption, all of which are directly counterproductive in a patient whose physiologic reserve is already narrowed. Fentanyl is the most commonly used transport analgesic, favored for its rapid onset, short duration, and relative hemodynamic stability compared to morphine, whose histamine-mediated vasodilation makes it less predictable in a volume-depleted or vasoplegic patient. Ketamine at sub-dissociative doses provides analgesic augmentation through a non-opioid mechanism that is particularly useful when opioid-related respiratory depression or hemodynamic compromise limits further fentanyl titration.

### Sedation Agent Selection for Transport: Propofol, Midazolam, and Dexmedetomidine

Propofol offers a rapidly titratable sedation depth that is attractive for shorter transports and for patients requiring frequent neurologic reassessment, since its rapid offset allows a brief lightening of sedation for examination without the prolonged emergence that characterizes longer-acting agents. Its principal transport-specific limitation is dose-dependent hypotension, which may be poorly tolerated in a hemodynamically marginal patient and which requires that any propofol infusion be paired with continuous arterial pressure monitoring and vasopressor readiness. Midazolam, while less hemodynamically destabilizing at typical doses, provides less predictable sedation depth and a longer, less controllable offset, and its amnestic properties, while sometimes desirable, can mask inadequate analgesia if the clinician mistakes the absence of recall for the absence of pain.

Dexmedetomidine provides sedation with preserved respiratory drive, a property that is specifically useful in patients who are spontaneously breathing or in whom a lighter sedation target is desired without the respiratory depression risk of opioid-benzodiazepine combinations. Its principal limitations in transport are a relatively slow onset that makes it poorly suited as a sole agent for acute agitation management, and a propensity for bradycardia that requires monitoring and may contraindicate its use in patients already at risk for bradycardic events, such as those with high-grade atrioventricular block or a spinal cord injury affecting cardiac sympathetic innervation.

### Neuromuscular Blockade: Indications, Monitoring, and Risks

Continuous neuromuscular blockade during transport is indicated in a narrow set of circumstances--severe ventilator dyssynchrony refractory to sedation optimization, refractory intracranial hypertension, or open-abdomen or severe burn patients requiring absolute immobility--and carries the non-trivial risk of awareness under paralysis if sedation depth is not rigorously maintained. A paralyzed patient cannot communicate pain, anxiety, or distress by any visible sign, and the crew must proactively ensure adequate sedation depth through scheduled assessment and anticipatory dosing rather than reactive titration triggered by signs that, in a paralyzed patient, simply cannot appear. Train-of-four monitoring, where available, provides objective assessment of the degree of neuromuscular blockade and should be used at regular intervals.

### THE IN-TRANSIT DETERIORATION SIGNATURE SYSTEM — Masked Hemodynamic Collapse Under Deep Sedation

**The Signature:** A gradual, progressive decline in blood pressure and cardiac output in a deeply sedated and possibly paralyzed patient that develops insidiously during transport, without the tachycardia, restlessness, or patient-initiated alerting behavior that would ordinarily signal early hemodynamic compromise.

**Movement Trigger:** The combination of deep sedation suppressing compensatory sympathetic responses with the transport environment's continuous, low-grade physiologic stressors--positional venous pooling, vibration-induced fluid shifts, and ongoing insensible losses--produces a cumulative hemodynamic burden that a deeply sedated patient cannot compensate for in the way an awake or lightly sedated patient would.

**Early Tell:** A narrowing pulse pressure or a subtle downward drift in mean arterial pressure on the arterial waveform, developing gradually over ten to twenty minutes, without any corresponding tachycardic response--the absence of tachycardia in the face of a falling pressure is itself the early tell, since it indicates that the normal sympathetic compensation is pharmacologically suppressed.

**Trap Logic:** This pattern is frequently attributed to "expected" hemodynamic effects of sedation rather than recognized as an evolving shock state, particularly because the slow pace of decline can fall below the threshold of attention when the crew is focused on other monitoring tasks. The discriminating feature is the trajectory: a brief, stable decrease in pressure after a sedation bolus is expected, but a sustained or progressive decline beyond the initial bolus effect is not.

**Signature Anchor:** In any deeply sedated or paralyzed patient, treat a sustained downward pressure trend that extends beyond the expected bolus effect of the most recent sedation dose as a hemodynamic event requiring volume assessment and vasopressor readiness, not as an expected pharmacologic effect to be observed.

## Drug-Environment Interactions in Transit

### Altitude Effects on Drug Metabolism and Distribution

Altitude induced hypoxemia, even when subclinical, reduces hepatic blood flow and can slow the clearance of medications metabolized through hepatic oxidative pathways, which includes many of the sedatives and opioids used routinely in transport. This effect is modest at typical cabin altitudes but can become clinically relevant in a patient with pre-existing hepatic dysfunction or one receiving multiple medications competing for the same metabolic pathways, and the practical implication is a lower threshold for dose reduction or extended dosing intervals in these populations during a flight at meaningful altitude, rather than assuming that the same dosing regimen used at sea level will produce the same pharmacokinetic behavior at altitude.

### Temperature and Vibration Effects on Infusion Accuracy

Infusion pump accuracy can be affected by ambient temperature extremes and by sustained vibration, both of which are common in the transport environment. Cold temperatures increase fluid viscosity, which can slow gravity-dependent infusion rates and alter the flow characteristics of syringe pumps calibrated at room temperature. Vibration can produce intermittent bolusing in syringe pumps if the syringe plunger is mechanically advanced by external oscillation, a phenomenon that has been documented in rotor-wing platforms and that can produce unpredictable dose delivery in vasoactive or sedative infusions where precision matters most. The practical countermeasure is to secure pumps against vibration-coupled surfaces, use anti-siphon tubing where available, and monitor for unexplained hemodynamic or sedation changes that may represent infusion-rate artifact rather than a change in the patient's underlying condition.

Figure 4.1: Multi-Line Infusion Setup and Labeling for Transport

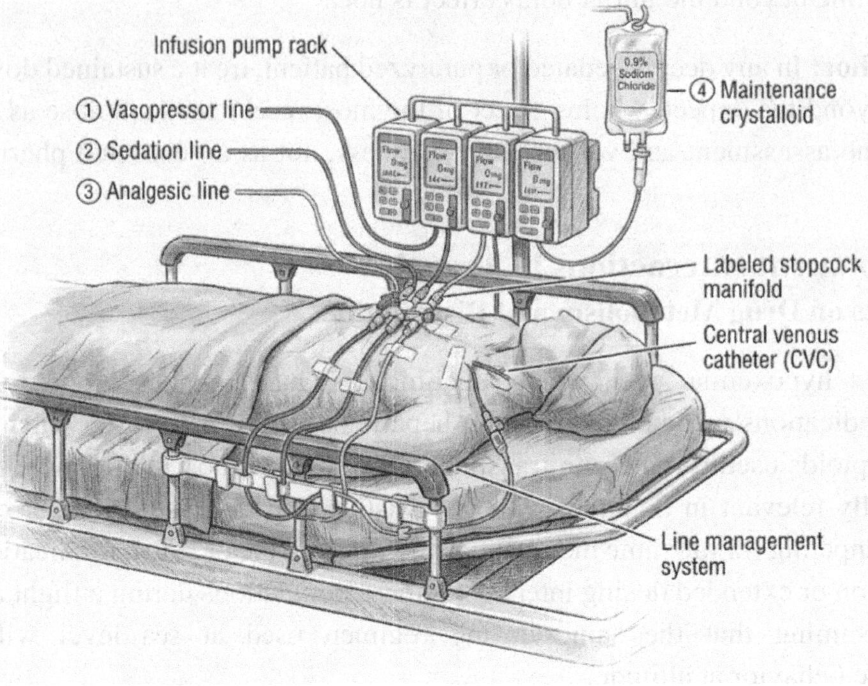


## Multi-Infusion Logistics and Pre-Departure Verification

### Line Labeling, Concentration Verification, and Pump Programming

A systematic pre-departure verification of every active infusion--confirming the labeled medication matches the bag or syringe, the programmed concentration matches the actual preparation, the programmed rate matches the intended dose, and the line is traced from pump to patient without crossing or confusion--is a non-negotiable safety step that should be completed before the patient leaves the sending facility's bedside, rather than during loading or after departure. Medication errors involving infusion pumps during interfacility transport are a recognized patient safety concern, and the majority of reported errors involve concentration mismatch between the programmed value and the actual preparation, a problem that originates at the moment of pump setup and is invisible thereafter unless actively verified.

### Battery Reserve and Supply Duration Planning

Every infusion pump's battery reserve must be independently confirmed for the full anticipated transport duration plus a safety margin for delay, following the same cold-weather derating logic introduced in Chapter 1 for all battery-dependent equipment. The volume of medication remaining in each syringe or bag should be verified against the programmed rate and the anticipated transport time, since running out of a vasoactive infusion mid-transport is an entirely preventable catastrophe that requires nothing more sophisticated than a volume-rate-time calculation performed before departure and a replacement syringe or bag pre-prepared and available if the calculation shows the current supply is marginal.

## Anticoagulation Management During Transport

Patients transported on continuous heparin infusions, whether for venous thromboembolism management, acute coronary syndromes, or mechanical circulatory support device anticoagulation, require particular attention to infusion continuity and dose verification during the sending-to-transport transition. Heparin dosing is weight-based and protocol-driven, and the transport clinician should confirm the current dose against the patient's weight, the most recent activated partial thromboplastin time or anti-factor Xa level, and the protocol in use at the sending facility, rather than simply continuing the displayed rate without verifying its appropriateness. Direct oral anticoagulants are not managed by continuous infusion, but the timing and dose of the most recent oral anticoagulant dose should be documented, since it directly informs reversal decisions if an acute hemorrhagic event occurs during transport.

## Controlled Substance Documentation and Chain of Custody

The handling of controlled substances during interfacility transport is subject to federal and state regulations that vary by jurisdiction, and transport programs must maintain a documentation and chain-of-custody system that accounts for every milligram of every controlled substance carried, administered, and wasted. This is not merely an administrative requirement; a discrepancy in controlled substance accounting can trigger regulatory investigation, program suspension, or individual licensure consequences for the crew members involved. Practically, this means that controlled substance quantities should be counted and documented at departure, that every dose administered should be witnessed and documented in real time rather than retrospectively, and that waste should be witnessed and documented at the earliest opportunity, ideally before the end of the specific transport during which it was generated.

## Medication Error Prevention in the Transport Environment

The transport environment carries a higher baseline risk for medication errors than a hospital setting, because many of the safeguards that reduce error rates at the bedside--pharmacy verification, barcode scanning, nurse double-checks, readily accessible drug references--are absent or attenuated during transport. The transport clinician's primary countermeasure is a set of deliberate, low-technology habits: verifying the five rights (right patient, right drug, right dose, right route, right time) verbally and out loud before every medication administration, even when working alone; using pre-calculated, weight-based dosing references rather than performing arithmetic under stress; and never administering a medication drawn up by someone else without independently verifying the label against the intended drug and dose. These habits are individually simple but collectively powerful, and their disciplined application is what compensates for the absence of the institutional safety nets available at the bedside.

| Error Type | Transport-Specific Risk Factor | Prevention Strategy |
|---|---|---|
| Concentration mismatch | Sending facility and transport team use different standard concentrations | Verify concentration on bag/syringe label before rate-equivalent transition |
| Wrong drug | Multiple syringes in low-light, confined cabin | Standardized labeling; verbal confirmation before administration |
| Wrong dose | Mental arithmetic under stress | Pre-calculated weight-based reference; avoid in-the-moment calculation |
| Infusion interruption | Line disconnection during loading/movement | Secure all connections before movement; verify flow immediately after |
| Supply exhaustion | Inadequate volume-rate-time calculation | Pre-departure calculation for every active infusion; replacement pre-prepared |

**KEY POINT:** A vasoactive infusion that runs dry mid-transport produces a predictable and potentially catastrophic hemodynamic collapse; the prevention is a simple volume-rate-time calculation performed before departure, with a replacement syringe pre-prepared if the margin is tight.

Consider a sixty-three-year-old man with septic shock on norepinephrine at a moderate dose, transferred by rotor-wing for source control at a tertiary center. During the pre-departure infusion transition, the transport nurse hangs her own norepinephrine preparation and matches the displayed rate from the sending facility's pump. However, the sending pharmacy had prepared the infusion at a higher concentration than the transport team's standard concentration, meaning the rate-equivalent transition actually delivers a lower dose per minute. Within eight minutes of switching lines, the patient's mean arterial pressure drifts from sixty-eight to fifty-four, and the arterial waveform shows a progressive narrowing of pulse pressure consistent with falling cardiac output rather than a vasodilatory event. Recognizing the temporal relationship to the infusion transition rather than attributing the change to disease progression, the nurse rechecks the concentration printed on the sending facility's bag against her own, identifies the mismatch, and adjusts the rate upward to achieve dose equivalence, with the pressure recovering over the subsequent five minutes. This case illustrates the chapter's central pharmacologic safety argument: concentration, not rate, determines dose, and an infusion transition that matches rate without verifying concentration can silently and immediately underdeliver a medication the patient depends on for hemodynamic survival.

## Advanced Vasoactive Pharmacology for Transport

### Angiotensin II: A Newer Vasopressor Option

Angiotensin II, approved for refractory distributive shock, provides a non-catecholamine vasoconstrictive mechanism that operates through the renin-angiotensin-aldosterone system rather than adrenergic receptors, and may be particularly useful in patients with catecholamine-refractory vasoplegia or those in whom escalating catecholamine doses are producing tachyarrhythmias or myocardial ischemia. Its transport-specific limitation is its relative unfamiliarity to many transport clinicians and its absence from most transport formularies, though its inclusion in some tertiary ICU protocols means that a transport clinician may inherit a patient already receiving it and must be prepared to continue the infusion during transport without interruption.

### Calcium Chloride Versus Calcium Gluconate: When the Distinction Matters

Calcium chloride delivers approximately three times as much elemental calcium per gram as calcium gluconate, making it the preferred agent when rapid calcium effect is clinically urgent--hyperkalemic cardiac toxicity, calcium channel blocker overdose, and severe symptomatic hypocalcemia. However, calcium chloride requires central venous access for safe administration, since peripheral infiltration produces severe tissue necrosis, while calcium gluconate can be safely administered through a peripheral vein. The transport clinician should carry both formulations and select based on the clinical urgency and the available access: calcium chloride through a confirmed central line for emergent indications, calcium gluconate through a peripheral line when the urgency permits the slower onset but safer peripheral route.

### Vasopressin Analogs and Terlipressin Considerations

Vasopressin is administered at a fixed, non-titrated dose as an adjunct to norepinephrine in septic and vasodilatory shock, but the transport clinician should be aware that its physiologic effects extend beyond vasoconstriction: it promotes water retention through V2 receptor activation (which can produce dilutional hyponatremia over hours to days), it can reduce splanchnic blood flow at higher doses, and its half-life of ten to thirty-five minutes means that its hemodynamic effect persists for a meaningful period after the infusion is stopped, which affects the timing of dose adjustments. Terlipressin, a synthetic vasopressin analog with a longer duration of action available in some countries, provides sustained vasoconstrictive effect from intermittent bolus dosing rather than continuous infusion, a logistical advantage for transport programs operating in settings where it is available.

## Sedation Depth Assessment Tools for Transport

### The Richmond Agitation-Sedation Scale in the Transport Environment

The Richmond Agitation-Sedation Scale provides a ten-point assessment of sedation depth from combative agitation (+4) through calm and cooperative (0) to unarousable (-5), and its transport application requires adaptation to the environmental constraints: the verbal stimulation component must account for cabin noise (the clinician must shout or use physical touch rather than speak at a normal volume), the eye-opening assessment must account for lighting conditions, and the motor response assessment must account for patient restraints that may limit movement independent of sedation depth. The RASS score should be documented at each reassessment interval as part of the transport monitoring bundle, and changes in the score between intervals should be interpreted in the context of recent sedation dose changes, procedure-related stimulation, and the transport-environment variables that might independently alter arousal.

### Processed EEG Monitoring: BIS and Sedline in Transport

Processed electroencephalographic monitoring devices, including the Bispectral Index and SedLine monitors, provide a continuous, numeric estimate of sedation depth that complements the clinical assessment scales, and some transport programs incorporate these devices for patients requiring deep sedation or neuromuscular blockade where clinical assessment is ablated. The transport-specific limitations include electrode adhesion on diaphoretic skin, signal artifact from vibration and electrical interference, and the cost and complexity of adding another monitoring device to an already-complex equipment set. For programs that do carry processed EEG monitoring, it is most valuable in the paralyzed patient, where clinical assessment of sedation depth is impossible and the risk of awareness under paralysis is the primary concern that the device addresses.

## Blood Product Administration During Transport

### Red Blood Cell Transfusion: Indications and Logistics

Red blood cell transfusion during transport is indicated for acute hemorrhage with hemodynamic instability, severe symptomatic anemia, and as part of massive transfusion protocol activation. The transport-specific logistics include blood product storage (packed red blood cells must be maintained at one to six degrees Celsius, which requires a validated cooler with temperature monitoring), compatibility verification (emergency-release O-negative blood can be transfused without crossmatching, but the crew should document that uncrossmatched blood was used for the receiving facility's transfusion service), and transfusion reaction monitoring, which is more challenging in the transport environment because the earliest signs of a transfusion reaction--fever, urticaria, and dyspnea--can be obscured by the patient's underlying condition and the transport environment's sensory constraints.

### Plasma, Platelet, and Cryoprecipitate Administration

Fresh frozen plasma requires thawing before administration, a process that takes twenty to thirty minutes and should be coordinated with the sending facility's blood bank before the transport crew's arrival so that thawed plasma is available for departure. Once thawed, plasma has a limited shelf life and must be administered promptly, making it a use-it-or-lose-it resource during transport. Platelets are stored at room temperature and do not require warming, but their availability at community sending facilities is often limited, and the transport crew should confirm platelet availability and request preparation before arrival. Cryoprecipitate, used for fibrinogen replacement in the coagulopathic bleeding patient, requires the same thawing process as plasma and the same pre-departure coordination with the blood bank.

### Whole Blood and Walking Blood Bank Considerations

Low-titer group O whole blood is increasingly available in military and civilian trauma transport programs as a balanced resuscitation product that provides red cells, plasma, and platelets in a single unit, simplifying the logistics of balanced resuscitation during transport. Programs that carry whole blood should maintain a cold-chain storage and verification system, and the crew should be trained in the specific administration protocols, compatibility requirements, and monitoring parameters for whole blood, which differ in some respects from component therapy. Walking blood bank protocols, in which crew members serve as emergency blood donors, exist in military transport medicine and some civilian remote-transport programs, but their implementation requires specific training, screening, and medical oversight that is beyond the scope of most civilian transport operations.

## Special Pharmacologic Populations in Transport

### Pediatric Pharmacokinetics and Weight-Based Dosing Verification

Pediatric patients in transport require weight-based dosing for every medication, and the pharmacokinetic differences between children and adults extend beyond simple dose scaling: neonates and infants have a proportionally larger volume of distribution for water-soluble drugs, immature hepatic enzyme systems that prolong the half-life of many medications, reduced protein binding that increases the free fraction of protein-bound drugs, and higher body water content that dilutes medications differently than in adults. The transport clinician managing a pediatric patient should use a length-based weight estimation system when actual weight is unavailable, should double-check every dose calculation against a pediatric reference before administration, and should be aware that the standard adult drug concentrations stocked in the transport kit may need to be diluted to achieve the precision required for pediatric dosing.

### Geriatric Pharmacology: Reduced Reserve and Polypharmacy

Older adults present the opposite end of the pharmacologic spectrum from pediatric patients: reduced hepatic and renal clearance prolongs drug half-lives, reduced cardiac output slows drug distribution, increased body fat percentage increases the volume of distribution for lipophilic drugs, and the polypharmacy typical of the geriatric population multiplies the risk of drug-drug interactions. The transport clinician should reduce initial doses of sedatives, opioids, and vasoactive agents in older patients, should extend dosing intervals to account for prolonged clearance, and should review the patient's home medication list for interactions with transport medications--a task that the sending facility's pharmacist has typically performed but that the transport crew should verify, since the sending facility's medication reconciliation may not have accounted for the transport-specific medications the crew will administer.

### Obesity and Drug Dosing: Which Weight to Use

Medication dosing in the obese patient is complicated by the fact that different drugs distribute differently in adipose versus lean tissue, and the appropriate dosing weight varies by drug class: succinylcholine is dosed on total body weight (because its rapid hydrolysis by pseudocholinesterase, which is proportional to plasma volume, scales with total body mass), while non-depolarizing neuromuscular blockers are dosed on ideal body weight (because they distribute primarily into lean tissue). Sedatives and opioids generally use adjusted body weight (a value between ideal and actual weight, calculated as ideal body weight plus forty percent of the difference between actual and ideal), and the transport clinician should have access to a dosing reference that specifies the appropriate weight basis for each medication rather than defaulting to actual body weight for all drugs, which will overdose lean-tissue-distributed medications and underdose plasma-volume-distributed ones.

**Pregnancy and Medication Safety During Transport**

Medication administration in the pregnant patient requires consideration of both maternal effect and fetal exposure, and the transport clinician should be familiar with the medications that are considered safe during pregnancy and those that carry known teratogenic or fetotoxic risks. For the most common transport medications: fentanyl is generally considered safe for short-term use in pregnancy (though prolonged use near delivery can produce neonatal respiratory depression), norepinephrine is the preferred vasopressor in pregnancy (phenylephrine can reduce uterine blood flow), and magnesium sulfate has an established safety profile for both tocolysis and seizure prophylaxis. Medications that should be avoided or used with extreme caution include ACE inhibitors (fetotoxic in the second and third trimesters), NSAIDs (risk of premature ductal closure in the third trimester), and benzodiazepines (neonatal sedation and respiratory depression if administered close to delivery).

The clinical scenarios addressed in this chapter illustrate a principle that recurs throughout the text: the transport environment does not merely add logistic complexity to the management of critical illness--it introduces specific physiologic stressors that interact with the patient's underlying condition to produce clinical changes that would not occur at the bedside. The altitude-related gas expansion, preload shifts, oxygenation challenges, and monitoring degradation described in Chapter 1, combined with the pharmacologic and equipment considerations from Chapters 4 and 5, create a modified clinical environment in which every bedside management principle must be re-examined through the lens of transport-specific risk. The disease-specific management recommendations in this chapter have been written with this re-examination already performed, incorporating the transport modifications into the clinical recommendations rather than presenting bedside management followed by a separate list of transport considerations, because the integration of disease knowledge and transport awareness is the competency that this text is designed to develop.

Inter-professional collaboration during the management of the conditions in this chapter deserves specific emphasis, because the complexity of many transport patients exceeds the capability of any single clinician acting alone. The nurse-paramedic team, the nurse-physician team, or whatever crew configuration the program uses represents a collaborative unit whose combined clinical capability exceeds the sum of its individual members, provided that the communication, role allocation, and shared mental model practices described in Chapter 24 are actively maintained throughout the transport. A transport in which one crew member manages the airway while the other manages hemodynamics, with both monitoring different aspects of the same clinical picture and cross-checking each other's assessments, produces a more complete and reliable clinical picture than either clinician could achieve alone, and this collaborative advantage is greatest during the high-workload, high-stress scenarios that the conditions in this chapter frequently produce.

Quality improvement in the management of these conditions during transport depends on systematic outcome tracking that links transport-specific management decisions to patient outcomes at the receiving facility. Did the patient who received a specific intervention during transport have a better or worse outcome than comparable patients who did not? Did a specific monitoring strategy detect deterioration earlier and allow more effective intervention? Did advance communication with the receiving facility produce measurably faster time-to-treatment on arrival? These questions can only be answered by programs that collect and analyze outcome data systematically, and the transport clinician's contribution to this process is meticulous, contemporaneous documentation of every clinical decision, every intervention, and every trajectory observation during the transport, since this documentation is the raw material from which quality improvement insights are derived. A transport program that does not analyze its outcomes cannot improve them, and a transport clinician who does not document their clinical reasoning cannot contribute to the program's learning.

**THE IN-TRANSIT DETERIORATION SIGNATURE SYSTEM — Pharmacologically Mediated Deterioration Patterns**

---

**Signature Introduced This Chapter:** Masked Hemodynamic Collapse Under Deep Sedation (insidious pressure decline without compensatory tachycardia in a deeply sedated or paralyzed patient).

**Pharmacologic Pattern Logic:** This Signature is distinct from the movement-triggered Signatures introduced in Chapter 1 because the primary mechanism is drug-mediated suppression of compensatory responses rather than a direct environmental stressor, though the transport environment's cumulative physiologic burden is the precipitating context that reveals the vulnerability. The absence of expected compensatory signs is itself the diagnostic clue.

**Cross-Reference Forward:** Chapter 11 (TBI and ICP Management) extends the sedation-depth monitoring discipline to neuroprotective sedation targets; Chapter 9 (MCS Devices) extends infusion logistics to anticoagulation management for mechanical support circuits.

## Summary and Key Concepts

Vasoactive agent selection in transport must account for both the patient's hemodynamic phenotype and the titratability constraints of the transport environment.

Sedation assessment in transit requires a standardized scale applied at fixed intervals, since environmental noise and restraint obscure the clinical cues used at the bedside.

Neuromuscular blockade suppresses all patient-initiated alerting behavior, requiring proactive rather than reactive sedation depth maintenance.

Altitude, temperature, and vibration each introduce specific drug-environment interactions that can alter drug metabolism, infusion accuracy, and dose delivery in ways invisible to standard monitoring.

Pre-departure infusion verification--medication identity, concentration, rate, line tracing, battery reserve, and supply duration--is a non-negotiable safety step that prevents entirely avoidable mid-transport catastrophes.

# CHAPTER 5: TRANSPORT EQUIPMENT, TECHNOLOGY, AND SAFETY SYSTEMS

**Learning Objectives**

1. Describe the operational characteristics and limitations of portable ventilators, monitors, and infusion pumps used in critical care transport.
2. Apply systematic equipment checks and battery reserve calculations adapted to specific mission profiles.
3. Recognize equipment failure patterns and distinguish them from patient-level clinical deterioration.
4. Configure stretcher, monitor, and device layouts to optimize clinical access and safety during loading and transit.
5. Integrate oxygen delivery systems, suction equipment, and communication devices into a cohesive transport platform.

**Chapter Outline**

This chapter addresses the equipment ecosystem that supports critical care transport as a clinical discipline in its own right, building directly on the altitude physiology introduced in Chapter 1, the monitoring principles established in Chapter 2, the ventilator management framework developed in Chapter 3, and the infusion logistics described in Chapter 4. Equipment is not merely the backdrop against which clinical decisions are made; it is itself a variable that can enable or constrain every intervention the clinician attempts, and a clinician who does not understand the specific performance characteristics, failure modes, and environmental vulnerabilities of the equipment they carry into transit is working with an incomplete clinical picture.

## Portable Ventilator Systems

### Transport Ventilator Categories and Mode Availability

Portable transport ventilators span a spectrum from simple, pneumatically driven devices offering only basic volume-controlled ventilation to sophisticated, turbine-driven platforms capable of modes and monitoring features that approach those of a full bedside ICU ventilator. The clinician's working knowledge of the specific device carried on their platform is not optional, because each device imposes its own set of mode availability constraints, alarm behavior, and waveform display limitations that directly affect the ventilator management strategies described in Chapter 3. A crew that arrives at a sending facility expecting to replicate a patient's complex pressure-support ventilation with automated leak compensation on a device that offers only volume-controlled assist-control will need to translate the ventilator strategy rather than copy it, and that translation must happen before departure, not during transit.

### Gas Supply Integration and Consumption Monitoring

Most transport ventilators consume compressed gas as a driving source, and the rate of gas consumption varies substantially across ventilator models, modes, and settings. A ventilator that uses compressed oxygen both as a driving gas and as the delivered gas consumes oxygen at a rate substantially higher than the patient's minute ventilation alone would suggest, since a portion of each breath cycle's gas supply is expended as mechanical work rather than delivered to the patient. This distinction is the basis for the oxygen supply calculation discussed in Chapter 1, but it carries an equipment-specific dimension: the crew must know the specific gas consumption characteristics of their device at the planned settings, not merely estimate consumption from the patient's ventilatory requirements alone, or the oxygen duration calculation will underestimate actual consumption and overestimate remaining supply.

### Ventilator Battery Performance and Backup Planning

Battery endurance for portable ventilators is typically specified by the manufacturer under controlled, room-temperature conditions at moderate settings, and actual endurance in the field frequently falls short of the published specification due to the cold-temperature derating effect described in Chapter 1, the higher-than-nominal settings required for many critically ill patients, and battery aging. The practical consequence is that a ventilator battery rated for four hours under ideal conditions may deliver substantially less than four hours on a cold tarmac with a patient requiring high minute ventilation, and the margin between actual battery endurance and planned transport duration must be verified rather than assumed for every mission. A manual resuscitation bag with an appropriate positive end-expiratory pressure valve, pre-assembled and immediately accessible, provides the ultimate backup for any ventilator battery failure and should be treated as a mandatory parallel system, not an emergency-only afterthought.

**CAUTION:** A manual resuscitation bag is the only ventilatory backup that requires no battery, no compressed gas source, and no electrical power; it should be pre-assembled, tested, and positioned for immediate access on every transport, regardless of ventilator battery status.

## Physiologic Monitors and Diagnostic Devices

### Multi-Parameter Monitor Configuration for Transport

The transport monitor serves as the clinician's primary sensory extension throughout transit, and its configuration--which parameters are displayed, which alarm thresholds are set, and how the display is physically positioned relative to the clinician's line of sight--directly affects the speed and reliability with which a developing problem is detected. Alarm thresholds should be set before departure based on the patient-specific baseline established in Chapter 2, narrow enough to detect meaningful deviation but wide enough to avoid the alarm fatigue that results from nuisance alarms triggered by normal transport-related artifact. The physical position of the monitor screen should allow the clinician to view waveforms and numeric trends without turning away from the patient or releasing a stabilizing grip on equipment, since a monitor that requires the clinician to lean across the cabin to read a number is functionally invisible during turbulence or a procedural emergency.

### Point-of-Care Testing and Laboratory Capabilities

Point-of-care blood gas analysis, glucose measurement, and basic metabolic panels, where carried by the transport program, provide real-time laboratory data that can meaningfully alter management decisions during transit, particularly for patients with evolving acid-base disturbances, diabetic emergencies, or electrolyte derangements whose trajectory cannot be reliably predicted from a single pre-departure laboratory draw. The decision to carry and deploy point-of-care testing equipment should be matched to mission profile and patient acuity: a routine, short-duration transport of a hemodynamically stable patient may not justify the setup time and supply cost, while a long-duration transport of a patient with diabetic ketoacidosis or a complex acid-base picture may make interval glucose and blood gas measurement genuinely decision-altering.

### Portable Ultrasound in the Transport Equipment Set

Portable ultrasound, introduced in Chapter 2 as a monitoring extension, carries equipment-specific considerations that affect its utility in transit: battery endurance under continuous or intermittent use, image quality degradation under vibration, probe durability during the mechanical stresses of loading and transport, and the storage and accessibility of the device within the cabin layout. Programs that include ultrasound in their standard transport equipment set should establish a specific storage location that protects the device during transit while allowing rapid deployment when needed, and should maintain a maintenance and quality-assurance schedule for the device that accounts for the harsher mechanical environment it experiences in transport compared to a hospital department.

**Figure 5.1: Transport Monitor and Equipment Layout on a Stretcher Configuration**

1 2 3 4

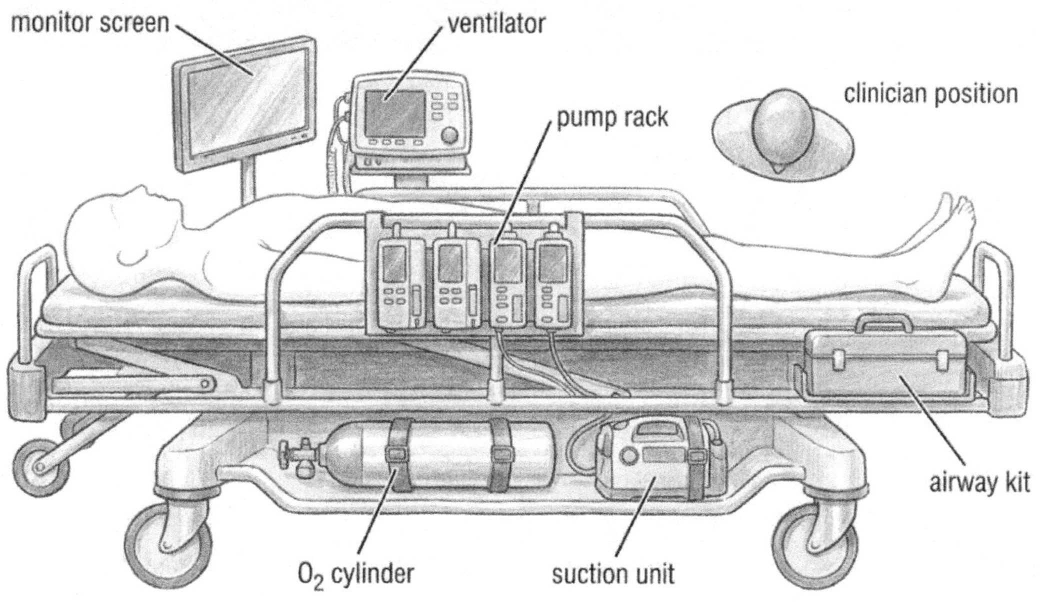

## Infusion Pump Systems and Power Management

### Syringe Pump Versus Volumetric Pump Selection

The choice between syringe-driver pumps and volumetric infusion pumps for transport is driven by the specific medications being administered: vasoactive infusions and sedation agents, which require precise, small-volume delivery, are best served by syringe pumps that deliver in fractions of a milliliter per hour, while larger-volume infusions such as maintenance crystalloid, blood products, or antibiotic solutions are better served by volumetric pumps that accommodate standard intravenous bags. Many transport programs carry both types, and the clinician should verify that each medication is matched to the appropriate pump type before departure, since programming a vasoactive infusion into a volumetric pump designed for larger volumes can produce clinically significant dose delivery inaccuracies at the low flow rates typical of vasopressor therapy.

### Power Management and Electrical Load Planning

The total electrical load of all battery-operated devices--ventilator, monitor, infusion pumps, suction, warming devices, and ultrasound--must be considered as a system rather than device by device, since some transport platforms provide a limited number of external power outlets, and exceeding the available electrical supply can force the crew to choose which devices run on external power and which run on internal battery, a triage decision that should be made deliberately during pre-departure planning rather than discovered mid-transport when a device unexpectedly exhausts its battery. A power management checklist, accounting for every device's power source, battery reserve, and priority ranking, ensures that the most clinically critical devices receive external power first and that battery-dependent devices have verified reserve for the full mission duration.

| Device | Typical Battery Endurance | Priority for External Power | Backup if Battery Fails |
|---|---|---|---|
| Portable ventilator | 2-8 hours (manufacturer/settings dependent) | Highest | Manual resuscitation bag with PEEP valve |
| Physiologic monitor | 2-6 hours | High | Manual assessment; intermittent pulse oximetry |
| Syringe infusion pump | 4-12 hours per pump | High (for vasoactive infusions) | Gravity drip with manual rate adjustment (imprecise) |
| Portable suction | 30-90 minutes continuous | Moderate | Manual suction device |
| Forced-air warmer | Variable; high power draw | Low (intermittent use) | Passive insulation; warmed blankets |

**THE IN-TRANSIT DETERIORATION SIGNATURE SYSTEM — Equipment-Masked Physiologic Deterioration**

---

**The Signature:** A change in monitored parameters--falling blood pressure, rising airway pressures, loss of capnography signal, or a new alarm pattern--that is initially attributed to an equipment malfunction, artifact, or transient signal disruption rather than to an actual change in the patient's physiology.

**Movement Trigger:** The transport environment generates a high background rate of equipment-related artifact--vibration-induced signal dropout, motion-triggered alarms, transient cable disconnections during repositioning--which creates a cognitive environment in which the crew's default explanation for any new alarm or parameter change is "equipment," not "patient."

**Early Tell:** A parameter change that persists beyond the typical duration of an equipment artifact, or that is accompanied by a concordant change in a second, independent monitoring modality, suggests a patient-level event rather than an isolated equipment issue.

**Trap Logic:** This pattern is the mirror image of the standard troubleshooting bias described in Chapter 3: where the airway chapter warned against checking the machine before the patient, this Signature warns against dismissing a real physiologic event as equipment noise. The discriminating feature is concordance--a genuine deterioration produces changes across multiple independent parameters, while an equipment artifact typically affects only one.

**Signature Anchor:** When any monitored parameter changes during transport, check for concordance across at least one additional independent monitoring modality before attributing the change to equipment artifact; a change visible in two independent systems is a patient event until proven otherwise.

## Oxygen Delivery Systems and Suction Equipment

### Cylinder, Liquid, and On-Board Oxygen Systems

Oxygen supply for transport is provided by compressed gas cylinders, portable liquid oxygen units, or, in some fixed-wing and rotor-wing platforms, on-board oxygen systems integrated into the aircraft. Each system has a specific capacity, flow-rate ceiling, and operational limitation that the clinician must understand for the specific platform and mission: compressed gas cylinders have a finite and calculable supply duration at a given flow rate, liquid oxygen units offer longer duration but require careful handling and venting procedures, and on-board systems provide the longest endurance but are available only on equipped aircraft and cannot be used during ground segments of a combined-mode transport. The oxygen supply calculation introduced in Chapter 1 should be performed using the actual supply system carried on the specific mission, not a generic estimate, and should account for the ventilator's gas consumption characteristics discussed earlier in this chapter.

### Portable and In-Line Suction Systems

Suction capability is essential for airway management and for managing gastric, thoracic, and wound drainage during transport, and the specific suction device carried--battery-powered portable unit, manual hand-pump suction, or in-line suction integrated into the vehicle or aircraft--determines both the suction pressure achievable and the duration of continuous use available. Battery-powered portable suction units have a limited continuous-use duration, typically thirty to ninety minutes depending on the device and battery charge, and should be tested for adequate suction pressure before departure rather than discovered to be inadequate during an acute airway emergency. A manual suction device, requiring no battery or power source, should accompany every transport as a backup, positioned for immediate access alongside the rescue airway equipment described in Chapter 3.

### Communication Devices and Connectivity in Transit

Reliable communication between the transport crew and both the sending and receiving facilities is a patient safety requirement, not a convenience, since the ability to provide advance notification of a deteriorating patient, request medical control guidance for a clinical decision that exceeds standing protocol authority, or redirect to an alternate receiving facility requires a functioning communication link throughout the transport. Cellular coverage is inconsistent over rural and mountainous terrain, satellite communication is available on some fixed-wing platforms but carries cost and latency limitations, and radio communication is platform-specific and may not be interoperable across different emergency medical services systems. The crew should confirm before departure that at least one communication modality is expected to remain functional throughout the planned route, and should have a contingency plan for communication loss, since a crew that cannot reach medical control during a transport that requires a diversion or escalation decision must be prepared to act within their standing protocols and clinical judgment rather than deferring to a consultation that cannot be reached.

### Equipment Decontamination and Infection Prevention Between Transports

Transport equipment, particularly the stretcher surface, monitor cables, and pump housings, is exposed to body fluids and pathogenic organisms from every patient transported, and the confined cabin environment limits the ability to perform thorough decontamination between consecutive transports to the same degree achievable in a hospital setting. Transport programs should maintain a standardized, timed decontamination protocol that specifies which surfaces require cleaning between every transport, which require terminal decontamination after known infectious exposures, and which disposable components--circuit tubing, suction catheters, single-use transducers--must be replaced rather than cleaned. This protocol is as much a patient safety intervention as any clinical skill, since a transport program that inadequately decontaminates between patients is functionally operating as an unrecognized vector for healthcare-associated infection.

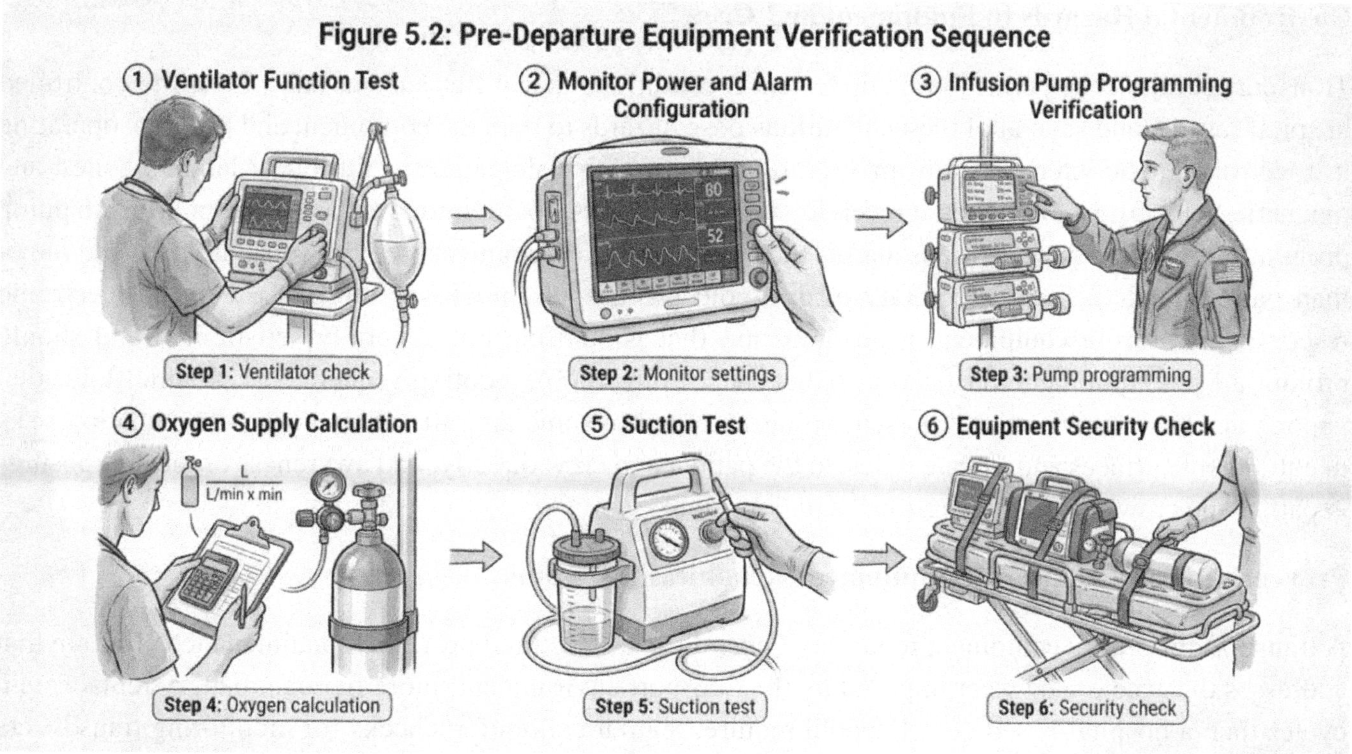


## Stretcher Configuration and Equipment Mounting

### Optimizing Clinical Access During Loading and Transit

The physical layout of equipment on and around the transport stretcher determines the clinician's ability to reach the patient, access monitoring displays, manipulate infusion pumps, and perform emergency procedures without obstruction. A layout that positions the monitor at the clinician's eye level, the ventilator and pump rack within arm's reach, and the airway and emergency equipment on the same side as the clinician's working position converts the confined cabin space into a functional workspace, while a poorly planned layout that places critical equipment behind or above the clinician, or on the opposite side of the patient, introduces delays and physical barriers that multiply under the stress of an in-transit emergency.

### Weight and Space Constraints Across Platform Types

Every transport platform--rotor-wing, fixed-wing, and ground ambulance--imposes specific weight and space limits that constrain the total equipment complement the crew can carry, and these limits interact with patient weight to determine the operational envelope for a given mission. A bariatric patient on a rotor-wing platform may consume enough of the aircraft's useful load to force a reduction in fuel carried, which in turn limits range and dictates routing decisions that would not apply to a lighter patient. The equipment loading plan should therefore be mission-specific rather than standardized, with the crew calculating total patient-plus-equipment weight against the platform's published useful load for the planned environmental conditions, including the density altitude and temperature adjustments that affect rotor-wing performance at altitude and in heat.

**Environmental Hazards to Equipment and Crew**

Transport equipment operates in environmental conditions that differ substantially from the controlled hospital setting, and several of these conditions pose hazards to both the equipment and the crew operating it. Electromagnetic interference from aircraft avionics, high-voltage power lines near landing zones, and magnetic fields from MRI suites at receiving facilities can disrupt monitor displays, corrupt infusion pump programming, or produce spurious alarms that the crew must recognize as environmentally induced rather than patient-related. Static electricity in dry, cold cabin environments can produce isolated electronic resets in monitoring equipment, a phenomenon that is startling but generally self-limited and should prompt a brief equipment verification rather than a full troubleshooting sequence. Hydraulic fluid, fuel vapors, and de-icing chemicals present on tarmacs and in some aircraft cabins pose contamination risks to equipment surfaces and, in rare cases, to the patient and crew directly, and awareness of these exposures is part of the crew's overall operational safety posture.

**Preventive Maintenance and Equipment Readiness Programs**

A transport program's equipment reliability depends on a structured preventive maintenance program that addresses the accelerated wear imposed by the transport environment: more frequent battery replacement cycles than a hospital-based device would require, regular calibration checks for monitoring transducers and flow sensors exposed to vibration, and systematic inspection of mechanical components such as stretcher locking mechanisms, equipment rail mounts, and cable connectors that are subject to repeated stress during loading and unloading. An equipment failure log, maintained across missions and reviewed periodically for patterns, can identify a specific device, device type, or operational condition associated with a disproportionate failure rate, allowing the program to address the root cause rather than repeatedly troubleshooting the same downstream symptom.

| Equipment Category | Common Transport-Specific Failure Mode | Preventive Strategy |
|---|---|---|
| Ventilator | Battery depletion beyond published spec; flow sensor drift from vibration | Cold-weather battery derating; pre-mission flow calibration check |
| Monitor | Signal dropout from cable disconnection during movement | Cable routing with slack; secure connectors before loading |
| Infusion pump | Vibration-induced syringe advance (bolusing); cold-slowed flow | Anti-vibration mounting; temperature-controlled pump compartment |
| Suction | Battery depletion during prolonged continuous use | Reserve manual suction always staged; fresh battery before each mission |

| | | |
|---|---|---|
| Stretcher mount | Equipment rail lock loosening from repeated loading cycles | Scheduled rail and lock inspection; torque verification |

### Equipment Security During Loading, Turbulence, and Deceleration

Every piece of equipment must be secured against the specific mechanical forces anticipated during the transport: the tilt and acceleration of stretcher loading, the sustained vibration of cruise, and the deceleration forces of landing or braking. Unsecured equipment is a projectile hazard during turbulence or a hard landing, and even equipment that does not become a projectile can shift sufficiently to disconnect a monitoring cable, dislodge an infusion line, or obstruct the clinician's access to the patient. Equipment mounting systems should be checked for security as part of the pre-departure verification, and any device that cannot be positively secured to the stretcher rail, equipment rack, or cabin mount should be positioned where it can do the least harm if it shifts, rather than balanced in a location that depends on the absence of turbulence to remain stable.

**KEY POINT:** Unsecured equipment in a transport cabin is not merely an inconvenience; during turbulence or a hard landing, it becomes a projectile that threatens both the patient and the crew. Every device must be positively secured before movement begins.

Consider a transport team preparing to load a ventilated, hemodynamically unstable patient onto a rotor-wing aircraft for a forty-minute flight. During the pre-departure equipment check, the crew discovers that the portable suction unit, which had been placed on the stretcher for the ground ambulance transfer to the helipad, was balanced on the patient's leg area rather than secured to the equipment rail. Additionally, the monitor cable connecting the arterial line transducer had been routed under the stretcher frame in a position that would become taut and likely disconnect during the head-up tilt of aircraft loading. By identifying and correcting both of these equipment-configuration issues before loading--securing the suction to the rail and rerouting the cable with adequate slack--the crew prevents what would have been a loss of arterial pressure monitoring data at the exact moment of the loading tilt, the same vulnerable transition described in Chapter 1. This case illustrates that equipment configuration is not a housekeeping task separate from clinical management but a direct patient safety intervention that determines whether the clinician will have the monitoring, airway, and intervention access they need at the moments they need them most.

## Advanced Equipment Troubleshooting During Transport

### Systematic Equipment Failure Response Protocol

When a piece of transport equipment fails during transit, the clinician must rapidly execute a three-step response: first, determine whether the failure affects patient safety immediately (a ventilator failure is immediately life-threatening; a warming device failure is not); second, activate the backup system for the failed device (manual resuscitation for ventilator failure, passive insulation for warmer failure); and third, decide whether the failure warrants a mission diversion, an unscheduled stop for repair, or continued transport with the backup system in use. This three-step sequence should be rehearsed as a team protocol, since the stress and time pressure of an equipment failure in transit degrades the structured decision-making that determines whether the response is measured and effective or chaotic and delayed.

### Redundancy Planning and Single Points of Failure

Every transport equipment configuration should be analyzed for single points of failure--components whose failure would produce an immediate, unrecoverable loss of a critical clinical capability. A ventilator with no manual resuscitation backup is a single point of failure; a single infusion pump running a life-sustaining vasopressor with no second pump available is a single point of failure; a monitor with a single cable connection that, if severed, eliminates all monitoring simultaneously is a single point of failure. The transport clinician should identify these single points of failure during the pre-departure equipment check and, wherever possible, establish a redundant capability: a pre-assembled manual resuscitation bag alongside the ventilator, a spare infusion pump loaded and ready, and a backup pulse oximeter independent of the primary monitor.

### Emergency Power Procedures and Generator Systems

Some transport platforms--particularly fixed-wing aircraft and specialized ground critical care units--are equipped with onboard generators or inverters that provide continuous AC power to transport equipment throughout the mission. The transport clinician should understand the specific power system on their platform: its capacity in watts, its fuel dependency and runtime, its behavior during engine shutdown and restart, and its failure mode. A generator failure during transport converts every AC-dependent device to battery operation simultaneously, and the combined battery drain of ventilator, monitor, and multiple infusion pumps can exhaust available battery reserves much faster than any single device would alone, making the power management prioritization from earlier in this chapter immediately critical.

### Equipment Interoperability and Standardization Challenges

Transport programs that operate across multiple platform types--ground ambulance, rotor-wing, and fixed-wing--frequently encounter equipment interoperability challenges: a monitor that fits the ground ambulance mount may not fit the helicopter mount, infusion pumps that connect to the fixed-wing aircraft's power system may require an adapter for the ground unit's outlets, and stretcher-to-aircraft loading systems may be incompatible across different aircraft types. These interoperability gaps are most dangerous when they are discovered during a mission rather than during pre-deployment planning, and the transport program's equipment standardization process should specifically test and verify cross-platform compatibility before any equipment change is implemented.

## Specialized Transport Equipment

### Mechanical Chest Compression Devices

Mechanical chest compression devices, whether piston-driven or load-distributing band systems, provide consistent, uninterrupted chest compressions during transport that are independent of rescuer fatigue, cabin space constraints, and the mechanical difficulty of performing effective manual compressions on a moving stretcher in a vibrating vehicle. Their principal advantage in transport is not superior compression quality per se--manual compressions by a fresh, well-positioned rescuer are equivalent--but rather the sustainability and consistency of compressions over the extended time period of a transport, during which manual rescuer fatigue, suboptimal positioning, and the interruptions required for rescuer rotation degrade compression quality progressively. Programs that carry mechanical compression devices should ensure that every crew member is trained in their application, troubleshooting, and the specific clinical scenarios in which they should and should not be used (they are generally contraindicated in traumatic cardiac arrest with suspected tension pneumothorax or cardiac tamponade, where the immediate management is addressing the reversible cause rather than providing chest compressions).

### Portable Blood Warmers and Rapid Infusers

Rapid infusion of cold blood products and crystalloid is a well-established cause of iatrogenic hypothermia that worsens coagulopathy and cardiac irritability, and portable blood warming devices are an essential component of the transport equipment set for any program that administers blood products during transport. Commercially available portable warmers range from battery-powered in-line warmers that heat fluid as it flows through the warming chamber to chemical heat packs applied around the infusion tubing, and the crew should understand the specific warming capacity and flow rate limitations of their device, since a warmer that functions adequately at a maintenance infusion rate may be unable to warm blood effectively at the high flow rates required during massive transfusion.

### Portable Ventilator Capabilities: Current Generation

Current-generation portable transport ventilators have closed much of the capability gap with bedside ICU ventilators, offering pressure-regulated volume control, pressure support with leak compensation, graphic waveform display, measured delivered tidal volume, FiO2 blending from 21 to 100 percent, and PEEP ranges adequate for ARDS management. The transport clinician should know the specific capabilities and limitations of their platform's ventilator model, including its maximum PEEP capability, its behavior during oxygen supply depletion, its alarm logic and how alarms are silenced or adjusted, and its battery endurance at the specific settings required for the patient being transported. Annual or semi-annual familiarization training with the transport ventilator, including simulated equipment failures and mode transitions, maintains the clinician's device-specific competence in a way that classroom-based instruction alone cannot achieve.

## Emerging Technology in Transport Medicine

### Artificial Intelligence and Decision Support in Transport

Artificial intelligence-driven clinical decision support systems are beginning to enter the transport medicine space, offering real-time analysis of continuous monitoring data to detect deterioration patterns earlier than human observation alone. These systems can analyze arterial waveform morphology, ventilator flow patterns, and multi-parameter trends to generate alerts for developing hemodynamic instability, ventilator dyssynchrony, or rhythm changes before they reach alarm thresholds, potentially operationalizing the same anticipatory detection that the Deterioration Signature System in this text teaches through clinical pattern recognition. The transport clinician should approach these systems as supplements to, rather than replacements for, clinical judgment, since the algorithms are only as good as the data they receive, and the transport environment's artifact-heavy monitoring data can produce false-positive alerts that the clinician must contextualize against their own assessment.

### Wearable Monitoring and Continuous Remote Oversight

Wearable biosensors that provide continuous monitoring of physiologic parameters beyond the traditional monitor-cable-electrode model are under development for transport applications, offering the potential for untethered patient monitoring that eliminates the cable-disconnection problem that plagues traditional monitoring systems during loading, movement, and repositioning. These devices, typically adhesive patches applied to the patient's torso, can continuously stream heart rate, respiratory rate, body temperature, and activity data to a central display, and some incorporate algorithms for early warning score calculation that flag deterioration before the clinician's next scheduled reassessment. Their current limitations include battery life, adhesion reliability on diaphoretic skin, and accuracy validation against clinical-grade monitors, but the trajectory of the technology suggests that they will become increasingly integrated into transport monitoring systems in the coming years.

### Drone-Delivered Medical Supplies to Transport Crews

Unmanned aerial vehicles (drones) are being piloted in several countries for delivery of blood products, medications, and defibrillators to remote locations and to transport crews who have exhausted a specific supply during a prolonged or complicated mission. The transport clinician should be aware that this capability exists in some systems and may become available in their program, since the ability to receive resupply mid-mission fundamentally changes the logistic calculation for prolonged transports: a crew that can receive additional blood products or medications via drone delivery is less constrained by the initial supply loaded at departure, and the go/no-go decision for a long-duration transport may be different when mid-mission resupply is available versus when the crew must carry everything needed for the entire mission from the start.

### Point-of-Care Imaging Advances for Transport

Handheld ultrasound devices, now available as smartphone-connected probes weighing less than a few hundred grams, have reduced the size, cost, and complexity barrier to carrying ultrasound capability on every transport platform. The image quality of these devices has reached a level sufficient for the focused assessments described throughout this text--cardiac function, IVC status, lung sliding, FAST examination--though they remain inferior to cart-based systems for detailed anatomic assessment. The transport clinician should view handheld ultrasound as a monitoring extension comparable to a stethoscope: a tool that should be immediately available on every transport, used routinely rather than reserved for emergencies, and that provides real-time anatomic and functional data that no other bedside assessment can offer.

The clinical scenarios addressed in this chapter illustrate a principle that recurs throughout the text: the transport environment does not merely add logistic complexity to the management of critical illness--it introduces specific physiologic stressors that interact with the patient's underlying condition to produce clinical changes that would not occur at the bedside. The altitude-related gas expansion, preload shifts, oxygenation challenges, and monitoring degradation described in Chapter 1, combined with the pharmacologic and equipment considerations from Chapters 4 and 5, create a modified clinical environment in which every bedside management principle must be re-examined through the lens of transport-specific risk. The disease-specific management recommendations in this chapter have been written with this re-examination already performed, incorporating the transport modifications into the clinical recommendations rather than presenting bedside management followed by a separate list of transport considerations, because the integration of disease knowledge and transport awareness is the competency that this text is designed to develop.

Inter-professional collaboration during the management of the conditions in this chapter deserves specific emphasis, because the complexity of many transport patients exceeds the capability of any single clinician acting alone. The nurse-paramedic team, the nurse-physician team, or whatever crew configuration the program uses represents a collaborative unit whose combined clinical capability exceeds the sum of its individual members, provided that the communication, role allocation, and shared mental model practices described in Chapter 24 are actively maintained throughout the transport. A transport in which one crew member manages the airway while the other manages hemodynamics, with both monitoring different aspects of the same clinical picture and cross-checking each other's assessments, produces a more complete and reliable clinical picture than either clinician could achieve alone, and this collaborative advantage is greatest during the high-workload, high-stress scenarios that the conditions in this chapter frequently produce.

Quality improvement in the management of these conditions during transport depends on systematic outcome tracking that links transport-specific management decisions to patient outcomes at the receiving facility. Did the patient who received a specific intervention during transport have a better or worse outcome than comparable patients who did not? Did a specific monitoring strategy detect deterioration earlier and allow more effective intervention? Did advance communication with the receiving facility produce measurably faster time-to-treatment on arrival? These questions can only be answered by programs that collect and analyze outcome data systematically, and the transport clinician's contribution to this process is meticulous, contemporaneous documentation of every clinical decision, every intervention, and every trajectory observation during the transport, since this documentation is the raw material from which quality improvement insights are derived. A transport program that does not analyze its outcomes cannot improve them, and a transport clinician who does not document their clinical reasoning cannot contribute to the program's learning.

**THE IN-TRANSIT DETERIORATION SIGNATURE SYSTEM — Equipment-Origin Deterioration Patterns**

---

**Signature Introduced This Chapter:** Equipment-Masked Physiologic Deterioration (a genuine patient-level event dismissed as equipment artifact because of the high background rate of transport-related noise and nuisance alarms).

**Equipment Pattern Logic:** This Signature inverts the Chapter 3 troubleshooting sequence: where Chapter 3 warned against troubleshooting the machine before assessing the patient, this chapter warns against the opposite error--dismissing a real physiologic change as "just equipment" because the transport environment generates so many transient equipment artifacts that the crew's default attribution becomes noise rather than signal. The concordance check across independent modalities is the tie-breaker.

**Cross-Reference Forward:** Chapter 9 (Mechanical Circulatory Support Devices in Transit) extends the equipment-patient attribution challenge to device alarms on ventricular assist devices, intra-aortic balloon pumps, and extracorporeal circuits, where the line between device behavior and patient physiology is even more blurred.

## Summary and Key Concepts

Portable ventilator mode availability, gas consumption, and battery endurance are device-specific and must be verified against the planned mission profile rather than assumed from generic specifications.

Monitor configuration, alarm thresholds, and physical display positioning directly affect how quickly a developing deterioration is detected.

Power management for all battery-dependent devices should be planned as a system, with the most critical devices prioritized for external power and verified battery reserve for the full mission.

Oxygen supply calculations must account for ventilator gas consumption characteristics specific to the device carried, not merely the patient's minute ventilation.

Equipment layout on the stretcher is a direct patient safety intervention, determining clinical access, monitoring visibility, and projectile risk during turbulence or emergency maneuvers.

# CHAPTER 6: ACUTE CORONARY SYNDROMES AND CARDIOGENIC SHOCK IN TRANSIT

**Learning Objectives**

1. Differentiate ST-elevation from non-ST-elevation acute coronary syndromes and apply transport-specific management priorities for each.
2. Recognize cardiogenic shock and initiate hemodynamic support using the vasoactive and monitoring framework established in earlier chapters.
3. Apply antiplatelet, anticoagulant, and thrombolytic therapy considerations specific to the time-sensitive interfacility transfer window.
4. Prioritize clinical actions for percutaneous coronary intervention-bound transfers to minimize door-to-balloon time.
5. Manage post-cardiac arrest patients during interfacility transport, including targeted temperature management and hemodynamic optimization.

**Chapter Outline**

This chapter applies the foundational assessment, monitoring, pharmacologic, and equipment principles from Chapters 1 through 5 to the specific challenge of transporting a patient with an acute coronary syndrome or cardiogenic shock. These patients are among the most time-sensitive in interfacility transport medicine: the clinical value of the transport itself is measured in minutes saved between symptom onset and definitive revascularization, and every decision made during transit either preserves or erodes that time advantage.

## ST-Elevation and Non-ST-Elevation Myocardial Infarction Management

### Electrocardiographic Recognition and Classification

The transport clinician must be independently capable of interpreting a 12-lead electrocardiogram for ST-elevation myocardial infarction, including recognition of ST-elevation equivalents such as a new left bundle branch block, posterior infarction pattern, and de Winter T-waves, since the transport team's interpretation is frequently the one that activates the receiving facility's catheterization laboratory and determines whether the patient arrives as an expected primary percutaneous coronary intervention case or as an undifferentiated chest pain transfer. Misinterpretation in either direction--missing true ST elevation or falsely identifying artifact or a benign variant as infarction--carries direct consequences for both the patient and the receiving facility's resource allocation.

### Non-ST-Elevation Acute Coronary Syndrome Risk Stratification

Non-ST-elevation acute coronary syndromes present a different transport management challenge: the clinical decision is less about the speed of transfer and more about the appropriateness of the level of monitoring and support during transit, the stability of the patient's hemodynamic and rhythm status, and the readiness to escalate if the patient's electrocardiographic or hemodynamic picture evolves during the transport window. A patient with a non-ST-elevation myocardial infarction and a rising troponin trend but stable hemodynamics requires a lower-intensity but still vigilant monitoring posture, while the same diagnosis with new hemodynamic instability, dynamic electrocardiographic changes, or recurrent symptoms despite medical therapy warrants the same urgency and resource commitment as an ST-elevation presentation.

### Serial Electrocardiographic Monitoring During Transport

A single pre-departure electrocardiogram is insufficient for a patient with an evolving coronary event, and the transport clinician should plan for repeat electrocardiographic acquisition at defined intervals during transit and immediately in response to any new symptom, rhythm change, or hemodynamic shift. This serial monitoring serves two purposes: it detects evolution from a non-ST-elevation to an ST-elevation pattern that would change the receiving facility's activation status, and it provides the receiving interventional team with a trajectory rather than a single snapshot, which directly informs their procedural planning and urgency assessment on arrival.

| ACS Classification | ECG Finding | Transport Priority | Key Transport Action |
|---|---|---|---|
| STEMI | ST elevation in contiguous leads or STEMI equivalent | Highest — time to reperfusion is the primary outcome driver | Activate catheterization laboratory immediately; direct-to-lab on arrival |
| High-risk NSTEMI | ST depression, dynamic T-wave changes, rising troponin with instability | High — escalation-ready transport | Continuous monitoring; serial ECGs; vasopressor and rhythm readiness |
| Low-risk NSTEMI/UA | Normal or nonspecific ECG with positive biomarkers or typical symptoms | Moderate — monitored transport | Serial ECGs; symptom-triggered reassessment |
| Post-arrest with STEMI | ROSC with ST elevation | Highest — dual priority: neuroprotection and reperfusion | Temperature management initiation; |

| | | | |
|---|---|---|---|
| | | | catheterization laboratory activation |

**Figure 6.1: ST-Elevation Patterns and Transport-Relevant Equivalents on 12-Lead ECG**

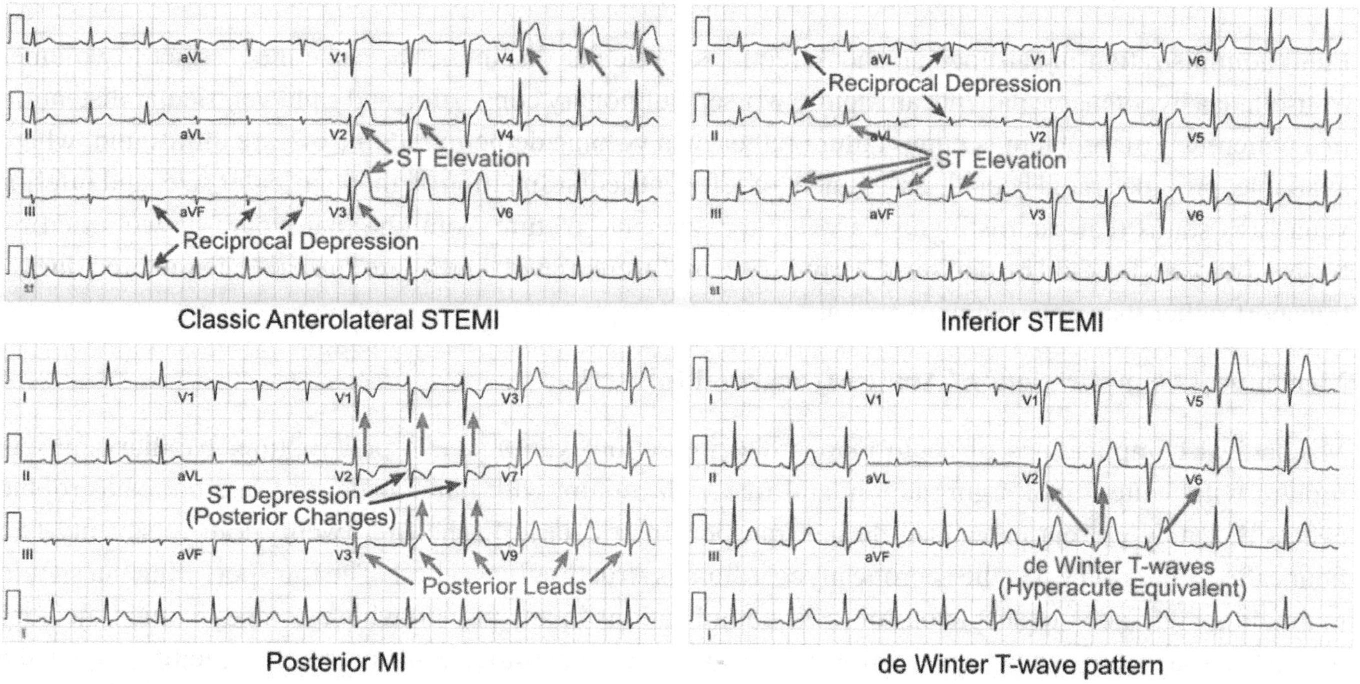


**Figure 6.1:** ST-Elevation Patterns and Transport-Rate-Relevant Equivalents on 12-Lead ECG

## Cardiogenic Shock Recognition and Hemodynamic Support

### Clinical Recognition of Cardiogenic Shock in the Transport Setting

Cardiogenic shock complicating acute myocardial infarction presents with the combination of sustained hypotension, evidence of end-organ hypoperfusion, and clinical or objective evidence of elevated left-sided filling pressures, a triad that should be assessed using the trend-based, patient-specific-baseline framework from Chapter 2 rather than a rigid numeric threshold. Cool, mottled extremities, altered mentation, declining urine output, and a rising lactate trend all contribute to the clinical picture, and the transport clinician's task is to assemble these into a working hemodynamic phenotype--predominantly cardiogenic, predominantly distributive, or mixed--that drives the correct vasoactive strategy from Chapter 4 rather than applying a default vasopressor without phenotyping.

### Vasoactive and Inotropic Support Strategies

Norepinephrine is the first-line vasopressor for cardiogenic shock with frank hypotension, providing afterload support through alpha-1 mediated vasoconstriction with modest inotropic augmentation, and should be titrated to a mean arterial pressure target that balances coronary perfusion pressure against the increased afterload burden on an already-failing ventricle. When the predominant problem is contractile failure rather than vasodilation, dobutamine added to norepinephrine or, in selected cases, low-dose epinephrine provides direct inotropic augmentation, though both carry the arrhythmogenic risk that requires the continuous rhythm monitoring already mandated for any transport patient on vasoactive support.

### Fluid Management in Cardiogenic Shock

Fluid administration in cardiogenic shock requires particular discipline, because the instinct to volume-resuscitate a hypotensive patient can rapidly worsen pulmonary congestion and right ventricular distention in a patient whose problem is pump failure rather than volume depletion. Point-of-care ultrasound, where available, provides rapid bedside assessment of left ventricular function, right ventricular size, and inferior vena cava status that can distinguish a volume-responsive picture from one that would be worsened by further fluid, and should be deployed early in any undifferentiated shock presentation encountered during transport rather than deferred until arrival.

### Mechanical Complications of Acute Myocardial Infarction

Mechanical complications of acute myocardial infarction--ventricular septal rupture, papillary muscle rupture with acute mitral regurgitation, and free wall rupture with tamponade--are rare but catastrophic events that may present or worsen during transport, particularly in the first twenty-four to seventy-two hours after infarction when the necrotic myocardium is structurally weakest. The transport clinician should maintain a high index of suspicion for these complications in any patient whose hemodynamic trajectory deteriorates abruptly and disproportionately to the electrocardiographic or rhythm picture, since the clinical presentation--sudden pulmonary edema, a new systolic murmur, or acute tamponade physiology--may initially mimic worsening cardiogenic shock from pump failure alone but requires an entirely different management pathway, typically emergent surgical intervention rather than further escalation of vasoactive support.

### Transport-Specific Arrhythmia Management in the Coronary Patient

Acute coronary syndrome patients are at heightened risk for both tachyarrhythmias and bradyarrhythmias during transport, and the transport clinician should have defibrillation pads pre-applied, a transcutaneous pacing capability confirmed, and antiarrhythmic medications drawn up or immediately accessible before departure. Ventricular tachycardia and ventricular fibrillation are the most immediately life-threatening rhythm emergencies, but accelerated idioventricular rhythm--a reperfusion arrhythmia that is generally benign and self-limited--must be distinguished from true ventricular tachycardia to avoid unnecessary treatment, since the clinical significance and management of the two are entirely different. High-degree atrioventricular block complicating inferior myocardial infarction is usually responsive to atropine and may resolve spontaneously, while the same block complicating anterior infarction typically reflects extensive septal necrosis and is more likely to require transcutaneous pacing as a bridge to a transvenous system at the receiving facility.

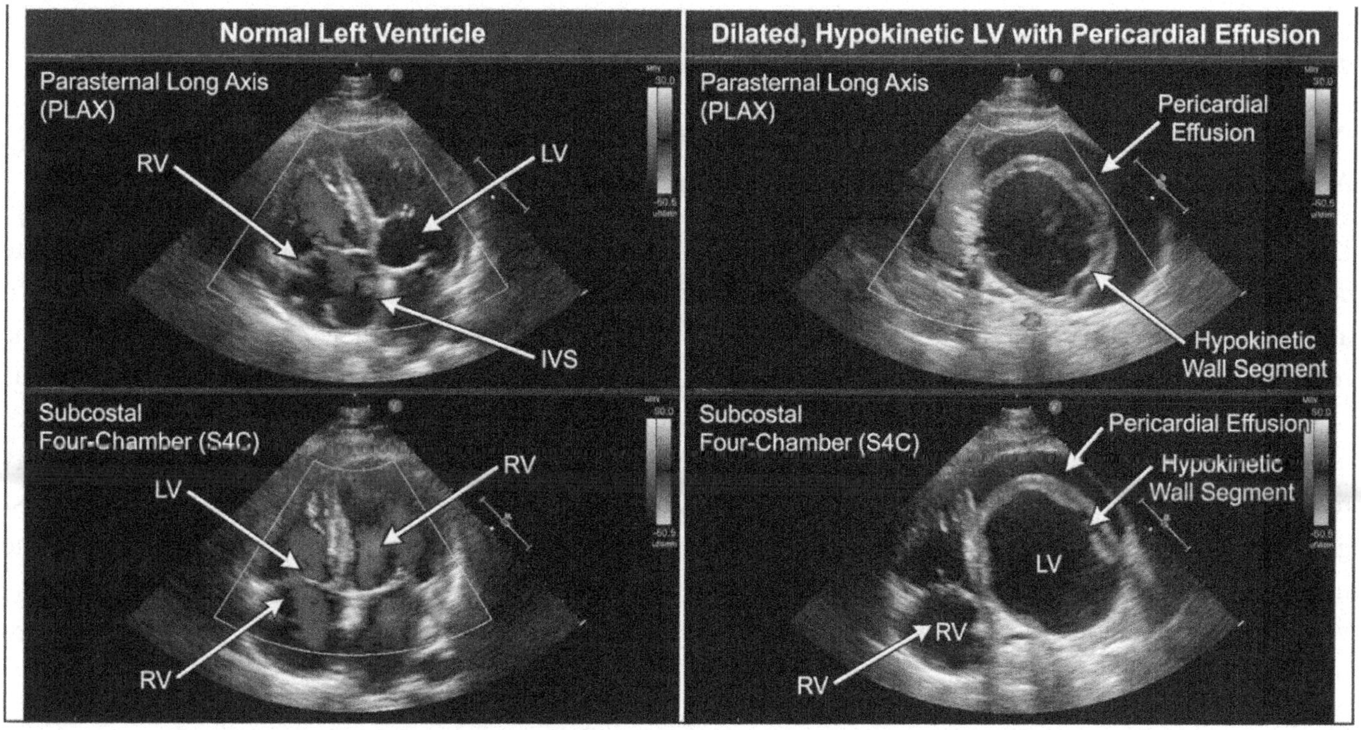


Figure 6.2: Point-of-Care Cardiac Ultrasound Views for Undifferentiated Shock in Transit

## THE IN-TRANSIT DETERIORATION SIGNATURE SYSTEM — Altitude-Exacerbated Myocardial Ischemia

**The Signature:** New or worsening electrocardiographic ischemic changes, chest pain, or hemodynamic instability that develop during ascent or at altitude in a patient with an acute coronary syndrome, in the absence of any change in antiplatelet or anticoagulant therapy.

**Movement Trigger:** The reduction in alveolar oxygen tension at altitude described in Chapter 1 produces a decrease in arterial oxygen content that, in a patient with an already compromised coronary blood flow from an acute plaque event, can tip the myocardial oxygen supply-demand balance toward ischemia at a threshold that would not have been crossed at sea level.

**Early Tell:** New ST-segment changes, a subtle worsening of existing ST deviation, or recurrence of chest pain temporally linked to the onset of climb or arrival at cruise altitude, detected through the serial electrocardiographic monitoring described earlier in this chapter.

**Trap Logic:** This pattern is easily attributed to natural disease progression rather than recognized as an altitude-potentiated event, because the electrocardiographic and symptomatic changes look identical to primary plaque instability. The discriminating feature is the temporal relationship to altitude change, which is the clinician's cue to consider cabin altitude restriction, increased supplemental oxygen, or descent as a therapeutic maneuver rather than solely escalating pharmacologic therapy.

**Signature Anchor:** In any patient with an active acute coronary syndrome transported by air, treat new ischemic changes temporally linked to ascent as a supply-demand mismatch exacerbated by altitude and respond with supplemental oxygen optimization and, where feasible, a request for lower cabin altitude or descent, in addition to standard anti-ischemic therapy.

## Antiplatelet, Anticoagulant, and Thrombolytic Considerations in Transit

### Antiplatelet Loading and Anticoagulation Timing

Dual antiplatelet therapy with aspirin and a P2Y12 receptor inhibitor is the standard of care for acute coronary syndromes, and the timing of loading doses relative to the transport window carries both benefit and risk considerations that the transport clinician must actively manage rather than defer entirely to the receiving facility. Aspirin should have been administered at the sending facility and confirmed by the transport crew during the inherited-workup verification described in Chapter 2. The P2Y12 inhibitor loading dose timing is more nuanced: loading before transport accelerates platelet inhibition and may reduce ischemic events during transit, but in a patient who may require emergent coronary artery bypass grafting rather than percutaneous intervention, early P2Y12 loading increases surgical bleeding risk and may delay the surgical option. The transport crew should confirm with the receiving interventional team, via the communication systems described in Chapter 5, whether pre-transport P2Y12 loading is desired or should be deferred to arrival.

### Thrombolytic Therapy in Transport

Prehospital or in-transport thrombolytic administration for ST-elevation myocardial infarction is a consideration when primary percutaneous coronary intervention is not available within guideline-recommended time windows, and the decision to administer a thrombolytic during transport involves weighing the time saved against the risks of bleeding complications in an environment where surgical rescue is unavailable. This decision should be made in consultation with medical control and with explicit verification of contraindications--recent surgery, active bleeding, history of hemorrhagic stroke, uncontrolled hypertension--before administration, and the crew must be prepared to manage the most serious complication, intracranial hemorrhage, with the limited resources available in transit.

| Contraindication Category | Specific Contraindication | Transport Implication |
|---|---|---|
| Absolute | Active internal bleeding (excluding menses) | Do not administer; prioritize rapid transport to PCI-capable facility |
| Absolute | History of hemorrhagic stroke at any time | Do not administer; document and communicate clearly to receiving team |
| Absolute | Intracranial neoplasm, AVM, or aneurysm | Do not administer; confirm with sending facility records |
| Relative | Severe uncontrolled hypertension (>180/110) | Treat hypertension first; reassess; if persistent, weigh risk-benefit carefully |

| | | |
|---|---|---|
| Relative | Major surgery or trauma within preceding 3 weeks | Weigh time-to-PCI against bleeding risk; consult medical control |
| Relative | Active peptic ulcer disease | Weigh risk-benefit; prepare for possible GI hemorrhage if administered |

**Right Ventricular Infarction Recognition and Volume-Sensitive Management**

Right ventricular infarction, typically accompanying inferior ST-elevation myocardial infarction, presents a transport management challenge that is the hemodynamic mirror image of left-sided cardiogenic shock: the failing right ventricle is preload-dependent, and the standard treatment is judicious volume administration rather than the volume restriction appropriate for left-sided pump failure. The transport clinician must actively screen for right ventricular involvement in any inferior myocardial infarction by obtaining right-sided precordial leads and assessing for the clinical triad of hypotension, clear lung fields, and elevated jugular venous pressure, since the management of right-sided failure--volume loading, avoidance of preload-reducing agents such as nitroglycerin and diuretics, and maintenance of atrioventricular synchrony--is directly opposite to the management of left-sided cardiogenic shock and applying the wrong strategy in the wrong direction will reliably worsen the patient.

**CAUTION:** Nitroglycerin administration in a patient with unrecognized right ventricular infarction can produce catastrophic, refractory hypotension by reducing the preload the failing right ventricle depends on; always screen for right ventricular involvement before administering nitroglycerin in any inferior STEMI.

## Percutaneous Coronary Intervention-Bound Transfer Priorities

**Minimizing Door-to-Balloon Time Through Transport Efficiency**

The transport team's contribution to overall door-to-balloon time is the interval between arrival at the sending facility and delivery of the patient to the receiving facility's catheterization laboratory, and every minute consumed by unnecessary delays at either end of the transport directly erodes the clinical benefit of the transfer. The most impactful time-saving measures are not speed-related but process-related: advance activation of the receiving catheterization laboratory based on the transport team's independent electrocardiographic interpretation, bypass of the receiving emergency department when a direct-to-lab pathway is available, and pre-departure completion of all consent, laboratory, and documentation requirements that would otherwise consume time at the receiving end.

**Communication With the Receiving Interventional Team**

Direct, real-time communication with the receiving interventional cardiologist during transport allows the transport team to transmit the electrocardiogram for remote review, receive guidance on antiplatelet and anticoagulant timing, confirm the direct-to-lab pathway, and provide an accurate estimated time of arrival that allows the catheterization team to be gowned and ready rather than summoned on arrival. This communication, facilitated by the systems described in Chapter 5, transforms the transport from a passive conveyance into an active extension of the receiving team's pre-procedural preparation.

## Post-Cardiac Arrest Care During Interfacility Transport

### Targeted Temperature Management Initiation and Maintenance

Post-cardiac arrest patients transferred for coronary intervention or advanced care may require initiation or maintenance of targeted temperature management during transport, which introduces specific logistical requirements: a cooling device or protocol (surface cooling with ice packs and cold saline, or a portable cooling device where available), continuous temperature monitoring, and sedation and paralysis sufficient to prevent shivering, which both generates heat and increases metabolic demand. The transport clinician should confirm the target temperature range and the timeline for achieving it with the receiving team before departure, since different institutions follow different protocols regarding target temperature and the speed of induction.

### Hemodynamic Optimization and Neuroprognostication Considerations

Post-cardiac arrest hemodynamic management during transport prioritizes maintaining adequate mean arterial pressure and cardiac output to support cerebral and end-organ perfusion, using the vasoactive framework from Chapter 4, while avoiding both hypotension and excessive hypertension. The transport clinician should document the neurologic examination performed at departure and repeat it at scheduled intervals, using the same trend-based framework from Chapter 2, since the neurologic trajectory observed during transport provides the receiving team with early prognostic information that a single arrival examination cannot supply.

Consider a fifty-eight-year-old man with an anterior ST-elevation myocardial infarction at a community hospital without catheterization capability, transferred by rotor-wing for primary percutaneous coronary intervention. The transport crew independently confirms anterolateral ST elevation on a repeat 12-lead, activates the receiving catheterization laboratory by direct communication during the flight, administers aspirin and heparin confirmed with the receiving interventional cardiologist, and withholds P2Y12 loading per the cardiologist's preference given concern for possible left main disease that might require surgical revascularization. During the twenty-five minute flight, the crew monitors serial rhythm strips and notes the development of an accelerated idioventricular rhythm consistent with reperfusion, which they document and communicate in real time. On arrival, the patient is delivered directly to the catheterization laboratory, bypassing the emergency department, with a total transport-related interval of thirty-eight minutes from sending facility departure to sheath insertion. The case illustrates that the transport team's contribution to door-to-balloon time operates primarily through process efficiency, advance activation, and real-time communication rather than through transport speed alone.

**KEY POINT:** Advance catheterization laboratory activation based on the transport team's own ECG interpretation, not deferred to arrival, is the single most impactful action the transport crew can take to reduce door-to-balloon time for STEMI transfers.

A second case illustrates the hemodynamic phenotyping challenge: a seventy-two-year-old woman with an inferior STEMI complicated by hypotension and bradycardia is initially managed with a norepinephrine infusion at the sending facility on the assumption that she is in cardiogenic shock. The transport crew, performing their own assessment, notes clear lung fields, elevated jugular venous pressure, and a right-sided ECG confirming ST elevation in V4R, consistent with right ventricular infarction rather than left-sided pump failure. Recognizing that the hemodynamic phenotype is preload-dependent right heart failure rather than vasodilatory or contractile left heart failure, the crew initiates a cautious fluid challenge, observes a prompt improvement in blood pressure and heart rate, and begins weaning the norepinephrine that was counterproductive in this specific hemodynamic context. This case demonstrates that the same vital sign abnormality--hypotension--requires entirely different management depending on the underlying hemodynamic phenotype, and that the transport clinician's independent assessment, applying the phenotyping framework from this chapter, can identify and correct a management mismatch inherited from the sending facility.

## Advanced Coronary Syndrome Management in Transport

### Killip Classification and Its Transport Application

The Killip classification stratifies acute myocardial infarction patients by the degree of heart failure present at presentation: Class I (no heart failure), Class II (mild heart failure with rales in the lower lung fields), Class III (frank pulmonary edema), and Class IV (cardiogenic shock). The transport clinician should assign a Killip class at departure and monitor for progression during transport, since upward movement through the Killip classes represents a worsening trajectory that should be communicated to the receiving team and that may change the urgency of the receiving facility's response. A patient who departs as Killip II and arrives as Killip III has developed new pulmonary edema during transport, a trajectory change that the receiving team needs to know about to adjust their initial management posture.

### Complicated STEMI: Mechanical Complications in Transit

Mechanical complications of acute myocardial infarction--ventricular septal rupture, papillary muscle rupture with acute mitral regurgitation, and free wall rupture with tamponade--are rare but catastrophic, and the transport clinician's ability to suspect these complications based on clinical findings is the critical link between a patient who arrives at the receiving facility with a provisional diagnosis and a prepared surgical team versus one who arrives with undifferentiated cardiogenic shock and a team that must diagnose the complication from scratch. A new, loud systolic murmur in a patient with worsening cardiogenic shock after myocardial infarction should raise immediate suspicion for ventricular septal rupture or acute mitral regurgitation; a sudden loss of pulse pressure with distended neck veins and muffled heart sounds should raise suspicion for tamponade from free wall rupture. Point-of-care ultrasound, if available and the clinician is trained, can provide immediate bedside confirmation of these mechanical complications during transport.

## Reperfusion Arrhythmias and Their Transport Management

Patients who receive thrombolytic therapy before or during transport, or who undergo spontaneous reperfusion, frequently develop reperfusion arrhythmias--most commonly accelerated idioventricular rhythm, which is a wide-complex rhythm at a rate of sixty to one hundred beats per minute that represents restored conduction through previously ischemic tissue rather than a malignant arrhythmia. The transport clinician must distinguish accelerated idioventricular rhythm from ventricular tachycardia, since the former is generally benign and self-limited (requiring only monitoring) while the latter requires antiarrhythmic therapy or cardioversion. The distinguishing features are rate (AIVR is typically below one hundred; VT is typically above one hundred twenty), hemodynamic stability (AIVR almost always maintains adequate perfusion), and temporal relationship to reperfusion therapy (AIVR typically appears within minutes to hours of thrombolytic administration or symptom improvement, while VT from ongoing ischemia typically appears without a reperfusion context).

## Anticoagulation Management in the ACS Transport Patient

Anticoagulation for acute coronary syndromes during transport typically involves unfractionated heparin administered as a weight-based bolus followed by a continuous infusion, with the specific dosing protocol determined by the receiving facility's preference and the planned intervention (PCI versus medical management). The transport clinician should confirm the specific heparin dose and protocol with the receiving interventional team whenever communication allows, since different catheterization laboratories use different heparin dosing strategies, and a patient who arrives with a subtherapeutic or supratherapeutic heparin level may require dose adjustment that delays the procedure. The infusion transition principles from Chapter 4 apply directly, with the additional consideration that the activated clotting time or aPTT at the time of arrival directly affects the procedural anticoagulation strategy.

## Glycoprotein IIb/IIIa Inhibitor Considerations

Glycoprotein IIb/IIIa inhibitors (abciximab, eptifibatide, tirofiban) may be initiated at the sending facility or during transport for high-risk non-ST-elevation acute coronary syndromes or as part of a facilitated PCI strategy, and the transport clinician should confirm the specific agent, dose, and timing of initiation, since these agents significantly increase bleeding risk and the receiving team must know exactly what antiplatelet and anticoagulant agents have been administered to plan their procedural approach. The transport clinician should monitor for signs of bleeding, particularly at vascular access sites, and should have the ability to discontinue the infusion if clinically significant bleeding develops during transport, recognizing that the platelet inhibition from abciximab persists for hours after discontinuation while the shorter-acting agents (eptifibatide, tirofiban) reverse more rapidly.

## Additional Clinical Considerations for Transport Management

The management of patients in Chapter 6 requires attention to several additional transport-specific clinical factors that extend the principles established in the main body of the chapter. The transport clinician should be aware that the disease processes covered here interact with the transport environment in ways that are specific to the combination of the underlying pathophysiology and the particular environmental stressor encountered during a given mission, and that a management approach that is adequate for a short ground transport may be insufficient for a longer air transport at altitude, or vice versa. The serial reassessment protocol established in Chapter 2 provides the framework for detecting these interactions as they develop, and the Deterioration Signature introduced in this chapter names the most characteristic pattern by which they declare themselves.

Each patient transport is a unique combination of a specific patient's physiology, a specific set of ongoing therapies, a specific transport platform with its own environmental characteristics, and a specific mission profile with its own altitude, duration, and route constraints. The anticipatory approach to transport medicine that this text teaches is not a set of memorized responses to predetermined scenarios but a cognitive framework for analyzing the specific combination of variables present in any given transport and identifying, before departure, the most likely points of vulnerability where the transport environment will test the patient's physiologic reserve. This chapter's clinical content provides the disease-specific knowledge needed to apply that framework to the conditions covered here, while the Deterioration Signature provides the named pattern that makes the most characteristic transport-specific vulnerability explicit, recognizable, and actionable.

The receiving team's ability to continue the patient's care seamlessly after the transport crew departs depends entirely on the quality and completeness of the clinical information the transport crew provides, and for the conditions covered in this chapter, the specific information that matters most includes: the trajectory of the patient's primary condition during transport (improving, stable, or worsening, with specific details), any interventions performed during transport and their response, any new clinical findings identified by the transport crew that were not present at the sending facility, and any anticipated needs that the receiving team should prepare for based on the transport crew's clinical assessment. This information, communicated through the structured handoff format established in Chapter 2 and supplemented by the trajectory communication emphasis that is a recurring theme throughout this text, is the final clinical act of the transport and the one that determines whether the transport adds value to the patient's care continuum or merely moves the patient from one location to another without preserving the clinical narrative that only the transport crew was positioned to observe.

The transport clinician managing the conditions addressed in this chapter should develop a systematic pre-departure assessment that specifically identifies the highest-risk transport-environment interaction for each patient's specific disease process, the monitoring parameters that will detect that interaction earliest, and the intervention that will address it most effectively. This pre-departure risk analysis, adapted from the general pre-mission physiologic risk profile introduced in Chapter 1, should be specific enough to generate a concrete prediction: what is the single most likely way this specific patient's condition will interact with the specific transport environment of this specific mission? Answering that question before departure, rather than discovering the answer during transit, is the practical application of the anticipatory transport medicine framework that this entire text is designed to develop.

Clinical case presentations embedded throughout this chapter illustrate the principle that transport-specific deterioration patterns are predictable rather than random, recognizable rather than mysterious, and preventable rather than inevitable, provided the clinician applies the systematic assessment, continuous monitoring, and named-pattern recognition framework that the Deterioration Signature System codifies. Each case demonstrates the same three-part sequence: a patient with a specific disease process encounters a specific transport-environment stressor, produces a specific clinical change that could be attributed to either the disease or the environment, and is correctly managed because the transport clinician recognized the specific named Signature and applied the correct transport-specific intervention rather than the generic disease-specific response that would have been appropriate at the bedside but is insufficient or incorrect in the transport context.

The evidence base for transport-specific management of the conditions in this chapter continues to evolve, with ongoing research into optimal monitoring strategies, transport-adapted treatment protocols, and outcome data that will refine the recommendations presented here. The transport clinician should maintain awareness of emerging evidence through continuing education, program-sponsored journal clubs, and the quality improvement processes described in Chapter 24, since the standard of care for transport medicine is not static and the recommendations in any textbook represent a snapshot of evidence at the time of writing rather than a permanent standard. The principles, however, are durable: anticipate rather than react, monitor trends rather than thresholds, communicate trajectories rather than snapshots, and recognize that the transport environment is a clinical variable that acts on every patient's physiology, not a neutral conduit between two points of care.

Finally, the transport clinician should recognize that the clinical expertise required to manage these conditions during transport represents a distinct competency that builds on but extends beyond the bedside critical care training that most transport clinicians bring to their role. A clinician who is expert in managing these conditions in the intensive care unit is not automatically expert in managing them during transport, because the environmental, equipment, monitoring, and resource constraints of transport introduce variables that bedside practice never encounters. Conversely, a transport clinician who has mastered the anticipatory, environment-aware management approach described in this text brings a perspective to patient care that the bedside clinician lacks: the ability to see the patient's physiology not as a fixed state being managed in a controlled environment, but as a dynamic process interacting continuously with an environment that is itself changing throughout the transport. This dual awareness--of the disease and of the environment acting on it--is the defining competency of transport critical care medicine, and it is what this text, from its first chapter through its last, is designed to develop.

The clinical scenarios addressed in this chapter illustrate a principle that recurs throughout the text: the transport environment does not merely add logistic complexity to the management of critical illness--it introduces specific physiologic stressors that interact with the patient's underlying condition to produce clinical changes that would not occur at the bedside. The altitude-related gas expansion, preload shifts, oxygenation challenges, and monitoring degradation described in Chapter 1, combined with the pharmacologic and equipment considerations from Chapters 4 and 5, create a modified clinical environment in which every bedside management principle must be re-examined through the lens of transport-specific risk. The disease-specific management recommendations in this chapter have been written with this re-examination already performed, incorporating the transport modifications into the clinical recommendations rather than presenting bedside management followed by a separate list of transport considerations, because the integration of disease knowledge and transport awareness is the competency that this text is designed to develop.

Inter-professional collaboration during the management of the conditions in this chapter deserves specific emphasis, because the complexity of many transport patients exceeds the capability of any single clinician acting alone. The nurse-paramedic team, the nurse-physician team, or whatever crew configuration the program uses represents a collaborative unit whose combined clinical capability exceeds the sum of its individual members, provided that the communication, role allocation, and shared mental model practices described in Chapter 24 are actively maintained throughout the transport. A transport in which one crew member manages the airway while the other manages hemodynamics, with both monitoring different aspects of the same clinical picture and cross-checking each other's assessments, produces a more complete and reliable clinical picture than either clinician could achieve alone, and this collaborative advantage is greatest during the high-workload, high-stress scenarios that the conditions in this chapter frequently produce.

Quality improvement in the management of these conditions during transport depends on systematic outcome tracking that links transport-specific management decisions to patient outcomes at the receiving facility. Did the patient who received a specific intervention during transport have a better or worse outcome than comparable patients who did not? Did a specific monitoring strategy detect deterioration earlier and allow more effective intervention? Did advance communication with the receiving facility produce measurably faster time-to-treatment on arrival? These questions can only be answered by programs that collect and analyze outcome data systematically, and the transport clinician's contribution to this process is meticulous, contemporaneous documentation of every clinical decision, every intervention, and every trajectory observation during the transport, since this documentation is the raw material from which quality improvement insights are derived. A transport program that does not analyze its outcomes cannot improve them, and a transport clinician who does not document their clinical reasoning cannot contribute to the program's learning.

**THE IN-TRANSIT DETERIORATION SIGNATURE SYSTEM — Coronary Ischemia Patterns During Transport**

**Signature Introduced This Chapter:** Altitude-Exacerbated Myocardial Ischemia (new or worsening ischemic changes temporally linked to ascent or altitude in a patient with an active acute coronary syndrome).

**Coronary Pattern Logic:** This Signature connects the altitude-physiology foundation from Chapter 1 (Dalton's law and reduced alveolar oxygen tension) to the specific clinical consequence of reduced myocardial oxygen supply in a patient with fixed coronary flow limitation, illustrating how the same environmental stressor produces different clinical presentations depending on the underlying disease process.

**Cross-Reference Forward:** Chapter 7 (Heart Failure and Hemodynamic Instability) extends the hemodynamic management principles to decompensated heart failure without acute coronary occlusion; Chapter 9 (Mechanical Circulatory Support Devices) addresses device-supported transport for refractory cardiogenic shock.

## Summary and Key Concepts

Independent ECG interpretation by the transport team, including recognition of ST-elevation equivalents, directly determines catheterization laboratory activation timing and receiving facility preparedness.

Cardiogenic shock phenotyping guides vasoactive strategy: norepinephrine for vasodilatory predominance, dobutamine or epinephrine for contractile failure, with point-of-care ultrasound to distinguish the phenotype.

P2Y12 inhibitor loading timing should be explicitly coordinated with the receiving interventional team, since early loading benefits percutaneous intervention but increases surgical bleeding risk.

Altitude-mediated reduction in arterial oxygen content can exacerbate myocardial ischemia in patients with fixed coronary lesions, making cabin altitude restriction a therapeutic maneuver in addition to pharmacologic anti-ischemic therapy.

Process efficiency, advance laboratory activation, and real-time communication with the receiving team contribute more to door-to-balloon time reduction than transport speed.

# CHAPTER 7: HEART FAILURE AND HEMODYNAMIC INSTABILITY IN TRANSIT

**Learning Objectives**

1. Recognize acute decompensated heart failure and differentiate it from other causes of respiratory distress and hypotension encountered during transport.
2. Titrate vasoactive and inotropic infusions for hemodynamic support using continuous arterial and central venous pressure monitoring.
3. Assess fluid responsiveness in the transport environment and apply it to guide volume management decisions.
4. Identify right ventricular failure and pulmonary hypertension as distinct hemodynamic entities requiring specific management approaches.
5. Manage hypertensive emergencies during transport with organ-specific blood pressure targets.

**Chapter Outline**

This chapter extends the cardiovascular framework from Chapter 6 to the broader population of patients with hemodynamic instability from heart failure and hypertensive crises, conditions that are among the most common reasons for critical care interfacility transport and that require continuous vasoactive titration throughout the transport window. Where Chapter 6 focused on the time-sensitive, reperfusion-driven management of acute coronary syndromes, this chapter addresses the hemodynamic stabilization and optimization challenge that defines heart failure transport.

## Acute Decompensated Heart Failure Management

### Clinical Presentation and Severity Stratification

Acute decompensated heart failure presents along a severity spectrum that ranges from isolated dyspnea with preserved blood pressure to frank cardiogenic shock with multi-organ hypoperfusion, and the transport clinician's initial task is to place the specific patient on this spectrum using the rapid assessment framework from Chapter 2, since the position on the spectrum determines both the monitoring intensity required and the vasoactive strategy applied during transit. A patient with pulmonary edema and a preserved or elevated blood pressure represents a predominantly congestive, afterload-mismatch phenotype amenable to vasodilator therapy, while the same degree of pulmonary edema in a hypotensive patient represents a low-output state requiring inotropic support and cautious diuresis, a distinction that carries directly opposite management implications.

### Diuretic Therapy and Volume Removal During Transport

Intravenous loop diuretic therapy initiated at the sending facility or during transport requires attention to urine output monitoring and electrolyte surveillance that is more challenging in the transport environment than at the bedside. The transport clinician should confirm urinary catheter placement and function before departure for any patient receiving aggressive diuretic therapy, since monitoring urine output by volume over fixed intervals is the most direct measure of diuretic response, and an obstructed or malpositioned catheter can falsely suggest diuretic resistance. Potassium and magnesium supplementation protocols should be established before departure, since diuretic-induced hypokalemia and hypomagnesemia predispose to arrhythmias in a patient population already at heightened rhythm risk.

**Noninvasive Positive Pressure Ventilation for Acute Pulmonary Edema**

Continuous positive airway pressure or bilevel positive airway pressure ventilation is a first-line treatment for acute cardiogenic pulmonary edema with preserved respiratory effort, and its transport-specific considerations include device compatibility with the transport ventilator platform, mask fit and tolerance in a patient who may be sitting at an unusual angle on a transport stretcher, and the crew's readiness to escalate to intubation if noninvasive ventilation fails to produce clinical improvement within a defined trial period. A noninvasive ventilation trial should not be initiated during the loading or climb phase of a flight, when the additive physiologic stress of altitude and acceleration makes it difficult to distinguish device failure from environmental worsening, but rather established and confirmed effective at the sending bedside before departure.

| Heart Failure Phenotype | Blood Pressure | Perfusion Status | Primary Transport Strategy |
|---|---|---|---|
| Wet-warm (congestion, preserved perfusion) | Normal or elevated | Adequate | Vasodilator + diuretic; noninvasive ventilation if hypoxemic |
| Wet-cold (congestion + hypoperfusion) | Low or borderline | Impaired | Inotrope + cautious diuresis; invasive monitoring strongly recommended |
| Dry-cold (hypoperfusion without congestion) | Low | Impaired | Cautious volume trial + inotrope; assess for RV failure |
| Hypertensive emergency with flash pulmonary edema | Severely elevated | Variable | Aggressive afterload reduction; noninvasive ventilation |

## Vasoactive and Inotropic Infusion Titration

### Matching the Vasoactive Agent to the Hemodynamic Phenotype

The vasoactive agent framework developed in Chapter 4 applies directly to heart failure management, with the critical transport-specific consideration that the hemodynamic phenotype may shift during transit as the patient responds (or fails to respond) to initial therapy, as altitude and positional changes alter preload and afterload, and as the underlying disease process evolves. A patient who departs the sending facility on a stable low-dose dobutamine drip for mild inotropic augmentation may require norepinephrine addition if blood pressure deteriorates during climb, or may conversely tolerate dobutamine weaning if afterload reduction and diuresis improve the hemodynamic profile during the transport window. The crew must monitor continuously and titrate to the patient's current hemodynamic state rather than a static dosing plan established at departure.

### Titration Endpoints and Monitoring Targets

The titration endpoint for vasoactive therapy in heart failure transport is not a single numeric target but a physiologic goal: adequate end-organ perfusion--assessed by mentation, urine output trend, and lactate clearance where point-of-care testing is available--at the lowest vasoactive support level achievable without hemodynamic compromise. Mean arterial pressure is a necessary but insufficient surrogate for perfusion, and the transport clinician should resist the temptation to fixate on a pressure number while ignoring the clinical perfusion assessment that determines whether the achieved pressure is actually translating into tissue oxygen delivery.

### Milrinone and Dobutamine Titration Considerations for Transport

Milrinone, favored for its combined inotropic and lusitropic (diastolic relaxation-enhancing) properties in heart failure, presents a specific transport challenge: its long half-life of two to three hours means that dose adjustments made during transport will not reach their full hemodynamic effect until well after the current transport window has ended, making milrinone a poor choice for reactive titration during a short flight but a reasonable choice for maintenance during a longer ground transport where a steady-state infusion established at the sending facility can be continued at a stable rate. Dobutamine, with its shorter half-life and more immediate dose-response relationship, is better suited to the titration flexibility required during the dynamic hemodynamic conditions of flight, though its vasodilatory beta-2 effect may necessitate concurrent norepinephrine to maintain adequate blood pressure, a dual-infusion strategy that is manageable but increases the complexity of line management and pump monitoring.

### Vasodilator Therapy for Congestion-Predominant Presentations

Nitroglycerin and nitroprusside provide afterload and preload reduction that directly targets the congestive component of acute heart failure, and in the patient with a preserved or elevated blood pressure, vasodilator therapy is often more effective than diuresis alone in producing rapid symptomatic improvement. Nitroglycerin is generally preferred in the transport setting for its more predictable dose-response and shorter half-life, while nitroprusside's potent arterial vasodilation produces more dramatic blood pressure reduction but carries a risk of cyanide accumulation with prolonged infusions and requires particularly close blood pressure monitoring that may strain the crew's attention during a complex transport. The transport clinician should be prepared for reflex tachycardia as afterload falls, and should have a clear plan for the common scenario in which vasodilator-mediated blood pressure reduction that was therapeutically desirable at the start of transport crosses into hemodynamically concerning territory as the patient's volume status shifts with diuresis during the transport window.

### Transition to Mechanical Circulatory Support: When to Escalate

When pharmacologic support fails to produce adequate hemodynamic stabilization--persistent hypotension despite escalating vasoactive and inotropic therapy, worsening end-organ perfusion markers, or a rising lactate trend despite maximal medical therapy--the transport clinician must recognize the threshold at which the patient has transitioned from pharmacologically manageable heart failure to refractory cardiogenic shock requiring mechanical circulatory support. This recognition is itself a clinical action, even when the mechanical support cannot be initiated during transport, because communicating this trajectory to the receiving facility in real time allows the receiving team to mobilize mechanical support resources--percutaneous ventricular assist device, intra-aortic balloon pump, or extracorporeal membrane oxygenation--before the patient's arrival rather than after, converting a reactive insertion into a proactive one that begins minutes earlier. Chapter 9 addresses the transport of patients already on mechanical support in detail.

**Figure 7.1:** Arterial and Central Venous Waveform Assessment of Volume Status

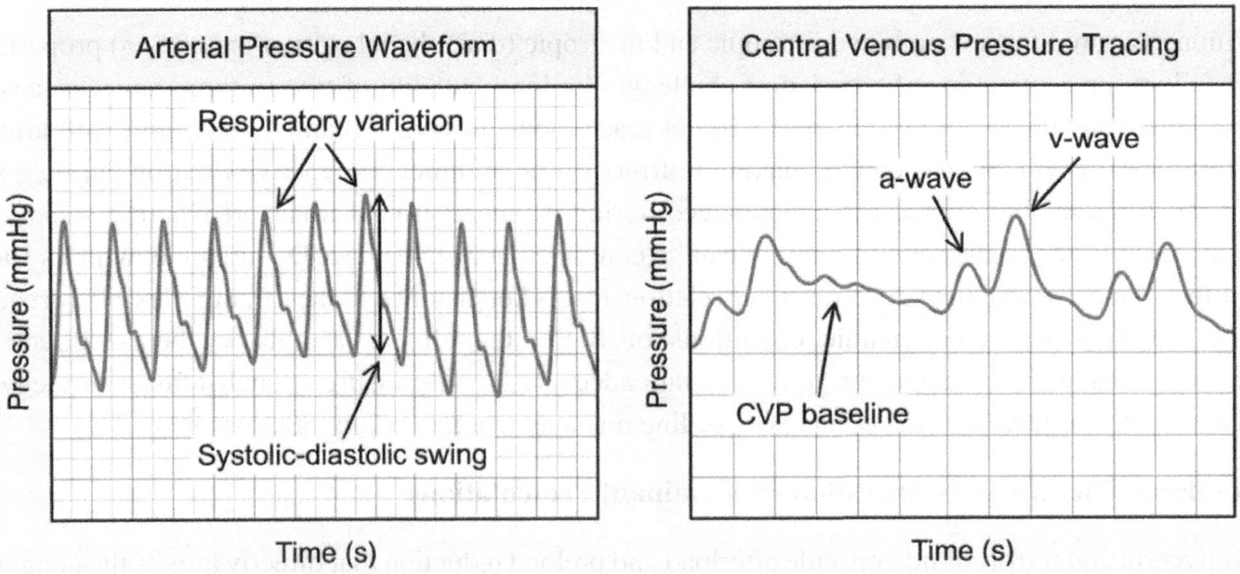

## Figure 7.2: Passive Leg Raise Test for Fluid Responsiveness Assessment.

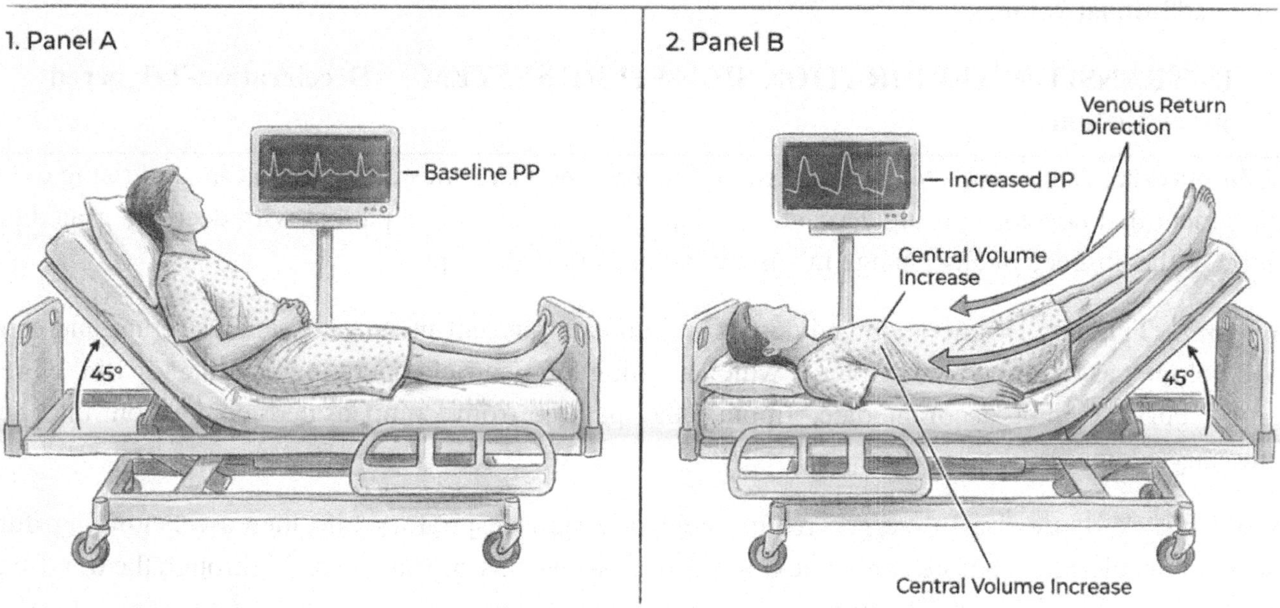


**Figure 7.2:** Passive Leg Raise Test for Fluid Responsiveness Assessment

## Fluid Responsiveness Assessment in the Transport Environment

### Dynamic Versus Static Indicators of Preload

Static measures of preload--central venous pressure and pulmonary artery occlusion pressure--have poor predictive value for volume responsiveness in the general critically ill population and are further degraded by the respiratory physiology variations introduced by positive pressure ventilation, spontaneous breathing effort, and the altitude-related intrathoracic pressure shifts described in Chapter 1. Dynamic measures of fluid responsiveness, including pulse pressure variation and stroke volume variation derived from the arterial waveform during controlled mechanical ventilation, provide substantially better prediction of whether a given patient will improve cardiac output in response to volume administration, and are measurable in the transport environment using the continuous arterial pressure monitoring recommended in Chapter 2.

### Passive Leg Raise as a Transport-Adapted Volume Assessment

Passive leg raise, which mimics the hemodynamic effect of a volume bolus by autotransfusing approximately three hundred milliliters of blood from the lower extremities into the central circulation, is a reversible, repeatable test of volume responsiveness that is particularly well suited to the transport environment because it does not require actual fluid administration and its hemodynamic effect can be assessed using the continuous arterial monitoring already in place. The test requires the clinician to observe the hemodynamic response--a rise in pulse pressure, cardiac output, or stroke volume variation--during the leg-raise maneuver and reverse the maneuver if no response is observed, avoiding the commitment of irreversible fluid administration in a patient whose hemodynamic phenotype may not tolerate additional volume.

**THE IN-TRANSIT DETERIORATION SIGNATURE SYSTEM — Deceleration-Triggered Pulmonary Edema**

**The Signature:** Acute worsening of respiratory distress, new crackles on auscultation, and rising oxygen requirement that develops during descent, deceleration, or landing in a patient with decompensated heart failure, in the absence of any change in vasoactive or diuretic therapy.

**Movement Trigger:** Deceleration and descent produce a transient increase in venous return and central blood volume, as described in Chapter 1, which a failing left ventricle operating near the top of the Frank-Starling curve cannot accommodate, tipping the patient from compensated congestion into acute pulmonary edema.

**Early Tell:** A subtle rise in oxygen requirement or a new respiratory rate increase beginning during descent or deceleration, before overt crackles or frothy secretions appear, detected through the trend-based monitoring framework from Chapter 2.

**Trap Logic:** This pattern is easily attributed to general disease progression or to the stress of the transport itself rather than recognized as a specific physiologic event triggered by the hemodynamic shift of deceleration. The discriminating feature is the temporal relationship to the descent or deceleration phase, which is the cue to apply afterload reduction and consider diuretic augmentation rather than simply increasing oxygen delivery.

**Signature Anchor:** In any patient with decompensated heart failure transported by air, anticipate the possibility of deceleration-triggered pulmonary edema during descent and have vasodilator and diuretic therapy immediately ready to deploy at the first sign of respiratory worsening during the descent phase, rather than waiting for full-blown pulmonary edema to develop before intervening.

## Right Ventricular Failure and Pulmonary Hypertension in Transit

### Recognizing the Right Ventricular Failure Phenotype

Right ventricular failure, whether from acute pulmonary embolism, decompensated pulmonary hypertension, or right-sided involvement in an acute myocardial infarction as discussed in Chapter 6, presents a hemodynamic phenotype that is fundamentally different from left-sided failure and requires a management approach tailored to the right ventricle's specific physiology: preload dependence, afterload sensitivity, and vulnerability to the altitude-related increases in pulmonary vascular resistance that occur with hypoxemia and hypercapnia. The transport clinician who applies the standard left-heart failure management--afterload reduction, diuresis, and fluid restriction--to a patient whose primary problem is right ventricular failure will reliably worsen the hemodynamic picture, because the failing right ventricle depends on adequate preload and cannot tolerate the reduction in pulmonary vascular resistance that left-sided afterload reduction provides only indirectly and often insufficiently.

### Altitude and Hypoxemia Effects on Pulmonary Vascular Resistance

Hypoxic pulmonary vasoconstriction--the physiologic response by which the pulmonary vasculature constricts in poorly ventilated lung regions to redirect blood flow toward better-oxygenated areas--becomes a pathologic stressor during transport at altitude, because the global reduction in alveolar oxygen tension described by Dalton's law in Chapter 1 can provoke diffuse pulmonary vasoconstriction in a patient who already has elevated pulmonary vascular resistance, acutely increasing the afterload against which the failing right ventricle must pump. This is the physiologic basis for maintaining generous oxygenation targets and requesting lower cabin altitudes in patients with known pulmonary hypertension or right ventricular failure, even when the patient's oxygen saturation appears acceptable at the current altitude, because the margin between acceptable saturation and the threshold for clinically significant hypoxic vasoconstriction may be narrower than the numeric display suggests.

### Inhaled Pulmonary Vasodilator Therapy During Transport

Inhaled nitric oxide and inhaled epoprostenol (prostacyclin) provide selective pulmonary vasodilation that reduces right ventricular afterload without producing the systemic hypotension associated with intravenous vasodilators, and are increasingly used in the transport of patients with severe pulmonary hypertension or right ventricular failure. The transport-specific challenge is logistical: inhaled nitric oxide requires a dedicated delivery system, a nitrogen dioxide scavenging mechanism, and continuous monitoring of delivered concentration and methemoglobin levels, all of which add weight, complexity, and battery draw to the transport equipment set. Inhaled epoprostenol can be delivered through a standard nebulizer attached to the ventilator circuit, offering a simpler alternative for programs that do not carry nitric oxide delivery systems, though it requires careful preparation and continuous administration because its effect dissipates rapidly if delivery is interrupted, producing an abrupt rebound increase in pulmonary vascular resistance that can precipitate acute right heart failure.

**CAUTION:** Abrupt interruption of an inhaled pulmonary vasodilator--whether from nebulizer malfunction, tank depletion, or inadvertent circuit disconnection--can produce a severe rebound pulmonary hypertensive crisis within minutes. Before initiating transport with an inhaled pulmonary vasodilator, verify supply duration against transport time and have a contingency plan for unplanned interruption.

| Inhaled Agent | Delivery Mechanism | Key Transport Advantage | Principal Transport Risk |
|---|---|---|---|
| Inhaled nitric oxide | Dedicated delivery system with scavenger | Selective pulmonary vasodilation; no systemic hypotension | Weight, complexity, $NO_2$ monitoring, methemoglobin risk |
| Inhaled epoprostenol | Standard nebulizer in ventilator circuit | Simpler setup; no specialized delivery system needed | Rebound PH crisis if interrupted; requires continuous nebulization |

A second case illustrates the right-sided phenotype: a thirty-one-year-old woman with known idiopathic pulmonary arterial hypertension on chronic inhaled and subcutaneous prostacyclin therapy, transferred by fixed-wing for evaluation of worsening functional class and possible lung transplant listing. During ascent, the crew notes a subtle increase in the patient's oxygen requirement and a new jugular venous distention not present at the sending bedside, consistent with altitude-exacerbated hypoxic pulmonary vasoconstriction superimposed on her baseline elevated pulmonary vascular resistance. The crew immediately optimizes oxygenation to target a saturation above ninety-five percent, requests a lower cabin altitude from the flight crew, and ensures the subcutaneous prostacyclin pump is functioning without interruption. The jugular venous distention resolves and oxygen requirement stabilizes within ten minutes of achieving the lower cabin altitude, confirming that the trigger was environmental rather than primary disease progression. This case reinforces the chapter's core principle: in right ventricular failure and pulmonary hypertension, the transport environment itself--specifically altitude-mediated hypoxia--is a modifiable therapeutic variable, not a fixed background condition, and treating the environment (cabin altitude, oxygenation) is as important as treating the patient.

## Hypertensive Emergencies During Transport

### Organ-Specific Blood Pressure Targets

Hypertensive emergencies requiring transport are defined not merely by the severity of the blood pressure elevation but by the presence of acute end-organ damage--encephalopathy, aortic dissection, acute heart failure with pulmonary edema, acute renal injury, or eclampsia--and the transport management of each involves a different blood pressure reduction target, rate of reduction, and agent selection. The transport clinician should confirm the specific target with the sending and receiving physicians before departure, since overly aggressive blood pressure reduction can precipitate cerebral or renal hypoperfusion that is as dangerous as the hypertension itself, and the target varies by end-organ: aortic dissection requires the most aggressive reduction, to a systolic target typically below one hundred twenty millimeters of mercury, while hypertensive encephalopathy requires a more gradual reduction of no more than twenty-five percent in the first hour to avoid watershed cerebral ischemia.

### Agent Selection for Blood Pressure Reduction in Transit

Nicardipine and clevidipine are titratable intravenous calcium channel blockers that provide smooth, predictable blood pressure reduction without the reflex tachycardia associated with some other vasodilators, and are well suited to the transport environment because their predictable dose-response relationship and short half-life allow the crew to approach the target gradually and hold at the desired level without overshooting. Esmolol, a short-acting beta-blocker, is specifically useful in the aortic dissection population where both heart rate and blood pressure reduction are therapeutic goals, and its rapid offset allows quick recovery if the blood pressure falls below the safe range. Labetalol, with its combined alpha- and beta-blocking properties, provides an alternative with a longer duration of action that may be appropriate for longer transports where the reduced titration frequency is an advantage rather than a limitation.

Consider a forty-five-year-old man transferred by ground critical care ambulance for management of a type B aortic dissection, initially stabilized at the sending facility with a nicardipine infusion targeting a systolic pressure below one hundred twenty. During a sixty-minute transport, the patient's blood pressure trends gradually upward from one hundred fifteen to one hundred thirty-five despite a stable nicardipine rate, and the crew, recognizing the trend rather than waiting for a threshold alarm, incrementally increases the nicardipine rate and adds a short-acting esmolol infusion targeting a heart rate below sixty-five. The blood pressure stabilizes at one hundred twelve, and the patient arrives at the receiving vascular surgery service with both pressure and heart rate within target. The case illustrates that hypertensive emergency management during transport is an active, continuous titration task rather than a set-and-forget infusion, and that the trend-based monitoring discipline from Chapter 2 is essential for detecting upward drift that would otherwise be missed by threshold-based alarm monitoring alone.

## Advanced Heart Failure Hemodynamic Management

### Differentiating Cardiogenic From Distributive Shock by Bedside Assessment

The hemodynamic overlap between cardiogenic and distributive shock can make bedside differentiation challenging, particularly in patients with mixed-etiology shock (such as septic shock with superimposed myocardial depression) where elements of both phenotypes coexist. The transport clinician's bedside assessment tools--point-of-care ultrasound for ventricular function and IVC status, arterial waveform analysis for pulse pressure and stroke volume variation, and clinical perfusion assessment for end-organ adequacy--collectively provide a hemodynamic picture that, while imperfect, is sufficient to guide vasoactive agent selection during the transport window. A hyperdynamic, well-contracting ventricle with a collapsible IVC points toward a distributive etiology requiring vasopressor support; a dilated, hypokinetic ventricle with a plethoric IVC points toward a cardiogenic etiology requiring inotropic support; and mixed findings require a combined approach with close monitoring for the response to each intervention.

### Pulmonary Artery Catheter Data Interpretation During Transport

Patients transferred with pulmonary artery catheters in place provide hemodynamic data--cardiac output, pulmonary artery pressures, pulmonary artery occlusion pressure, and mixed venous oxygen saturation--that directly informs vasoactive management but that must be interpreted with awareness of the transport-specific artifacts that can degrade data quality. Pulmonary artery catheter pressure readings are affected by the same transducer leveling and altitude-related atmospheric pressure changes that affect arterial and central venous pressure readings, and the continuous mixed venous oxygen saturation reading can be affected by catheter migration or wedging that the transport environment's vibration and position changes can produce. The transport clinician should treat pulmonary artery catheter data as a valuable but not infallible data source, verifying its plausibility against the clinical picture and re-zeroing the transducer at the same intervals used for other invasive pressure monitoring.

### Mechanical Support Escalation Criteria During Transport

Recognizing when pharmacologic support has reached its therapeutic ceiling and mechanical circulatory support is needed is a critical transport judgment that requires explicit criteria rather than gestalt. Objective indicators of pharmacologic failure include: a rising lactate despite escalating vasopressor and inotropic support, a falling mixed venous oxygen saturation below a critical threshold despite maximized cardiac output support, progressive multi-organ dysfunction markers (rising creatinine, rising liver enzymes, worsening coagulopathy) despite apparently adequate blood pressure, and a norepinephrine-equivalent dose above a recognized high-dose threshold without hemodynamic improvement. When these criteria are met during transport, the transport clinician's primary action is communication: alerting the receiving facility to mobilize mechanical support resources (IABP, Impella, ECMO) before the patient's arrival, so that the transition from pharmacologic to mechanical support begins minutes earlier.

### Acute Valvular Emergencies in Transport

Acute valvular emergencies--prosthetic valve thrombosis, acute endocarditis with valvular insufficiency, and acute native valve rupture--present during transport as sudden hemodynamic deterioration that may not respond to standard vasoactive therapy because the hemodynamic problem is structural rather than functional. The transport clinician should suspect a valvular etiology when hemodynamic instability is accompanied by a new or changing murmur, when the patient has a prosthetic valve and presents with embolic phenomena, or when the degree of hemodynamic compromise is disproportionate to the patient's volume status and myocardial function. Point-of-care echocardiography can identify gross valvular pathology, prosthetic valve immobility or rocking, and severe valvular regurgitation, though definitive diagnosis requires formal echocardiography at the receiving facility. The management during transport is supportive--hemodynamic optimization with vasoactive agents and volume management--while communicating the suspected diagnosis to the receiving team for surgical or interventional planning.

### Aortic Dissection: Blood Pressure and Heart Rate Dual-Target Management

Acute aortic dissection management during transport focuses on the dual-target reduction of both blood pressure and heart rate to reduce aortic wall shear stress, which is the primary driver of dissection propagation. The target is typically a systolic pressure below one hundred twenty millimeters of mercury and a heart rate below sixty beats per minute, achieved through combined beta-blocker (esmolol infusion for its rapid onset and short half-life, allowing precise titration) and vasodilator therapy (nicardipine or nitroprusside added if blood pressure remains above target after adequate beta-blockade). The sequence matters: beta-blockade must precede vasodilator therapy, because vasodilator-induced reflex tachycardia in the absence of beta-blockade increases aortic wall shear stress and can worsen the dissection. The transport clinician should confirm this sequencing was followed at the sending facility and should maintain both targets continuously throughout transport using the continuous arterial monitoring that is mandatory for any dissection transport.

### Additional Clinical Considerations for Transport Management

The management of patients in Chapter 7 requires attention to several additional transport-specific clinical factors that extend the principles established in the main body of the chapter. The transport clinician should be aware that the disease processes covered here interact with the transport environment in ways that are specific to the combination of the underlying pathophysiology and the particular environmental stressor encountered during a given mission, and that a management approach that is adequate for a short ground transport may be insufficient for a longer air transport at altitude, or vice versa. The serial reassessment protocol established in Chapter 2 provides the framework for detecting these interactions as they develop, and the Deterioration Signature introduced in this chapter names the most characteristic pattern by which they declare themselves.

Each patient transport is a unique combination of a specific patient's physiology, a specific set of ongoing therapies, a specific transport platform with its own environmental characteristics, and a specific mission profile with its own altitude, duration, and route constraints. The anticipatory approach to transport medicine that this text teaches is not a set of memorized responses to predetermined scenarios but a cognitive framework for analyzing the specific combination of variables present in any given transport and identifying, before departure, the most likely points of vulnerability where the transport environment will test the patient's physiologic reserve. This chapter's clinical content provides the disease-specific knowledge needed to apply that framework to the conditions covered here, while the Deterioration Signature provides the named pattern that makes the most characteristic transport-specific vulnerability explicit, recognizable, and actionable.

The receiving team's ability to continue the patient's care seamlessly after the transport crew departs depends entirely on the quality and completeness of the clinical information the transport crew provides, and for the conditions covered in this chapter, the specific information that matters most includes: the trajectory of the patient's primary condition during transport (improving, stable, or worsening, with specific details), any interventions performed during transport and their response, any new clinical findings identified by the transport crew that were not present at the sending facility, and any anticipated needs that the receiving team should prepare for based on the transport crew's clinical assessment. This information, communicated through the structured handoff format established in Chapter 2 and supplemented by the trajectory communication emphasis that is a recurring theme throughout this text, is the final clinical act of the transport and the one that determines whether the transport adds value to the patient's care continuum or merely moves the patient from one location to another without preserving the clinical narrative that only the transport crew was positioned to observe.

The clinical scenarios addressed in this chapter illustrate a principle that recurs throughout the text: the transport environment does not merely add logistic complexity to the management of critical illness--it introduces specific physiologic stressors that interact with the patient's underlying condition to produce clinical changes that would not occur at the bedside. The altitude-related gas expansion, preload shifts, oxygenation challenges, and monitoring degradation described in Chapter 1, combined with the pharmacologic and equipment considerations from Chapters 4 and 5, create a modified clinical environment in which every bedside management principle must be re-examined through the lens of transport-specific risk. The disease-specific management recommendations in this chapter have been written with this re-examination already performed, incorporating the transport modifications into the clinical recommendations rather than presenting bedside management followed by a separate list of transport considerations, because the integration of disease knowledge and transport awareness is the competency that this text is designed to develop.

Inter-professional collaboration during the management of the conditions in this chapter deserves specific emphasis, because the complexity of many transport patients exceeds the capability of any single clinician acting alone. The nurse-paramedic team, the nurse-physician team, or whatever crew configuration the program uses represents a collaborative unit whose combined clinical capability exceeds the sum of its individual members, provided that the communication, role allocation, and shared mental model practices described in Chapter 24 are actively maintained throughout the transport. A transport in which one crew member manages the airway while the other manages hemodynamics, with both monitoring different aspects of the same clinical picture and cross-checking each other's assessments, produces a more complete and reliable clinical picture than either clinician could achieve alone, and this collaborative advantage is greatest during the high-workload, high-stress scenarios that the conditions in this chapter frequently produce.

Quality improvement in the management of these conditions during transport depends on systematic outcome tracking that links transport-specific management decisions to patient outcomes at the receiving facility. Did the patient who received a specific intervention during transport have a better or worse outcome than comparable patients who did not? Did a specific monitoring strategy detect deterioration earlier and allow more effective intervention? Did advance communication with the receiving facility produce measurably faster time-to-treatment on arrival? These questions can only be answered by programs that collect and analyze outcome data systematically, and the transport clinician's contribution to this process is meticulous, contemporaneous documentation of every clinical decision, every intervention, and every trajectory observation during the transport, since this documentation is the raw material from which quality improvement insights are derived. A transport program that does not analyze its outcomes cannot improve them, and a transport clinician who does not document their clinical reasoning cannot contribute to the program's learning.

## THE IN-TRANSIT DETERIORATION SIGNATURE SYSTEM — Heart Failure Hemodynamic Patterns

**Signature Introduced This Chapter:** Deceleration-Triggered Pulmonary Edema (acute worsening of congestive symptoms during descent or deceleration in a patient with decompensated heart failure, driven by a transient increase in venous return that the failing left ventricle cannot accommodate).

**Heart Failure Pattern Logic:** This Signature is the hemodynamic complement of the Ascent-Triggered Device Flow Compromise from Chapter 1: where ascent reduces preload and unmasks preload-dependent problems, descent increases preload and unmasks afterload-intolerant or volume-intolerant problems. Recognizing which phase of flight poses the greater threat for a specific patient's hemodynamic phenotype is the practical takeaway.

**Cross-Reference Forward:** Chapter 9 (Mechanical Circulatory Support Devices) extends the preload-afterload interaction to VAD-supported patients whose flow characteristics respond to these same flight-phase-dependent hemodynamic shifts; Chapter 13 (ARDS) addresses the overlap between cardiogenic and noncardiogenic pulmonary edema differentiation in the transport setting.

## Summary and Key Concepts

Heart failure phenotyping--wet-warm, wet-cold, dry-cold--determines the correct vasoactive, diuretic, and volume strategy for transport; applying the wrong phenotype-specific management reliably worsens the patient.

Dynamic fluid responsiveness assessment, including passive leg raise and pulse pressure variation, provides better volume management guidance in transit than static preload measures.

Right ventricular failure and pulmonary hypertension require a management approach opposite to left-sided failure, with particular attention to the altitude-mediated increase in pulmonary vascular resistance from hypoxic vasoconstriction.

Hypertensive emergency management during transport requires organ-specific blood pressure targets, titratable agents, and continuous trend-based monitoring rather than threshold-based alarms.

Descent and deceleration produce a preload surge that can precipitate acute pulmonary edema in a heart failure patient operating near the top of the Frank-Starling curve, making the descent phase an anticipatable moment of vulnerability.

# CHAPTER 8: ARRHYTHMIAS AND ELECTRICAL EMERGENCIES IN TRANSIT

**Learning Objectives**

1. Recognize and manage tachyarrhythmias requiring emergent intervention during transport.
2. Identify bradyarrhythmias and apply transcutaneous pacing in the transport environment.
3. Perform cardioversion and defibrillation safely in the confined cabin of a vehicle or aircraft.
4. Manage patients with implantable cardiac devices during transport, including troubleshooting inappropriate shocks.
5. Recognize electrolyte-driven arrhythmias and initiate targeted correction during transit.

**Chapter Outline**

This chapter addresses rhythm emergencies as they present in the transport environment, where the confined space, limited backup, and continuous vibration-related artifact challenge both rhythm recognition and intervention. The transport clinician must be independently capable of interpreting rhythm disturbances and initiating definitive electrical or pharmacologic therapy without the immediate support of a cardiologist or electrophysiologist, because the time between rhythm deterioration and hemodynamic collapse in the most dangerous arrhythmias is measured in seconds to minutes, far shorter than any consultation or diversion timeline.

## Tachyarrhythmia Recognition and Management

### Narrow-Complex Tachycardias in Transit

Narrow-complex tachycardias encountered during transport include supraventricular tachycardia, atrial fibrillation with rapid ventricular response, atrial flutter, and sinus tachycardia, and the transport clinician's first task is to distinguish sinus tachycardia--which is a physiologic response to an underlying cause such as pain, hypovolemia, hypoxemia, or fever and should not be treated as a primary rhythm problem--from a primary supraventricular arrhythmia requiring rate or rhythm control. Adenosine remains the first-line diagnostic and therapeutic agent for regular narrow-complex tachycardia of uncertain mechanism, and its ultra-short half-life makes it safe to administer in the transport environment, though the crew should be prepared for the brief period of asystole or marked bradycardia that follows successful termination.

The administration technique for adenosine requires rapid intravenous push followed immediately by a saline flush, ideally through a proximal intravenous site or a central line to ensure that the drug reaches the heart before its ultra-short half-life degrades it in the peripheral circulation. In a transport patient with only a distal peripheral line, the rapid push-flush technique becomes even more critical, since a slow or uncoordinated administration produces subtherapeutic drug delivery and a false impression of adenosine failure. The crew should prepare both the adenosine syringe and a flush syringe on a stopcock assembly before attempting the push, so that the transition from drug to flush is seamless and the full dose is delivered in a single bolus rather than an attenuated drip.

Vagal maneuvers--including the modified Valsalva technique with leg elevation, which has demonstrated superior conversion rates compared to the standard Valsalva maneuver in emergency department studies--should be attempted before adenosine in a hemodynamically stable patient with regular narrow-complex tachycardia, since successful vagal termination avoids the brief but uncomfortable period of asystole that adenosine produces and confirms the re-entrant mechanism without requiring any medication. The modified Valsalva is performed by having the patient strain against a closed glottis for fifteen seconds in a semi-recumbent position, then immediately repositioning the patient supine with passive leg elevation to forty-five degrees for fifteen seconds, a sequence that is feasible even in the confined space of a transport stretcher.

### Wide-Complex Tachycardias and the Default-to-VT Principle

A wide-complex tachycardia should be treated as ventricular tachycardia until proven otherwise, because the consequences of misidentifying ventricular tachycardia as a supraventricular tachycardia with aberrant conduction and treating it with a calcium channel blocker or other AV-nodal blocking agent can be catastrophic--specifically, hemodynamic collapse from inappropriate vasodilation in a rhythm that requires electrical conversion. In the transport environment, where detailed electrophysiologic analysis is unavailable, the default-to-VT principle is a conservative and life-preserving cognitive rule: if the rhythm is wide and fast and the clinician is uncertain, treat it as ventricular tachycardia with synchronized cardioversion if hemodynamically stable or immediate defibrillation if pulseless or hemodynamically unstable.

### Atrial Fibrillation and Flutter Rate Control During Transport

Atrial fibrillation and atrial flutter with rapid ventricular response are among the most common arrhythmias encountered during interfacility transport, and the transport management priority is rate control rather than rhythm conversion. Diltiazem is the most commonly used rate-control agent for atrial fibrillation with rapid ventricular response in patients with preserved ventricular function, delivered as a bolus followed by a continuous infusion titrated to a heart rate target. In patients with reduced ejection fraction, amiodarone provides both rate control and potential rhythm conversion without the negative inotropic effects of calcium channel blockers, though its slower onset and multiple potential side effects require close monitoring.

Amiodarone loading during transport requires specific attention to its infusion-related complications: hypotension from the polysorbate 80 solvent in the intravenous formulation, phlebitis from peripheral infusion (which argues for central access when available for a loading dose), and the potential for QT prolongation that can paradoxically precipitate the very arrhythmias it is intended to treat. A loading dose is typically administered as a slow intravenous push or short infusion over ten to twenty minutes, followed by a maintenance infusion, and the crew should monitor blood pressure continuously during the loading period and be prepared to slow or hold the infusion if significant hypotension develops. The aqueous formulation of intravenous amiodarone, where available, produces less hypotension and phlebitis than the polysorbate-based formulation, a distinction that may be relevant for programs selecting their transport formulary.

**Post-Conversion Monitoring and Recurrence Planning**

After successful termination of any tachyarrhythmia during transport, whether by pharmacologic or electrical means, the crew should anticipate the possibility of recurrence during the remainder of the transport window rather than assuming the arrhythmia has been definitively resolved. This means maintaining defibrillation pads in place, keeping antiarrhythmic infusions running if initiated, and continuing the same monitoring intensity as before conversion rather than downgrading surveillance. Recurrence of a tachyarrhythmia that was initially terminated successfully is common, particularly in the setting of an ongoing metabolic or ischemic trigger that has not been corrected, and a crew that has already returned equipment to storage or reduced monitoring intensity will be slower to respond to a recurrence than one that maintains readiness throughout the transport.

| Arrhythmia | First-Line Transport Intervention | Key Transport Consideration |
|---|---|---|
| SVT (regular narrow-complex) | Vagal maneuvers, then adenosine | Brief asystole after conversion expected; have TCP ready |
| Atrial fibrillation (rapid response) | Diltiazem (preserved EF); amiodarone (reduced EF) | Avoid CCB if EF <40%; monitor for hypotension |
| Monomorphic VT (stable) | Amiodarone; synchronized cardioversion if unstable | Default to VT for any uncertain wide-complex; never use CCB |
| Polymorphic VT / Torsades | IV magnesium; defibrillation if pulseless | Check QTc; correct hypokalemia/hypomagnesemia |
| VF / Pulseless VT | Immediate defibrillation + ACLS | Cabin space limits CPR quality; consider mechanical CPR |

**Figure 8.1: Rhythm Strip Differentiation of Transport-Relevant Tachyarrhythmias**

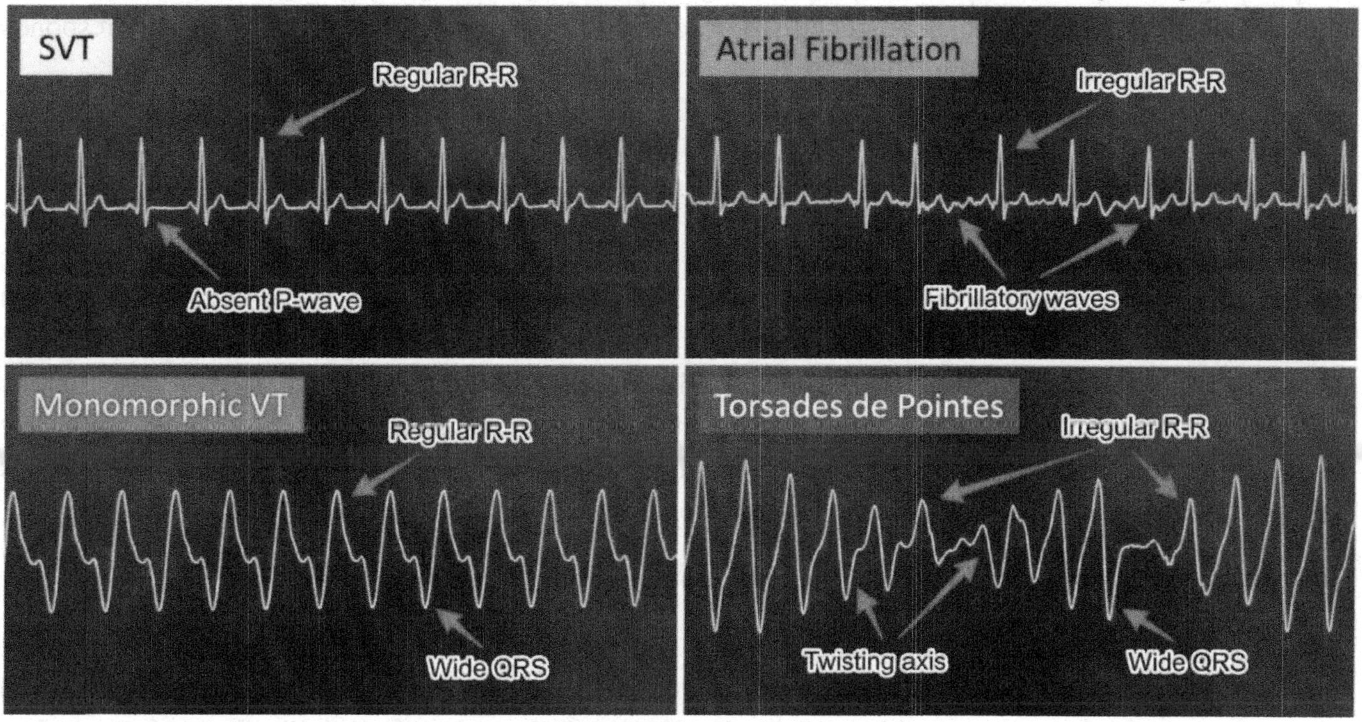


## Bradyarrhythmia and Pacing Considerations

### Identifying Hemodynamically Significant Bradycardia

Not every bradycardia encountered during transport requires intervention; the clinical decision point is whether the slow rate is producing hemodynamic compromise--hypotension, altered mentation, signs of shock, or worsening heart failure. The transport clinician should be particularly vigilant for high-degree AV block in the setting of acute anterior myocardial infarction, where the block typically reflects extensive septal necrosis and is unlikely to respond to atropine alone, requiring transcutaneous pacing as a bridge to transvenous pacing at the receiving facility.

### Transcutancous Pacing in the Transport Environment

Transcutaneous pacing should be initiated before departure in any patient with a hemodynamically significant bradycardia or a high-risk block pattern, rather than deferred to a reactive deployment mid-transport. Electrical and mechanical capture must both be confirmed: electrical capture is visible on the monitor as a pacing spike followed by a wide QRS complex, but mechanical capture--confirmed by a palpable pulse or an arterial waveform that corresponds to the paced rhythm--is the clinically meaningful endpoint, since electrical capture without mechanical capture provides no hemodynamic benefit.

### Pharmacologic Temporizing Agents for Bradycardia

Atropine is the first-line pharmacologic agent for symptomatic sinus bradycardia and low-degree AV block, but it is frequently ineffective in high-degree block and in denervated or transplanted hearts. For atropine-refractory bradycardia, a dopamine or epinephrine infusion provides chronotropic support as a temporizing measure. Isoproterenol, a pure beta-agonist, is rarely used in transport but may be considered in beta-blocker or calcium channel blocker overdose-related bradycardia where the mechanism responds specifically to beta-agonist stimulation.

## Cardioversion and Defibrillation in the Transport Setting

### Safety Considerations for Electrical Therapy in a Confined Cabin

Delivering an electrical shock in the confined cabin of an aircraft or ground ambulance introduces safety considerations absent from a hospital resuscitation bay: all crew members must be clearly warned and physically verified as not in contact with the patient, the stretcher frame, or any conductive surface before energy is delivered, and the oxygen flow should be directed away from the defibrillation pads to eliminate the ignition risk in an oxygen-enriched environment. In a rotor-wing aircraft, the decision to defibrillate during flight must also account for the brief distraction of the clinical crew during the charge-clear-shock sequence, which temporarily removes both clinicians from other monitoring and intervention tasks.

### Synchronized Cardioversion Versus Defibrillation: Decision Framework

The decision between synchronized cardioversion and unsynchronized defibrillation follows the same hemodynamic stability framework used at the bedside: synchronized cardioversion for organized tachyarrhythmias with a pulse and identifiable R-wave, and unsynchronized defibrillation for pulseless ventricular tachycardia, ventricular fibrillation, and any tachyarrhythmia producing cardiovascular collapse. The transport defibrillator should be pre-checked for synchronization capability and pad placement verified before departure for any patient at risk for arrhythmia deterioration.

### Cardiopulmonary Resuscitation in the Confined Transport Environment

If a cardiac arrest occurs during transport, the confined cabin space limits the mechanical efficiency of manual chest compressions, since the rescuer may lack the overhead clearance, stable platform, or body positioning required to deliver compressions at adequate depth and rate. A mechanical chest compression device, where carried, provides consistent compression quality independent of rescuer positioning and fatigue, and should be strongly considered for any transport program that routinely carries patients at high risk for in-transit cardiac arrest. Programs that do not carry a mechanical device should have a rehearsed plan for optimizing manual compressions within their specific cabin configuration, including which crew member performs compressions, how they position themselves, and at what interval they rotate.

The decision to initiate or continue resuscitation during active flight or ground transport versus requesting a stop introduces an additional layer of complexity: in a ground ambulance, pulling to the side of the road to improve CPR quality is a viable and often recommended option, since the delay in arrival is typically small relative to the improvement in compression quality. In a rotor-wing aircraft, landing for CPR is a more consequential operational decision that involves the pilot, affects the mission timeline, and may place the aircraft in an unplanned landing zone, and the decision must balance the clinical benefit of improved compression quality against the operational risks and delays of an unplanned landing. Each transport program should have a pre-established protocol for this decision, agreed upon with the flight crew, so that the clinical team is not making an operational safety decision under the acute stress of a cardiac arrest.

### Post-Resuscitation Care and Transport Continuation Decisions

When return of spontaneous circulation is achieved during transport, the post-resuscitation care priorities mirror those described in Chapter 6 for post-cardiac arrest management: hemodynamic optimization with vasoactive support, targeted temperature management if indicated and feasible, ventilator adjustment to avoid both hyperoxia and hypocapnia, and continuous rhythm monitoring for recurrent arrest. The crew must also make a real-time decision about whether to continue to the originally planned receiving facility, divert to a closer facility, or, if the arrest occurred before departure, return to the sending facility, a decision that should be guided by the patient's post-resuscitation stability, the time remaining to each potential destination, and the specific capabilities needed at the receiving end.

### Drug Overdose-Related Arrhythmias

Toxic ingestions of tricyclic antidepressants, sodium channel-blocking drugs, and cardiotoxic substances produce arrhythmias whose management differs from the standard ACLS algorithms and requires specific pharmacologic interventions that the transport clinician must recognize and initiate. Tricyclic antidepressant toxicity produces a characteristic wide-complex tachycardia with a rightward axis deviation and a terminal R-wave in lead aVR, findings that should trigger intravenous sodium bicarbonate administration as the first-line antiarrhythmic intervention rather than the amiodarone or lidocaine that would be appropriate for a non-toxic wide-complex tachycardia. Beta-blocker and calcium channel blocker overdoses produce bradycardia and hypotension that may be refractory to standard doses of atropine and vasopressors, requiring high-dose insulin with glucose therapy, intravenous calcium, and, in the case of beta-blocker toxicity, glucagon as specific antidotal interventions. These toxicologic arrhythmia presentations are addressed in greater depth in Chapter 20 (Toxicologic Emergencies), but the transport clinician's ability to recognize the electrocardiographic and clinical patterns of common cardiotoxic ingestions and initiate specific therapy without waiting for toxicology consultation is a genuine life-saving skill in the transport setting.

**CLINICAL PEARL:** A terminal R-wave in lead aVR in the context of a wide-complex tachycardia should immediately raise suspicion for sodium channel blocker toxicity, and the appropriate first-line treatment is intravenous sodium bicarbonate, not amiodarone.

A second case illustrates the implantable device challenge: a fifty-four-year-old woman with a biventricular ICD for ischemic cardiomyopathy, transferred by ground critical care ambulance for device evaluation after receiving three shocks at home, two of which her cardiologist suspects were inappropriate based on remote monitoring data. During the thirty-minute transport, the patient receives a fourth shock that produces visible distress but no hemodynamic change, and the monitor shows a narrow-complex tachycardia at a rate just above the device's programmed detection threshold, consistent with sinus tachycardia misclassified as ventricular tachycardia by the device. The transport nurse applies a magnet over the device, which suspends tachyarrhythmia therapy and prevents further inappropriate shocks, documents the time and clinical context of the magnet application, and confirms that external defibrillation pads are applied and the defibrillator is charged and ready in case a genuine ventricular arrhythmia occurs while device therapy is suspended. The patient arrives at the receiving electrophysiology service without further shocks, and the magnet is removed only after the device has been interrogated and reprogrammed. This case illustrates both the value and the risk of magnet application: it stopped the inappropriate shocks that were causing the patient distress and could have triggered a genuine arrhythmia through repeated myocardial stimulation, but it also disabled the device's ability to treat a genuine event, requiring the crew to maintain external defibrillation readiness for the remainder of the transport.

**THE IN-TRANSIT DETERIORATION SIGNATURE SYSTEM — Vibration-Obscured Rhythm Deterioration**

**The Signature:** A progressive rhythm deterioration--such as widening QRS morphology, increasing ectopy, or transition from a stable tachycardia to an unstable one--that develops during transport but is initially missed because vibration-induced baseline artifact on the monitor obscures the morphologic changes that would be apparent on a clean bedside tracing.

**Movement Trigger:** Continuous engine and airframe vibration produces baseline artifact on the cardiac monitor that can mimic or mask ectopy, obscure subtle morphologic changes, and degrade the signal-to-noise ratio.

**Early Tell:** A persistent or recurring artifact alarm on the cardiac monitor, combined with a concurrent change in a second modality--hemodynamic instability on the arterial tracing, a capnography change, or a clinical change in the patient--suggesting the rhythm change is real.

**Trap Logic:** The high background rate of vibration-induced artifact conditions the crew to interpret monitor irregularities as noise. The discriminating feature is concordance with a second monitoring modality: genuine rhythm deterioration produces concordant hemodynamic changes that vibration artifact alone will not.

**Signature Anchor:** When a cardiac monitor alarm persists during transport, check for concordance with the arterial waveform or a brief manual pulse assessment before dismissing it as artifact; a genuine rhythm deterioration will produce concordant hemodynamic changes.

## Implantable Device Management in Transit

### Pacemaker and ICD Troubleshooting During Transport

Patients with implantable pacemakers or cardioverter-defibrillators present specific transport challenges: inappropriate shocks triggered by electromagnetic interference, artifact, or supraventricular tachycardias misclassified by the device; pacing failure in a pacemaker-dependent patient; and the transport crew's inability to interrogate or reprogram the device without a manufacturer-specific programmer. The practical transport management relies on external measures: application of a magnet over an ICD suspends tachyarrhythmia therapy and stops inappropriate shocks, while application over a pacemaker typically produces asynchronous pacing at a fixed rate.

### Magnet Application and Its Limitations

A magnet should be carried on every critical care transport platform and its use understood by every crew member. However, magnet application over an ICD disables tachyarrhythmia therapy entirely, meaning that a genuine ventricular fibrillation event while the magnet is in place will not be treated by the device, and the crew must provide external defibrillation manually. The response varies by manufacturer and programming, and the crew should document the time of application, the clinical indication, and the observed device response for the receiving electrophysiology team.

**KEY POINT:** A magnet applied to an ICD stops inappropriate shocks but also disables the device's ability to treat genuine ventricular fibrillation; the crew must have external defibrillation capability immediately available whenever a magnet is in place.

## Electrolyte-Driven Arrhythmias

### Hyperkalemia and Its Cardiac Manifestations

Hyperkalemia is the most immediately dangerous electrolyte-driven arrhythmia trigger encountered in transport, producing a predictable sequence of electrocardiographic changes--peaked T-waves, PR prolongation, QRS widening, sine-wave pattern, and ultimately ventricular fibrillation or asystole. Intravenous calcium is the first intervention, providing immediate membrane stabilization within minutes, buying time for definitive potassium-lowering therapies to take effect. Point-of-care potassium measurement, where available, should be obtained in any patient with new electrocardiographic changes suggestive of hyperkalemia.

### Hypokalemia, Hypomagnesemia, and Torsades De Pointes

Hypokalemia and hypomagnesemia, frequently coexisting, predispose to QT prolongation and torsades de pointes, characteristically responsive to intravenous magnesium sulfate regardless of measured magnesium level. The transport clinician should review the patient's medication list for QT-prolonging agents that may compound electrolyte-driven risk, and should ensure magnesium sulfate is immediately accessible for any patient with a known or suspected prolonged QT interval.

**Figure 8.2: Electrocardiographic Progression of Hyperkalemia**

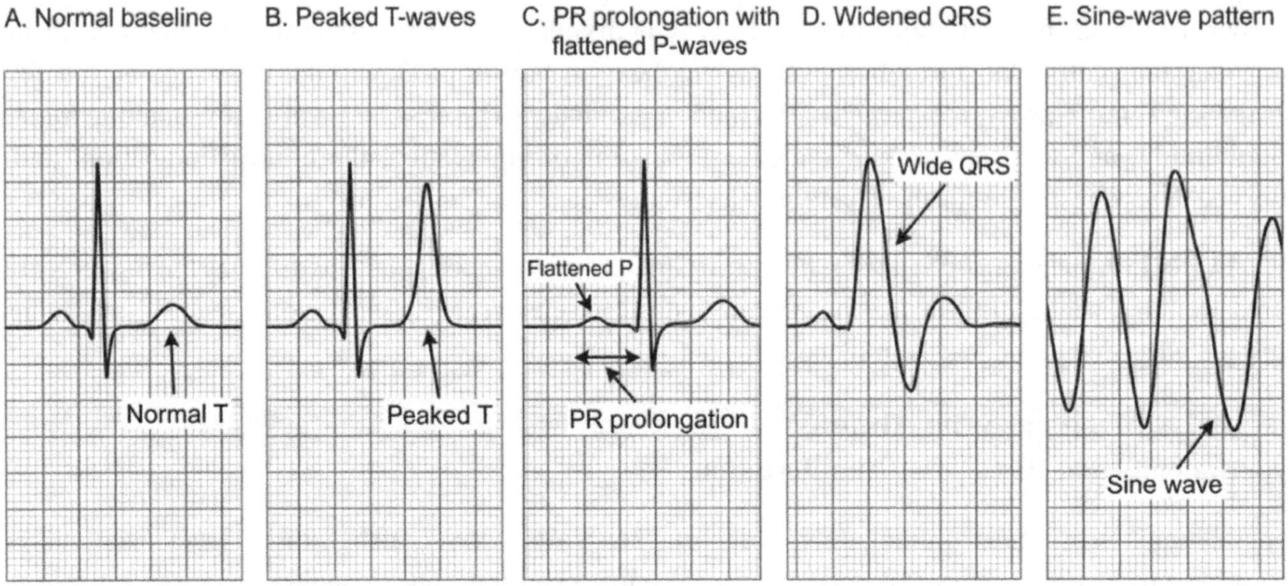


**A.** Normal baseline **B.** Peaked T-waves **C.** PR prolongation with flattened P-waves **D.** Widened QRS **E.** Sine-wave pattern

Consider a sixty-seven-year-old man with end-stage renal disease and a missed dialysis session, transferred by ground critical care ambulance for emergent dialysis access, whose pre-departure ECG shows peaked T-waves and a QRS duration at the upper limit of normal. During a forty-five-minute transport, the crew notes progressive QRS widening on the continuous monitor and, recognizing the hyperkalemic progression pattern rather than attributing the widening to artifact, administers intravenous calcium chloride, insulin with dextrose, and nebulized albuterol. The QRS narrows within minutes of calcium administration, and point-of-care potassium confirms severe hyperkalemia. This case illustrates that electrocardiographic recognition of the hyperkalemic progression is a transport survival skill because the progression from widened QRS to cardiac arrest can be measured in minutes, and that the empiric treatment triad can be safely delivered during transport without waiting for laboratory confirmation.

## Advanced Arrhythmia Management in Transport

### Pre-Excited Atrial Fibrillation: The Lethal Exception to Standard Rate Control

Atrial fibrillation conducted through an accessory pathway (pre-excited atrial fibrillation, or Wolff-Parkinson-White syndrome with atrial fibrillation) presents as an irregularly irregular wide-complex tachycardia that can be fatal if treated with standard rate-control agents. AV-nodal blocking drugs--diltiazem, beta-blockers, adenosine, and digoxin--are absolutely contraindicated because they preferentially slow conduction through the AV node while leaving the accessory pathway unopposed, which can paradoxically increase the ventricular rate through the pathway and trigger ventricular fibrillation. The correct management is either electrical cardioversion (for any hemodynamic instability) or procainamide (for the hemodynamically stable patient), which slows conduction through the accessory pathway itself. The transport clinician must recognize this pattern--an irregular wide-complex tachycardia with varying QRS morphology and extremely rapid rates sometimes exceeding three hundred beats per minute--and avoid the reflexive administration of diltiazem or a beta-blocker that would be appropriate for typical atrial fibrillation but is potentially lethal in pre-excited atrial fibrillation.

### Hypothermic Arrhythmias and Their Transport-Specific Management

Hypothermia below thirty degrees Celsius produces arrhythmias--most characteristically the Osborn wave (J wave) on ECG, progressing through atrial fibrillation to ventricular fibrillation as core temperature falls further--that are refractory to standard pharmacologic and electrical treatment until the patient is rewarmed. The transport clinician managing an arrhythmia in a hypothermic patient should prioritize active rewarming over repeated defibrillation attempts or antiarrhythmic drug administration, since the cold myocardium is physiologically incapable of sustaining a stable rhythm regardless of pharmacologic or electrical intervention. One defibrillation attempt is reasonable in hypothermic ventricular fibrillation, but repeated shocks in a patient whose core temperature remains below thirty degrees are unlikely to achieve sustained conversion and should be deferred until active rewarming has raised the core temperature above thirty degrees, at which point the myocardium becomes progressively more responsive to standard therapies.

### Supraventricular Tachycardia in the Pediatric Transport Patient

Supraventricular tachycardia in infants and young children can produce hemodynamic compromise more rapidly than in adults because the pediatric myocardium is more rate-dependent for cardiac output and less able to compensate for the reduced diastolic filling time of a rapid tachycardia. The management sequence follows the same priorities as in adults--vagal maneuvers first, then adenosine--but the techniques differ: the diving reflex, elicited by applying a cold, wet cloth or ice bag to the infant's face for fifteen to thirty seconds, is the most effective vagal maneuver in infants and young children, replacing the Valsalva maneuver used in older patients. Adenosine dosing is weight-based, and the rapid-push technique with immediate flush is even more critical in pediatric patients, where the smaller peripheral veins and longer transit time to the heart make slow administration ineffective. Cardioversion, at the weight-based energy dose of 0.5 to 1 joule per kilogram for the initial attempt, should be performed without delay if the infant or child is hemodynamically compromised.

### Pacemaker Malfunction: Failure to Pace, Failure to Capture, Failure to Sense

Permanent pacemaker malfunction presents during transport in three recognizable patterns: failure to pace (no pacing spike visible on the monitor despite a bradycardic rate below the programmed lower rate limit), failure to capture (pacing spikes visible but not followed by a QRS complex, indicating that the electrical stimulus is not producing mechanical contraction), and failure to sense (inappropriate pacing spikes delivered during the native rhythm, indicating that the device is not detecting the patient's intrinsic beats). Each pattern has a different significance: failure to pace may indicate lead fracture, battery depletion, or electromagnetic interference; failure to capture may indicate lead displacement, threshold elevation, or metabolic derangement affecting myocardial excitability; and failure to sense may indicate lead insulation failure or programming issues. The transport clinician's management for all three patterns, when producing hemodynamic compromise, is transcutaneous pacing as the immediate backup, with the specific malfunction pattern documented and communicated to the receiving electrophysiology team for device interrogation.

### Amiodarone Toxicity During Extended Transport

Amiodarone, while the most broadly effective antiarrhythmic agent in the transport formulary, carries a risk of acute toxicity during loading that the transport clinician must monitor for: hypotension from the polysorbate solvent, QT prolongation that can paradoxically produce torsades de pointes, and phlebitis from peripheral infusion. The hypotensive effect is most pronounced during the initial loading bolus and can be mitigated by slowing the infusion rate, administering through a central line where available, and having a small fluid bolus ready to support blood pressure during the loading period. The QT-prolonging effect is cumulative and may not manifest during a short transport, but the transport clinician should be aware that a patient who has received multiple antiarrhythmic agents (amiodarone plus another QT-prolonging drug) is at heightened risk for proarrhythmic events, and should monitor the QT interval if serial ECGs are obtained.

## Cardiac Arrest Management Specific to Transport Populations

### In-Transit Cardiac Arrest: Decision to Continue Versus Stop

A cardiac arrest during transport forces an immediate operational decision: continue CPR during movement (accepting the degraded compression quality and limited intervention capability of a moving vehicle) or stop the vehicle and perform resuscitation under more controlled conditions (accepting the delay in reaching the receiving facility). The answer depends on the specific circumstances: the proximity to the receiving facility (if arrival is imminent, continuing movement with CPR in progress may be appropriate), the suspected cause of the arrest (a treatable cause that requires capabilities only available at the receiving facility favors continued movement, while a cause that is treatable in the field favors stopping), and the quality of CPR achievable during movement on the specific platform. Ground ambulances should generally stop for cardiac arrest management because the improvement in CPR quality is immediate and significant; rotor-wing aircraft face a more complex decision because an unplanned landing introduces its own risks and delays.

### Reversible Causes of Cardiac Arrest in the Transport Setting

The standard H's and T's mnemonic for reversible causes of cardiac arrest takes on transport-specific significance because several reversible causes are more likely in the transport environment than at the bedside: tension pneumothorax from altitude-related expansion of an occult pneumothorax (connecting directly to the Chapter 1 Signature), cardiac tamponade from a worsening pericardial effusion during transport movement, hypovolemia from rebleeding of a tamponaded hemorrhage source (connecting to the Chapter 15 Signature), hyperkalemia in a renal failure patient who has missed dialysis, hypothermia from environmental exposure during transport, and toxins from a delayed-onset ingestion declaring itself during the transport window. The transport clinician should systematically consider each transport-specific reversible cause during any in-transit cardiac arrest rather than defaulting to a standard ACLS algorithm that may not address the actual precipitant.

**Additional Clinical Considerations for Transport Management**

The management of patients in Chapter 8 requires attention to several additional transport-specific clinical factors that extend the principles established in the main body of the chapter. The transport clinician should be aware that the disease processes covered here interact with the transport environment in ways that are specific to the combination of the underlying pathophysiology and the particular environmental stressor encountered during a given mission, and that a management approach that is adequate for a short ground transport may be insufficient for a longer air transport at altitude, or vice versa. The serial reassessment protocol established in Chapter 2 provides the framework for detecting these interactions as they develop, and the Deterioration Signature introduced in this chapter names the most characteristic pattern by which they declare themselves.

Each patient transport is a unique combination of a specific patient's physiology, a specific set of ongoing therapies, a specific transport platform with its own environmental characteristics, and a specific mission profile with its own altitude, duration, and route constraints. The anticipatory approach to transport medicine that this text teaches is not a set of memorized responses to predetermined scenarios but a cognitive framework for analyzing the specific combination of variables present in any given transport and identifying, before departure, the most likely points of vulnerability where the transport environment will test the patient's physiologic reserve. This chapter's clinical content provides the disease-specific knowledge needed to apply that framework to the conditions covered here, while the Deterioration Signature provides the named pattern that makes the most characteristic transport-specific vulnerability explicit, recognizable, and actionable.

The receiving team's ability to continue the patient's care seamlessly after the transport crew departs depends entirely on the quality and completeness of the clinical information the transport crew provides, and for the conditions covered in this chapter, the specific information that matters most includes: the trajectory of the patient's primary condition during transport (improving, stable, or worsening, with specific details), any interventions performed during transport and their response, any new clinical findings identified by the transport crew that were not present at the sending facility, and any anticipated needs that the receiving team should prepare for based on the transport crew's clinical assessment. This information, communicated through the structured handoff format established in Chapter 2 and supplemented by the trajectory communication emphasis that is a recurring theme throughout this text, is the final clinical act of the transport and the one that determines whether the transport adds value to the patient's care continuum or merely moves the patient from one location to another without preserving the clinical narrative that only the transport crew was positioned to observe.

The clinical scenarios addressed in this chapter illustrate a principle that recurs throughout the text: the transport environment does not merely add logistic complexity to the management of critical illness--it introduces specific physiologic stressors that interact with the patient's underlying condition to produce clinical changes that would not occur at the bedside. The altitude-related gas expansion, preload shifts, oxygenation challenges, and monitoring degradation described in Chapter 1, combined with the pharmacologic and equipment considerations from Chapters 4 and 5, create a modified clinical environment in which every bedside management principle must be re-examined through the lens of transport-specific risk. The disease-specific management recommendations in this chapter have been written with this re-examination already performed, incorporating the transport modifications into the clinical recommendations rather than presenting bedside management followed by a separate list of transport considerations, because the integration of disease knowledge and transport awareness is the competency that this text is designed to develop.

Inter-professional collaboration during the management of the conditions in this chapter deserves specific emphasis, because the complexity of many transport patients exceeds the capability of any single clinician acting alone. The nurse-paramedic team, the nurse-physician team, or whatever crew configuration the program uses represents a collaborative unit whose combined clinical capability exceeds the sum of its individual members, provided that the communication, role allocation, and shared mental model practices described in Chapter 24 are actively maintained throughout the transport. A transport in which one crew member manages the airway while the other manages hemodynamics, with both monitoring different aspects of the same clinical picture and cross-checking each other's assessments, produces a more complete and reliable clinical picture than either clinician could achieve alone, and this collaborative advantage is greatest during the high-workload, high-stress scenarios that the conditions in this chapter frequently produce.

Quality improvement in the management of these conditions during transport depends on systematic outcome tracking that links transport-specific management decisions to patient outcomes at the receiving facility. Did the patient who received a specific intervention during transport have a better or worse outcome than comparable patients who did not? Did a specific monitoring strategy detect deterioration earlier and allow more effective intervention? Did advance communication with the receiving facility produce measurably faster time-to-treatment on arrival? These questions can only be answered by programs that collect and analyze outcome data systematically, and the transport clinician's contribution to this process is meticulous, contemporaneous documentation of every clinical decision, every intervention, and every trajectory observation during the transport, since this documentation is the raw material from which quality improvement insights are derived. A transport program that does not analyze its outcomes cannot improve them, and a transport clinician who does not document their clinical reasoning cannot contribute to the program's learning.

**THE IN-TRANSIT DETERIORATION SIGNATURE SYSTEM — Electrical Deterioration Patterns**

**Signature Introduced This Chapter:** Vibration-Obscured Rhythm Deterioration (progressive rhythm deterioration masked by vibration-induced monitor artifact, detected through concordance with a second monitoring modality).

**Electrical Pattern Logic:** This Signature extends the Equipment-Masked Deterioration framework from Chapter 5 into the specific domain of cardiac rhythm monitoring, where the consequences of delayed recognition are uniquely time-critical because the interval between arrhythmia onset and hemodynamic collapse can be seconds.

**Cross-Reference Forward:** Chapter 9 (MCS Devices) addresses the overlap between device-generated electrical artifacts and genuine rhythm deterioration; Chapter 19 (Electrolyte Derangements) extends hyperkalemia and hypokalemia management.

## Summary and Key Concepts

Wide-complex tachycardias should be treated as ventricular tachycardia until proven otherwise; administration of AV-nodal blockers to misidentified VT can produce cardiovascular collapse.

Transcutaneous pacing should be established before departure for any patient with hemodynamically significant bradycardia, confirmed by both electrical and mechanical capture.

Cardioversion and defibrillation in a confined cabin require explicit safety verification, including oxygen redirection and crew clearance confirmation.

Vibration-induced monitor artifact can mask genuine rhythm deterioration; concordance with a second monitoring modality is the tie-breaker.

A magnet is the only universally available tool for modifying implantable device behavior during transport, but its use disables the device's own defibrillation capability.

Hyperkalemia produces a predictable ECG progression that the transport clinician must treat empirically with calcium, insulin-glucose, and beta-agonist without waiting for laboratory confirmation.

# CHAPTER 9: MECHANICAL CIRCULATORY SUPPORT DEVICES IN TRANSIT

**Learning Objectives**

1. Describe the physiology and flow characteristics of intra-aortic balloon pumps, continuous-flow ventricular assist devices, and extracorporeal membrane oxygenation circuits relevant to transport.
2. Anticipate altitude and acceleration effects on device performance using the gas-law and hemodynamic principles from Chapter 1.
3. Troubleshoot common device alarms during transport and distinguish device-level problems from patient-level hemodynamic events.
4. Manage anticoagulation for mechanical support circuits during the transport window.
5. Coordinate transport logistics including power management, equipment mounting, and team composition for device-supported patients.

**Chapter Outline**

This chapter addresses the transport of patients supported by mechanical circulatory devices--intra-aortic balloon pumps, continuous-flow ventricular assist devices, and extracorporeal membrane oxygenation circuits--as a distinct clinical and logistical discipline that integrates the hemodynamic management from Chapters 6 and 7, the device physiology introduced in Chapter 1, the equipment and power management framework from Chapter 5, and the pharmacologic anticoagulation considerations from Chapter 4. These transports carry the highest equipment complexity and the narrowest margin for error of any critical care transport, and the crew's familiarity with the specific device, its alarm logic, and its environmental vulnerabilities is the primary determinant of patient safety during transit.

## Intra-Aortic Balloon Pump Management During Transport

### Timing, Triggering, and Augmentation Assessment

The intra-aortic balloon pump augments cardiac output by inflating during diastole to improve coronary perfusion pressure and deflating immediately before systole to reduce left ventricular afterload, a timing sequence that depends on accurate ECG or arterial pressure triggering to deliver its hemodynamic benefit. During transport, vibration-induced artifact can degrade the quality of the ECG trigger signal, producing mistimed inflation-deflation cycles that reduce or eliminate the device's hemodynamic benefit without generating an obvious alarm, since the pump is still cycling--just not at the correct point in the cardiac cycle. The transport clinician should verify timing by inspecting the augmented arterial waveform for appropriate diastolic augmentation and systolic unloading at regular intervals during transport, not merely confirming that the pump is cycling.

### Helium Supply and Console Management

The balloon pump console uses helium as the inflation gas due to its low viscosity and rapid diffusion, and the helium tank carried with the console has a finite supply that must be verified against the planned transport duration before departure. Helium leak alarms, which indicate that gas is escaping from the balloon or the drive line, should prompt immediate investigation for balloon perforation, which can introduce helium into the arterial circulation and, more importantly, allow blood to enter the balloon membrane, producing a catastrophic device failure. A helium leak alarm during transport that is confirmed as a genuine leak rather than a transient alarm artifact is an indication to cease balloon pump operation and transition to pharmacologic hemodynamic support for the remainder of the transport.

### Positioning and Immobilization of the Catheterized Leg

The balloon pump catheter is typically inserted through the femoral artery, and the catheterized leg must be immobilized in a straight position to prevent catheter migration, kinking, or vascular injury during loading and transit. This immobilization requirement interacts with the stretcher configuration and cabin space constraints described in Chapter 5, and should be addressed during the equipment layout planning phase rather than discovered as a problem during loading. Limb perfusion distal to the insertion site should be assessed at each reassessment interval, since the catheter occupies a significant portion of the femoral artery lumen and can compromise distal flow, particularly in a patient with peripheral vascular disease or a small-caliber artery.

| IABP Alarm | Most Likely Cause | Transport Action |
|---|---|---|
| Timing error | Trigger signal degradation from vibration artifact | Switch to arterial pressure trigger; verify augmented waveform manually |
| Helium leak | Balloon perforation or drive-line leak | Confirm genuine leak; if confirmed, cease pump operation and transition to pharmacologic support |
| Low augmentation | Catheter migration, hypovolemia, or arrhythmia | Verify catheter depth; assess volume status; check rhythm for irregularity affecting timing |
| Console battery low | Extended operation on battery without external power | Connect to external power; verify remaining battery if external power unavailable |

## Ventricular Assist Device Physiology and Altitude Effects

### Continuous-Flow VAD Hemodynamics During Transport

Continuous-flow ventricular assist devices, now the predominant long-term mechanical support platform, generate flow by spinning an internal impeller at a set rotational speed, and the actual flow delivered depends on the pressure differential across the pump--specifically, on the preload presented to the inflow cannula and the afterload against which the outflow cannula discharges. This preload and afterload dependence is the physiologic basis for the Ascent-Triggered Device Flow Compromise Signature introduced in Chapter 1: when altitude-related preload reduction decreases the pressure presented to the inflow cannula, device flow falls even though the pump speed has not changed, producing a flow alarm that is frequently and incorrectly attributed to pump malfunction or thrombus rather than recognized as a predictable hemodynamic event.

### Altitude-Related Flow and Suction Events

At the extreme end of preload reduction during ascent, the left ventricle can collapse around the inflow cannula, producing a suction event that is signaled by intermittent flow alarms, a characteristic oscillating pattern in the power consumption tracing, and, if sustained, by hemodynamic instability. Suction events are managed by reducing pump speed temporarily to allow the ventricle to refill, correcting the underlying preload deficit with volume or positioning, and then gradually returning to the previous speed, a sequence that the transport clinician must be prepared to execute independently since the device manufacturer's clinical support is typically unavailable in real time during transport. The Chapter 1 discussion of proactive leg elevation and euvolemia confirmation before ascent is specifically designed to prevent suction events in the first place.

### Controller and Driveline Management During Transport

The VAD controller, which houses the device's operating software and displays flow, power, and speed parameters, is powered by two batteries that provide a redundant power supply, and the transport crew must verify that both batteries are fully charged before departure and that spare batteries are carried for the full anticipated transport duration plus a delay margin. The driveline--the percutaneous cable connecting the internal pump to the external controller--is vulnerable to mechanical stress during loading and movement, and must be secured against traction, kinking, and inadvertent disconnection with the same deliberate attention given to any other life-sustaining line. Driveline damage or disconnection is a non-recoverable emergency that no in-transit intervention can correct, making prevention through meticulous line management the only viable strategy.

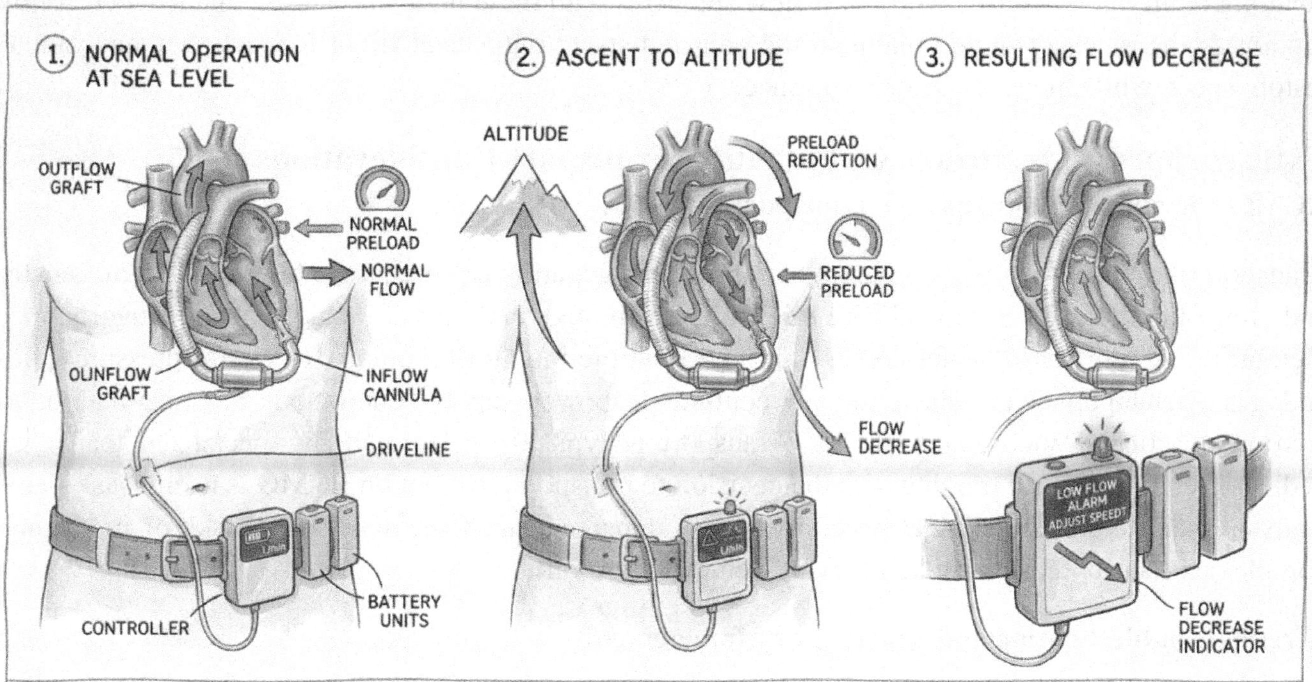


Figure 9.1: VAD Console and Cannula Configuration With Altitude-Related Flow Effects

## THE IN-TRANSIT DETERIORATION SIGNATURE SYSTEM — Suction-Event Cascade at Altitude

**The Signature:** Intermittent, escalating flow alarms accompanied by oscillating power consumption and progressive hemodynamic instability in a VAD-supported patient during or shortly after ascent, progressing from mild flow reduction to a fully developed suction event with ventricular collapse.

**Movement Trigger:** Altitude-related preload reduction, as described in Chapter 1, reduces the filling volume presented to the left ventricle and the VAD inflow cannula. If the pump speed is not reduced or preload is not augmented, the ventricle progressively empties until the ventricular wall collapses around the cannula, obstructing inflow.

**Early Tell:** The earliest signal is an intermittent, self-resolving flow dip rather than a sustained alarm--a brief drop in displayed flow followed by a return to baseline, occurring in a pattern that coincides with the respiratory cycle or with transient positional shifts, suggesting that the ventricle is cycling between adequate and marginal filling.

**Trap Logic:** This pattern is frequently attributed to pump thrombus because the flow alarm and power oscillation can superficially resemble the hemodynamic signature of an impeller clot. The discriminating feature is timing: a suction event that begins precisely during ascent and improves with leg elevation or volume administration points to a preload mechanism, while pump thrombus typically presents as a persistent, position-independent power elevation that does not respond to volume or positioning.

**Signature Anchor:** At the first sign of an intermittent flow alarm during ascent in a VAD-supported patient, reduce pump speed by a small increment, elevate the patient's legs, and assess volume status before pursuing a thrombus-focused workup. If flow stabilizes with these preload-restoring maneuvers, confirm suction as the mechanism and maintain the adjusted speed until level flight is reached, then gradually restore speed while monitoring for recurrence.

## Extracorporeal Membrane Oxygenation Transport Considerations

### ECMO Circuit Components and Transport Logistics

Transport of a patient on extracorporeal membrane oxygenation represents the highest level of logistical and clinical complexity in critical care transport, involving a circuit that includes a centrifugal pump, a membrane oxygenator, a heater-cooler unit, and multiple monitoring points for circuit pressures, flow, and gas exchange, all of which require continuous power supply, continuous anticoagulation, and continuous clinical surveillance. ECMO transport is typically performed by specialized teams with dedicated equipment and training, and the decision to transport a patient on ECMO is itself a risk-benefit analysis that weighs the clinical necessity of the transfer against the substantial risks of managing a complex extracorporeal circuit in a moving vehicle or aircraft.

### Circuit Troubleshooting and Emergency Management

The most immediately life-threatening ECMO circuit emergencies during transport are air entrainment into the circuit, circuit decannulation, and pump failure, each of which requires a rehearsed, team-based response that has been practiced before the transport begins. Air entrainment produces a characteristic chattering sound from the pump and a visible air-fluid interface in the circuit tubing, and the immediate response is to clamp the circuit, stop the pump, de-air the circuit if possible, and transition to conventional cardiopulmonary support until the circuit is confirmed air-free. Decannulation is a catastrophic event producing massive hemorrhage from the cannulation site and immediate loss of ECMO support, and the response is direct pressure on the site, emergent recannulation if feasible, and transition to conventional support. Pump failure, while alarming, is managed by clamping the circuit to prevent retrograde flow and initiating conventional support until the pump can be replaced or restarted.

### Gas Exchange Management and Oxygenator Function at Altitude

The membrane oxygenator's gas exchange efficiency is affected by the same altitude-related changes in partial pressure described in Chapter 1, since the sweep gas flowing through the oxygenator operates at the ambient cabin pressure rather than at sea-level pressure, which can reduce the efficiency of carbon dioxide removal and, to a lesser degree, oxygen delivery at significant cabin altitudes. The transport perfusionist or managing clinician should anticipate the need to increase sweep gas flow during ascent to maintain carbon dioxide clearance, and should monitor post-oxygenator blood gas values at intervals to confirm adequate gas exchange throughout the flight.

**CAUTION:** ECMO circuit air entrainment can produce a fatal air embolism within seconds; any chattering sound or visible air in the circuit requires immediate circuit clamping and pump stop before any other troubleshooting step.

## Team Composition and Competency Requirements for ECMO Transport

ECMO transport requires a team composition that exceeds the standard critical care transport crew, typically including a perfusionist or ECMO specialist responsible for circuit management in addition to the transport nurse or paramedic responsible for patient-level clinical care, and a physician either present on the transport or available by real-time communication for clinical decisions that exceed the crew's standing protocols. The division of labor between the circuit manager and the patient clinician must be explicitly defined before departure, since a single clinician attempting to manage both the patient's hemodynamics and the ECMO circuit's parameters simultaneously will inevitably prioritize one at the expense of the other during a moment of crisis. Transport programs initiating or expanding ECMO transport capability should require device-specific training, including simulated emergency scenarios performed in the actual transport platform, before credentialing any crew member to participate in ECMO transports.

## Patient Assessment in the Absence of a Palpable Pulse

Patients supported by continuous-flow ventricular assist devices frequently have a nonpulsatile or minimally pulsatile circulation, which eliminates or severely attenuates the palpable pulse, rendering standard pulse checks unreliable for assessing hemodynamic status and creating a specific challenge for distinguishing cardiac arrest from device-supported circulation. The transport clinician must rely on alternative indicators of adequate circulation: the device's flow and power parameters, the arterial waveform (which may show a low-amplitude pulsatile pattern superimposed on a mean pressure), end-tidal capnography as a surrogate for cardiac output, and the patient's level of consciousness and skin perfusion. A VAD-supported patient who becomes unresponsive should not have resuscitation withheld on the assumption that "the device is running"--a cardiac arrest can occur despite an operating VAD if the native ventricle fibrillates or if the device develops a flow-limiting malfunction--but the assessment must use the non-pulse-dependent indicators listed above rather than a traditional pulse check.

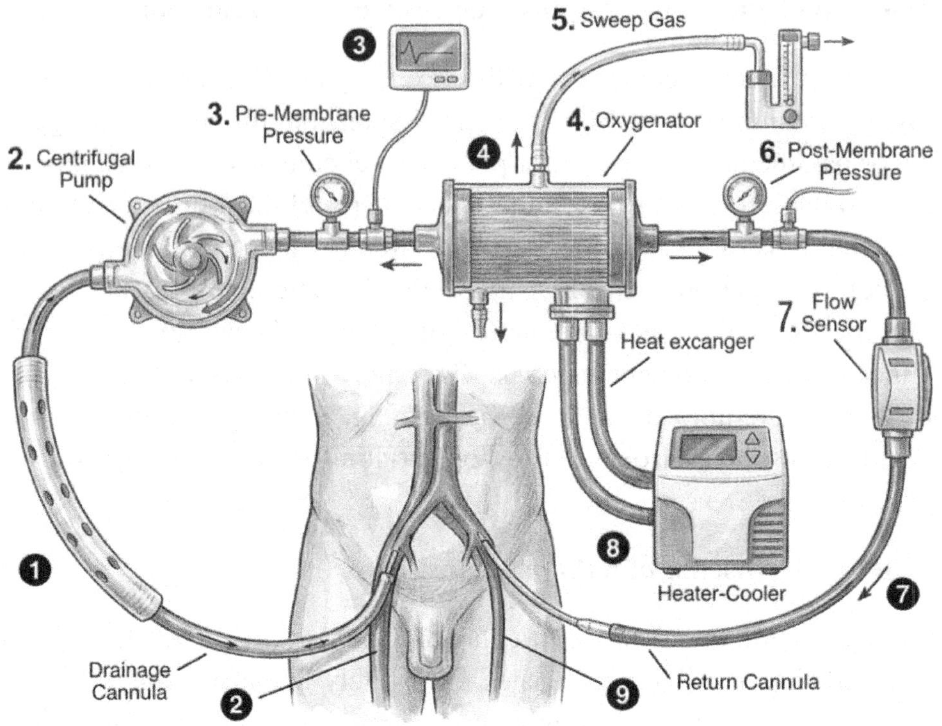


| Device Type | Power Source Requirement | Battery Endurance | External Power Priority |
|---|---|---|---|
| IABP console | AC or internal battery | 30-90 min depending on model | High -- connect to vehicle power immediately |
| Continuous-flow VAD controller | Dual battery system | 4-12 hours per battery pair | Carry spare batteries for full transport + margin |
| ECMO pump/console | AC or internal battery | 30-60 min on most consoles | Highest -- essential uninterrupted AC power or generator |
| Heater-cooler unit | AC only (most models) | None -- requires continuous AC | Required for temperature management; no battery backup |

## Device Alarm Troubleshooting En Route

### Systematic Alarm Interpretation Across Device Types

Every mechanical circulatory support device generates alarms for a range of conditions, from immediately life-threatening (air in circuit, decannulation, pump failure) to operational (low battery, minor flow variation, temperature drift), and the transport clinician must be able to triage alarm urgency rapidly rather than treating every alarm with equal priority. A systematic approach--assessing the patient's clinical status first, then correlating the alarm with the hemodynamic trend and the device's displayed parameters, then checking for environmental or positional triggers--parallels the general equipment-versus-patient troubleshooting framework from Chapter 5 but applies it to the specific, higher-stakes context of a life-sustaining mechanical device.

### Documentation and Communication of Device Events

Every device alarm, parameter change, and intervention during transport should be documented with a timestamp and communicated to the receiving team in the structured handoff format established in Chapter 2, since the receiving team's ability to manage the device safely depends on knowing exactly what happened during transit, what interventions were performed, and what the current device parameters are. This documentation is particularly important for VAD patients, whose device data is typically downloaded and reviewed by the VAD coordinator or manufacturer representative at the receiving facility, and who will rely on the transport crew's documentation to fill the gap between the last device download at the sending facility and the first at the receiving facility.

## Anticoagulation Management for Mechanical Support Devices

### Heparin Infusion Continuity and Monitoring

Continuous heparin anticoagulation is required for most mechanical circulatory support circuits to prevent thrombotic complications, and the transport clinician's primary responsibility is ensuring uninterrupted infusion delivery throughout the transport window. The infusion transition considerations from Chapter 4 apply with particular force here, since even a brief interruption of heparin delivery in a patient with an ECMO circuit or a pulsatile VAD can precipitate circuit thrombosis that is immediately and potentially irreversibly device-disabling. Point-of-care activated clotting time measurement, where available, provides real-time assessment of anticoagulation adequacy that allows dose adjustment during transport rather than waiting for laboratory-based activated partial thromboplastin time results at the receiving facility.

### Bleeding Complications and Anticoagulation Reversal Decisions

The opposite risk--hemorrhagic complications from over-anticoagulation or from the acquired coagulopathy associated with mechanical circulatory support--presents the transport clinician with a challenging risk-benefit decision: reducing or reversing anticoagulation to manage active bleeding risks device thrombosis, while continuing full anticoagulation in the face of active bleeding risks exsanguination. This decision should be made in consultation with the receiving mechanical support team whenever communication allows, and should be guided by the severity and source of bleeding, the type of device and its thrombotic sensitivity, and the remaining transport time, with the general principle that immediately life-threatening hemorrhage takes precedence over thrombotic risk during the acute transport window.

## Percutaneous Ventricular Assist Devices: Impella Considerations

The Impella family of percutaneous microaxial ventricular assist devices, increasingly used as short-term hemodynamic support in cardiogenic shock and high-risk percutaneous coronary intervention, presents transport-specific challenges distinct from both the IABP and durable VADs discussed above. The device's catheter-based design means that migration of the device tip out of its optimal position across the aortic valve can produce acute hemodynamic compromise without any external alarm, detectable only by a change in the device's position signal on the controller display, a waveform that the transport clinician must be trained to interpret. The console's purge system, which delivers a heparin-containing solution through the catheter to prevent thrombosis at the motor housing, must be maintained and its fluid volume verified before departure, since purge system failure leads to device thrombosis within a short timeframe. Additionally, the console's display of hemodynamic waveforms and motor current provides real-time functional information that the crew should monitor continuously, since a progressive increase in motor current can signal impeller obstruction from thrombus or positional malfunction before any hemodynamic change becomes apparent on the patient's arterial line.

## Pre-Departure Device Readiness Verification

Before departing the sending facility with any mechanical circulatory support device, the transport crew should complete a structured device readiness verification that confirms: all device batteries are fully charged and spare batteries are carried, all console alarms are functioning and appropriately set, the anticoagulation infusion has adequate volume for the full transport duration, the device is physically secured to the stretcher or equipment rack in a position that does not compromise clinical access or line integrity, and a brief verbal handoff from the sending device specialist confirms the current device parameters, recent alarm history, and any anticipated issues specific to this patient's device interaction. This verification is distinct from the general pre-departure equipment check described in Chapter 5 because it addresses device-specific parameters that a general checklist would not capture, and it should be performed in addition to, not instead of, the standard equipment verification.

A second case illustrates the ECMO transport complexity: a twenty-eight-year-old man with fulminant myocarditis on veno-arterial ECMO, transported by specialized ground critical care unit from a community hospital to a transplant center, a distance of ninety minutes. During the transport, the perfusionist notes a gradual increase in pre-membrane pressure on the circuit, suggesting early oxygenator clotting, and communicates this to the transport physician by mobile phone. The physician authorizes a small heparin bolus and an increase in the maintenance infusion rate, and the pressure trend stabilizes. Simultaneously, the transport nurse notes a subtle decline in the patient's native cardiac contribution to the arterial waveform, suggesting either worsening myocardial function or a positional shift affecting LV filling. Point-of-care echocardiography through the transport ultrasound confirms a new pericardial effusion not present at the sending facility, and the receiving surgical team is notified before arrival, allowing them to prepare for possible pericardiocentesis or surgical drainage on arrival rather than discovering the effusion during the initial post-arrival workup. This case illustrates the dual-track surveillance required for ECMO transport: the circuit and the patient are two separate clinical problems being managed simultaneously, and a team that monitors only the device or only the patient will miss events originating in the other domain.

Consider a forty-one-year-old man with a continuous-flow LVAD transported by fixed-wing aircraft for transplant evaluation. Approximately six minutes into climb, the VAD flow display shows a progressive decline from 5.2 to 4.4 liters per minute, accompanied by an intermittent low-flow alarm that resolves and recurs every fifteen to twenty seconds. The crew, recognizing the Suction-Event Cascade pattern from the Deterioration Signature System, immediately reduces pump speed by two hundred revolutions per minute, elevates the patient's legs, and administers a two-hundred-milliliter crystalloid bolus. Flow stabilizes at 4.8 liters per minute within ninety seconds, and the intermittent alarm pattern resolves. The crew maintains the reduced speed for the remainder of the climb and gradually restores the original speed during level cruise, monitoring for recurrence. Had the crew instead interpreted the alarm pattern as pump thrombus and initiated a thrombolytic evaluation or attempted to increase pump speed to compensate for the apparent flow reduction, both responses would have worsened a suction event that was being caused by inadequate preload, not by pump obstruction, illustrating why the correct first response to a flow alarm during ascent is always a preload-directed intervention.

## Advanced VAD Management During Transport

### VAD Hemodynamic Assessment Without Palpable Pulse

Assessment of hemodynamic adequacy in a patient supported by a continuous-flow VAD requires adaptation of the standard clinical examination because the traditional indicators of circulation--palpable pulse, auscultated blood pressure by cuff, and pulse oximetry waveform quality--are attenuated or absent in the setting of non-pulsatile flow. Mean arterial pressure, measured by a Doppler-assisted technique over the radial or brachial artery and an appropriately sized cuff, provides the best noninvasive hemodynamic assessment in the non-pulsatile patient, though invasive arterial monitoring provides continuous data and is strongly recommended for any VAD transport. The arterial waveform in a VAD patient typically shows a flat or minimally pulsatile tracing at a mean pressure that represents the combined output of the device and any residual native cardiac function, and changes in the mean pressure or in the degree of pulsatility provide hemodynamic trend information that serves the same function as the standard arterial waveform analysis described in Chapter 2.

### Right Heart Failure in the LVAD Patient

Left ventricular assist devices unload the failing left ventricle, which can unmask or precipitate right ventricular failure by several mechanisms: the sudden increase in cardiac output produced by the LVAD increases venous return to the right heart beyond its capacity, the interventricular septum shifts leftward as the LV decompresses and reduces the right ventricle's contribution to its own output, and pre-existing right ventricular dysfunction that was masked by the low-output state becomes apparent once left-sided output is restored. The transport clinician should monitor for right heart failure in any LVAD patient, particularly one recently implanted, by assessing for rising central venous pressure, hepatomegaly, and new edema, and should be prepared to support the right ventricle with inotropic therapy (milrinone is preferred for its pulmonary vasodilatory effect) and optimization of pulmonary vascular resistance through adequate oxygenation and ventilation.

### VAD-Specific Cardiac Arrest Management

Cardiac arrest in a VAD patient does not follow the standard ACLS algorithm because the device provides mechanical circulatory support independent of the native cardiac rhythm, meaning that a VAD patient in ventricular fibrillation may still be conscious and hemodynamically supported if the device flow is adequate. The assessment of cardiac arrest in a VAD patient must therefore rely on clinical indicators of perfusion rather than pulse check: level of consciousness, blood pressure (by Doppler), and device flow parameters. If the patient is truly in cardiac arrest with loss of consciousness and inadequate device flow, the management includes defibrillation for shockable rhythms (which may restore a native rhythm that augments device function), vasopressor support to maintain preload and afterload, and chest compressions only as a last resort, since external compressions in a patient with an intracorporeal device carry a risk of dislodging the inflow or outflow cannula. The receiving VAD coordinator should be contacted immediately for device-specific guidance.

### Driveline Infection and Emergency Management

Driveline infections are the most common long-term complication of implantable VADs, and a patient being transported with an active driveline infection requires specific wound management: sterile dressing maintained over the exit site, antimicrobial therapy continued without interruption, and avoidance of traction or manipulation of the driveline that could worsen the infection or introduce additional organisms. The transport clinician should inspect the driveline exit site as part of the pre-departure assessment, document the current wound appearance, and communicate any acute changes to the receiving team. An acutely displaced driveline--pulled partially out of the subcutaneous tunnel--is a surgical emergency that cannot be corrected in the field, and the transport clinician's role is to stabilize the driveline in its current position, apply a sterile dressing, and expedite transport to the receiving surgical team.

### ECMO Cannula Site Management and Limb Perfusion Monitoring

Veno-arterial ECMO cannulation, typically through the femoral artery and femoral vein, can produce distal limb ischemia from the arterial cannula's occlusion of flow to the ipsilateral leg, and many patients have a distal perfusion cannula in place that provides retrograde flow to the leg beyond the arterial cannulation site. The transport clinician should confirm the presence and function of the distal perfusion cannula before departure, should monitor the ipsilateral limb for signs of ischemia (pallor, coolness, absent pulses, cyanosis) at each reassessment interval, and should report any change in limb perfusion immediately to the receiving surgical team. A limb ischemia event during transport is a surgical problem that cannot be corrected in transit, but early recognition and communication can reduce the ischemic time by allowing the receiving team to prepare for decannulation or perfusion cannula adjustment on arrival.

## Additional Clinical Considerations for Transport Management

The management of patients in Chapter 9 requires attention to several additional transport-specific clinical factors that extend the principles established in the main body of the chapter. The transport clinician should be aware that the disease processes covered here interact with the transport environment in ways that are specific to the combination of the underlying pathophysiology and the particular environmental stressor encountered during a given mission, and that a management approach that is adequate for a short ground transport may be insufficient for a longer air transport at altitude, or vice versa. The serial reassessment protocol established in Chapter 2 provides the framework for detecting these interactions as they develop, and the Deterioration Signature introduced in this chapter names the most characteristic pattern by which they declare themselves.

Each patient transport is a unique combination of a specific patient's physiology, a specific set of ongoing therapies, a specific transport platform with its own environmental characteristics, and a specific mission profile with its own altitude, duration, and route constraints. The anticipatory approach to transport medicine that this text teaches is not a set of memorized responses to predetermined scenarios but a cognitive framework for analyzing the specific combination of variables present in any given transport and identifying, before departure, the most likely points of vulnerability where the transport environment will test the patient's physiologic reserve. This chapter's clinical content provides the disease-specific knowledge needed to apply that framework to the conditions covered here, while the Deterioration Signature provides the named pattern that makes the most characteristic transport-specific vulnerability explicit, recognizable, and actionable.

The receiving team's ability to continue the patient's care seamlessly after the transport crew departs depends entirely on the quality and completeness of the clinical information the transport crew provides, and for the conditions covered in this chapter, the specific information that matters most includes: the trajectory of the patient's primary condition during transport (improving, stable, or worsening, with specific details), any interventions performed during transport and their response, any new clinical findings identified by the transport crew that were not present at the sending facility, and any anticipated needs that the receiving team should prepare for based on the transport crew's clinical assessment. This information, communicated through the structured handoff format established in Chapter 2 and supplemented by the trajectory communication emphasis that is a recurring theme throughout this text, is the final clinical act of the transport and the one that determines whether the transport adds value to the patient's care continuum or merely moves the patient from one location to another without preserving the clinical narrative that only the transport crew was positioned to observe.

The clinical scenarios addressed in this chapter illustrate a principle that recurs throughout the text: the transport environment does not merely add logistic complexity to the management of critical illness--it introduces specific physiologic stressors that interact with the patient's underlying condition to produce clinical changes that would not occur at the bedside. The altitude-related gas expansion, preload shifts, oxygenation challenges, and monitoring degradation described in Chapter 1, combined with the pharmacologic and equipment considerations from Chapters 4 and 5, create a modified clinical environment in which every bedside management principle must be re-examined through the lens of transport-specific risk. The disease-specific management recommendations in this chapter have been written with this re-examination already performed, incorporating the transport modifications into the clinical recommendations rather than presenting bedside management followed by a separate list of transport considerations, because the integration of disease knowledge and transport awareness is the competency that this text is designed to develop.

Inter-professional collaboration during the management of the conditions in this chapter deserves specific emphasis, because the complexity of many transport patients exceeds the capability of any single clinician acting alone. The nurse-paramedic team, the nurse-physician team, or whatever crew configuration the program uses represents a collaborative unit whose combined clinical capability exceeds the sum of its individual members, provided that the communication, role allocation, and shared mental model practices described in Chapter 24 are actively maintained throughout the transport. A transport in which one crew member manages the airway while the other manages hemodynamics, with both monitoring different aspects of the same clinical picture and cross-checking each other's assessments, produces a more complete and reliable clinical picture than either clinician could achieve alone, and this collaborative advantage is greatest during the high-workload, high-stress scenarios that the conditions in this chapter frequently produce.

Quality improvement in the management of these conditions during transport depends on systematic outcome tracking that links transport-specific management decisions to patient outcomes at the receiving facility. Did the patient who received a specific intervention during transport have a better or worse outcome than comparable patients who did not? Did a specific monitoring strategy detect deterioration earlier and allow more effective intervention? Did advance communication with the receiving facility produce measurably faster time-to-treatment on arrival? These questions can only be answered by programs that collect and analyze outcome data systematically, and the transport clinician's contribution to this process is meticulous, contemporaneous documentation of every clinical decision, every intervention, and every trajectory observation during the transport, since this documentation is the raw material from which quality improvement insights are derived. A transport program that does not analyze its outcomes cannot improve them, and a transport clinician who does not document their clinical reasoning cannot contribute to the program's learning.

**THE IN-TRANSIT DETERIORATION SIGNATURE SYSTEM — Mechanical Circulatory Support Deterioration Patterns**

---

**Signature Introduced This Chapter:** Suction-Event Cascade at Altitude (intermittent, escalating flow alarms with oscillating power consumption during ascent, progressing toward ventricular collapse if preload is not restored).

**Device Pattern Logic:** This Signature extends the Ascent-Triggered Device Flow Compromise from Chapter 1 to its most severe expression: where Chapter 1 described a mild, self-limited flow decline, this chapter describes the progressive cascade from mild reduction through intermittent suction events to full ventricular collapse, emphasizing that early intervention at the first intermittent alarm prevents progression to the catastrophic endpoint.

**Cross-Reference Forward:** The anticoagulation management principles extend to any device-dependent patient; Chapter 12 (Pneumothorax and Thoracic Emergencies) addresses the interaction between ECMO cannulation and thoracic decompression in the multiply injured patient.

## Summary and Key Concepts

IABP timing depends on clean trigger signal quality, which vibration can degrade; the augmented arterial waveform must be inspected visually at regular intervals rather than assumed correct from pump cycling alone.

Continuous-flow VAD flow is preload- and afterload-dependent, making altitude-related preload reduction a predictable and manageable cause of flow alarms that should not be reflexively attributed to pump thrombus.

ECMO transport is the highest-complexity critical care transport, requiring dedicated team training, rehearsed emergency protocols, and uninterrupted anticoagulation and power supply.

Device alarms should be triaged by assessing the patient first, correlating the alarm with hemodynamic trend and environmental context, and checking for positional or altitude-related triggers before pursuing device-focused troubleshooting.

Heparin infusion continuity is non-negotiable for mechanical support circuits; even brief interruption can precipitate circuit thrombosis that is immediately device-disabling.

# CHAPTER 10: ACUTE STROKE AND NEUROVASCULAR EMERGENCIES IN TRANSIT

**Learning Objectives**

1. Recognize ischemic stroke presentations including large vessel occlusion screening findings relevant to transport triage decisions.
2. Apply blood pressure management guidelines specific to acute ischemic and hemorrhagic stroke during interfacility transport.
3. Manage patients with subarachnoid hemorrhage and identify vasospasm-related deterioration during transit.
4. Prioritize time-sensitive interventions for thrombectomy-bound and thrombolytic-eligible stroke transfers.
5. Perform serial neurologic reassessment during transport using a structured, reproducible method.

**Chapter Outline**

This chapter addresses the transport of patients with acute cerebrovascular emergencies, the most time-sensitive neurologic conditions encountered in interfacility transport. The clinical value of these transports is measured in minutes: every minute of delay between symptom onset and revascularization in acute ischemic stroke with large vessel occlusion translates directly into measurable loss of neural tissue, and the transport team's contribution to outcome operates primarily through the same process-efficiency and advance-activation framework developed for acute coronary syndrome transfers in Chapter 6.

## Ischemic Stroke Recognition and Thrombolytic/Thrombectomy-Bound Transfer

### Large Vessel Occlusion Screening for Transport Triage

The critical triage decision for acute ischemic stroke in the transport setting is whether the patient has a large vessel occlusion amenable to endovascular thrombectomy, since this determination dictates the receiving facility selection: a patient with a suspected large vessel occlusion should be transported to a comprehensive stroke center with thrombectomy capability rather than a primary stroke center that can administer thrombolytics but cannot perform catheter-based intervention. Validated prehospital and interfacility screening scales--assessing for cortical signs such as gaze deviation, neglect, aphasia, and the severity of contralateral motor deficit--provide a structured method for estimating the probability of a large vessel occlusion at the bedside, even without confirmatory imaging, and should be applied systematically for every acute stroke transfer rather than relying on an unstructured clinical impression.

**Thrombolytic Administration and Monitoring During Transport**

Intravenous thrombolytic therapy (alteplase or tenecteplase) for acute ischemic stroke may be initiated at the sending facility before transport, during transport if the sending facility lacks the capability or if the time window favors in-transit administration, or deferred to the receiving facility if the remaining time window allows and the transport time is short. When thrombolytic therapy is administered before or during transport, the crew must monitor for the most serious complication--symptomatic intracranial hemorrhage--through serial neurologic assessment and blood pressure monitoring, since a sudden worsening in neurologic examination during or after thrombolytic administration should be treated as intracranial hemorrhage until proven otherwise, with immediate cessation of the thrombolytic infusion, blood pressure management, and communication with the receiving facility to prepare for emergent imaging and possible neurosurgical intervention on arrival.

**Advance Activation of the Receiving Stroke Team**

The transport team's single most impactful contribution to time-to-treatment for stroke transfers, paralleling the catheterization laboratory activation described for STEMI in Chapter 6, is advance activation of the receiving facility's stroke response: notifying the neurointervention team, transmitting imaging or clinical data for remote review, confirming the patient meets thrombectomy or thrombolytic criteria based on the transport team's own assessment, and providing an accurate estimated time of arrival that allows the receiving team to have the angiography suite staffed and ready on arrival. Every minute saved through advance activation translates directly into preserved neural tissue, making this communication step as clinically consequential as any medication or procedure the crew administers during transit.

**KEY POINT:** For thrombectomy-eligible stroke transfers, advance activation of the receiving neurointervention team is as clinically consequential as any medication administered during transit; every minute of delay between arrival and arterial access translates into measurable neural tissue loss.

| Stroke Transfer Type | Time Priority | Key Transport Action | Receiving Facility Requirement |
|---|---|---|---|
| LVO with thrombectomy eligibility | Highest -- time = brain tissue | Advance neurointervention activation; direct to angiography suite | Comprehensive stroke center |
| Thrombolytic-eligible, no LVO | High -- treatment within time window | Administer or continue thrombolytic; monitor for hemorrhagic conversion | Primary or comprehensive stroke center |

| | | | |
|---|---|---|---|
| Hemorrhagic stroke | High -- neurosurgical evaluation | Blood pressure management; ICP precautions | Facility with neurosurgical capability |
| SAH with suspected vasospasm | High -- definitive aneurysm management | Hemodynamic augmentation; nimodipine continuation | Comprehensive stroke/neurovascular center |

## Hemorrhagic Stroke and Blood Pressure Management

### Intracerebral Hemorrhage and Hematoma Expansion Prevention

Acute intracerebral hemorrhage management during transport centers on blood pressure control to reduce the risk of ongoing hematoma expansion, the primary modifiable driver of early neurologic deterioration. Current evidence supports intensive blood pressure lowering to a systolic target below one hundred forty millimeters of mercury within the first hours of symptom onset, using the titratable intravenous agents described in Chapter 7--nicardipine and clevidipine are preferred for their predictable dose-response and short half-life, which allow the crew to approach the target gradually without overshooting into the hypotensive range that would compromise cerebral perfusion.

### Coagulopathy Reversal in Anticoagulant-Associated Hemorrhage

Intracerebral hemorrhage in a patient receiving anticoagulation therapy--whether warfarin, a direct oral anticoagulant, or heparin--is a particularly urgent subset because the ongoing coagulopathy drives continued hematoma expansion and worsens the neurologic prognosis. Reversal of warfarin with four-factor prothrombin complex concentrate, reversal of dabigatran with idarucizumab, and reversal of factor Xa inhibitors with andexanet alfa or, where unavailable, four-factor prothrombin complex concentrate should be initiated at the earliest opportunity, ideally at the sending facility before transport but during transport if the sending facility did not administer it. The transport clinician should confirm whether reversal has been given, what agent was used, and whether the effect has been confirmed by a post-reversal coagulation study, since incomplete or unverified reversal changes the urgency and management on arrival.

### Neuroprotective Positioning and Environmental Management

Head-of-bed elevation to thirty degrees, midline head positioning to optimize jugular venous drainage, avoidance of cervical collar over-tightening that can impede venous outflow, and maintenance of normothermia and normoglycemia are standard neuroprotective measures that should be applied to every patient with acute intracranial hemorrhage during transport. These positioning requirements interact with the stretcher configuration and loading constraints described in Chapter 5, and should be verified after every patient repositioning during the transport, since the tilt and movement of loading can inadvertently alter head position.

## Glucose Management and Hypoglycemia Exclusion

Hypoglycemia can mimic or worsen the neurologic deficits of acute stroke, and point-of-care glucose measurement should be obtained early in the assessment of any patient with acute neurologic change, both at the sending facility and at fixed intervals during transport if the patient is receiving insulin or has a history of diabetes. Hyperglycemia, which is common in acute stroke and is associated with worse neurologic outcomes, should be treated with insulin therapy targeting a glucose range that avoids both extremes, since overcorrection into hypoglycemia is at least as dangerous as the hyperglycemia itself and can produce a neurologic decline that is indistinguishable from stroke progression without a glucose check.

## Temperature Management and Fever Prevention

Fever in acute stroke is associated with worse outcomes through mechanisms that include increased metabolic demand in ischemic tissue, enhanced excitotoxicity, and blood-brain barrier disruption, and should be treated aggressively with antipyretic therapy and active cooling measures during transport. The transport environment can contribute to temperature dysregulation in both directions: hypothermia from cabin exposure in cooler conditions, and hyperthermia from inadequate cabin cooling in warm environments or from covering the patient with insulation intended for the opposite extreme. Temperature should be monitored continuously, ideally via an esophageal or bladder probe rather than an axillary or forehead sensor, since core temperature is the clinically relevant measure and surface temperature can be misleading in a patient exposed to the variable thermal environment of a transport cabin.

## Seizure Surveillance and Management During Stroke Transport

Seizures complicate approximately five to ten percent of acute strokes, particularly hemorrhagic strokes and cortical ischemic events, and can produce secondary neurologic injury through increased metabolic demand in already-compromised brain tissue, aspiration risk, and hemodynamic instability. The transport clinician should be prepared to administer first-line benzodiazepine therapy for any witnessed seizure, and should maintain a heightened index of suspicion for nonconvulsive seizure activity--manifesting as unexplained fluctuations in level of consciousness, subtle repetitive movements, or gaze deviation that is out of proportion to the known stroke territory--since nonconvulsive seizures are clinically invisible without electroencephalographic monitoring and can only be suspected from the clinical pattern during transport. Any suspected seizure during a stroke transport should be communicated to the receiving team, since it may change the receiving team's priorities to include emergent electroencephalography and anticonvulsant loading on arrival.

## Airway Protection Decisions in Acute Stroke

The decision to intubate a stroke patient before transport involves weighing the airway protection benefit against the risks of the procedure itself and the loss of the neurologic examination that intubation with sedation and paralysis produces. A patient with a severely depressed level of consciousness, absent protective airway reflexes, or active vomiting should be intubated before transport, since managing these airway threats reactively during transit is substantially more dangerous than securing the airway proactively at a stationary bedside. However, a patient with a moderate neurologic deficit and preserved consciousness and airway reflexes should generally not be intubated prophylactically, since the neurologic examination during transport is the primary clinical tool available to the crew and the receiving team, and ablating it through sedation eliminates the trajectory information that Chapter 2 established as the transport clinician's most valuable contribution.

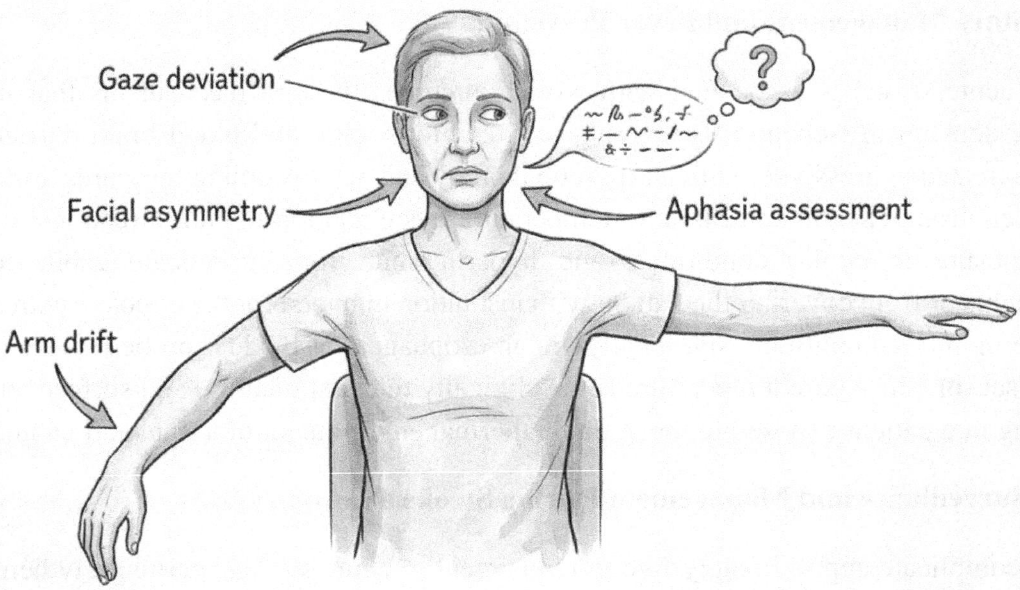


Figure 10.1: Large Vessel Occlusion Screening Assessment

**THE IN-TRANSIT DETERIORATION SIGNATURE SYSTEM — Altitude-Potentiated Intracranial Pressure Elevation**

**The Signature:** New or worsening signs of elevated intracranial pressure--declining level of consciousness, new pupillary asymmetry, progressive hypertension with bradycardia, or new vomiting--that develop during ascent or at altitude in a patient with acute intracranial hemorrhage or cerebral edema.

**Movement Trigger:** The gas-law expansion described in Chapter 1 can increase the volume of any intracranial air (pneumocephalus from recent surgery, trauma, or a small air collection associated with the hemorrhage itself) and, through the reduction in atmospheric pressure, alter the transmural pressure gradients that govern cerebral venous drainage, potentially contributing to a net increase in intracranial volume and pressure.

**Early Tell:** A subtle decline in Glasgow Coma Scale score or a new-onset headache worsening temporally linked to the ascent phase, detected through the serial neurologic reassessment framework described later in this chapter, before any pupillary or vital sign changes appear.

**Trap Logic:** This pattern is easily attributed to natural disease progression rather than recognized as an altitude-potentiated event, because the clinical signs of elevated intracranial pressure look identical regardless of the cause. The discriminating feature is the temporal relationship to altitude change, which should prompt consideration of cabin altitude restriction or descent as a therapeutic maneuver.

**Signature Anchor:** In any patient with acute intracranial pathology transported by air, treat new neurologic deterioration temporally linked to ascent as potentially altitude-potentiated and respond with a request for lower cabin altitude, head-of-bed elevation confirmation, and hyperosmolar therapy readiness, in addition to standard neuroprotective interventions.

## Subarachnoid Hemorrhage and Vasospasm Considerations

### Securing the Aneurysm: Transport Priority and Rebleeding Prevention

Patients with aneurysmal subarachnoid hemorrhage are typically transferred for definitive aneurysm securing--either surgical clipping or endovascular coiling--at a comprehensive neurovascular center, and the transport management priority is preventing rebleeding during transit, which carries a catastrophic mortality risk. Blood pressure management targets for unsecured aneurysmal subarachnoid hemorrhage are typically more conservative than for intracerebral hemorrhage, targeting a systolic pressure below one hundred sixty millimeters of mercury or below the patient's known chronic baseline, whichever is lower, to reduce the transmural pressure across the aneurysm dome while maintaining adequate cerebral perfusion.

### Vasospasm Recognition and Hemodynamic Augmentation

Cerebral vasospasm, the delayed narrowing of intracranial arteries that produces secondary ischemia days to weeks after the initial hemorrhage, is primarily a concern for patients transferred during the vasospasm window rather than in the acute phase, but the transport clinician should be aware that a patient presenting with new or worsening focal neurologic deficits during the vasospasm-risk period may be experiencing vasospasm-mediated ischemia rather than rebleeding, and the management of these two complications is opposite: vasospasm is treated with hemodynamic augmentation (volume expansion and induced hypertension to drive flow through narrowed vessels), while rebleeding is treated with blood pressure reduction. Differentiating these two complications during transport without access to advanced imaging requires close clinical assessment and, where the clinical picture is ambiguous, communication with the receiving neurosurgical team for guidance on which management strategy to prioritize.

Hemodynamic augmentation for vasospasm during transport involves raising the mean arterial pressure above the patient's baseline using vasopressor therapy, typically with norepinephrine or phenylephrine, while maintaining euvolemia through crystalloid infusion. The target blood pressure for augmentation is typically individualized based on the patient's neurologic response: the pressure is raised incrementally until neurologic improvement is observed or a predefined ceiling is reached, and the transport crew should communicate with the receiving team to establish the specific augmentation target before departure. Overshoot beyond the target carries a risk of exacerbating cerebral edema or precipitating rebleeding from an unsecured aneurysm, making continuous arterial pressure monitoring a requirement rather than an option for any vasospasm patient undergoing hemodynamic augmentation during transport.

### Posterior Circulation Stroke and Diagnostic Challenges in Transport

Posterior circulation strokes involving the vertebrobasilar system present a specific diagnostic challenge during transport because their clinical presentation--vertigo, diplopia, dysarthria, ataxia, and altered level of consciousness--can be subtle, fluctuating, and easily mistaken for a non-stroke etiology such as vestibular disease or metabolic encephalopathy, particularly in a transport environment where a comprehensive neurologic examination is difficult to perform. A basilar artery occlusion producing progressive brainstem dysfunction is among the most rapidly lethal stroke presentations, and the transport clinician's clinical suspicion for this diagnosis should be high in any patient with acute-onset posterior circulation symptoms, even when the presentation appears initially mild, because the trajectory from mild brainstem symptoms to coma and respiratory arrest can be measured in minutes to hours. Serial reassessment during transport should specifically include assessment of brainstem function--pupillary reactivity, corneal reflexes, and the oculocephalic response where appropriate--in addition to the standard Glasgow Coma Scale and motor assessment.

### Nimodipine Administration and Monitoring

Nimodipine, a calcium channel blocker with relative selectivity for cerebral vasculature, is standard prophylactic therapy against vasospasm following aneurysmal subarachnoid hemorrhage and should be continued without interruption during transport. The principal transport-specific consideration is the hypotension that nimodipine can produce, which may be compounded by the altitude-related preload reduction and positional hemodynamic shifts described in Chapter 1, and the crew should be prepared to manage this with volume support or vasopressor therapy rather than by discontinuing a medication that has evidence-based neuroprotective benefit.

## Large Vessel Occlusion Screening for Transport Triage

### Validated Screening Scales and Their Transport Application

Several validated prehospital and interfacility screening scales have been developed specifically to identify patients with a high probability of large vessel occlusion who should bypass a primary stroke center in favor of a comprehensive stroke center with thrombectomy capability. These scales typically assess a combination of cortical signs and motor deficit severity, and while none has perfect sensitivity or specificity, their systematic application produces more accurate triage decisions than unstructured clinical judgment alone, particularly when applied by clinicians whose primary training is in critical care transport rather than neurology. The transport clinician should be trained in the specific scale used by their regional stroke system and should apply it to every acute ischemic stroke transfer to ensure that the receiving facility selection matches the patient's likely intervention needs.

Figure 10.2: Head Positioning and Neuroprotective Stretcher Configuration

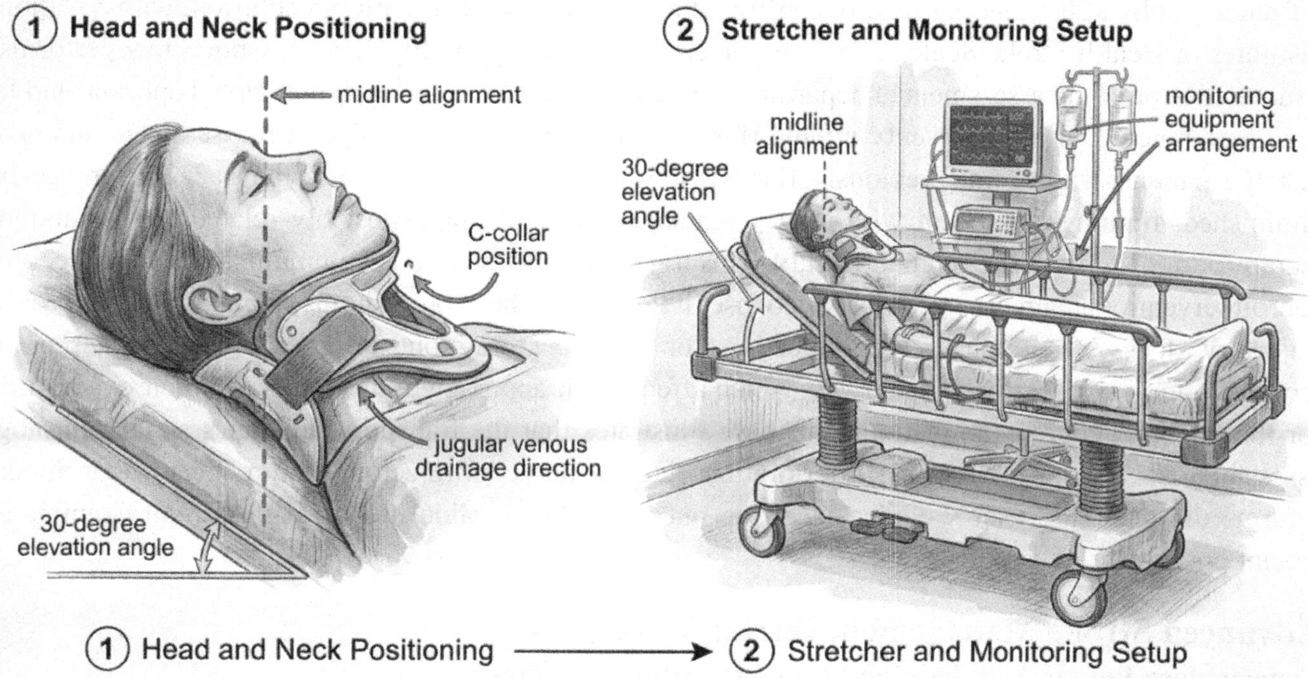


## Neurologic Reassessment During Transit

### Structured Serial Neurologic Examination

Serial neurologic reassessment during stroke transport follows the same trend-based monitoring principle established in Chapter 2, applied to the neurologic domain: the Glasgow Coma Scale score, pupillary size and reactivity, motor response in all extremities, and any lateralizing findings should be assessed at fixed intervals and documented with timestamps, so that the receiving team receives a trajectory rather than a single arrival examination. A worsening Glasgow Coma Scale score, new pupillary asymmetry, or loss of a previously present motor response during transport is a clinically decisive finding that should trigger immediate communication with the receiving team and consideration of whether the deterioration reflects a potentially reversible cause--such as hypoglycemia, hypotension, or a new seizure--or represents primary neurologic progression requiring emergent intervention on arrival.

### Challenges of Neurologic Assessment in the Transport Environment

Neurologic assessment during transport is more challenging than at the bedside because ambient noise obscures verbal responses, cabin lighting may be inadequate for pupillary assessment without a dedicated penlight, and the patient's position on the transport stretcher may limit the clinician's ability to assess motor strength symmetrically. A dedicated penlight should be immediately accessible for pupillary assessment at every reassessment interval, and the clinician should establish a consistent verbal assessment technique--loud, clear, and repeated commands adapted to the noise level--to ensure that apparent verbal unresponsiveness represents a genuine neurologic finding rather than the patient's inability to hear the examiner over cabin noise.

Consider a seventy-one-year-old woman transferred by rotor-wing for endovascular thrombectomy after CT angiography at the sending facility confirmed a left middle cerebral artery occlusion, with a National Institutes of Health Stroke Scale score of eighteen at the sending facility. The transport crew performs a structured neurologic assessment at departure, confirming right-sided hemiplegia, global aphasia, and left gaze preference. During the twenty-minute flight, the crew performs a midpoint reassessment and notes that the patient's right arm, previously flaccid, now withdraws to pain, and the gaze preference has diminished, findings consistent with early spontaneous improvement possibly related to thrombolytic therapy administered at the sending facility. This trajectory information is communicated to the receiving neurointervention team in real time, who use it to adjust their procedural planning: the improving trajectory does not eliminate the indication for thrombectomy but informs the team that partial recanalization may already be underway, which affects their approach to the vessel and their expectations for the post-procedure examination. This case illustrates that the transport clinician's serial neurologic assessment serves not merely as a deterioration detector but as a trajectory communicator that directly informs the receiving team's clinical decision-making, adding value that a single arrival examination cannot provide.

## Advanced Stroke Management During Transport

### Tenecteplase Versus Alteplase for Transport Administration

Tenecteplase, a modified tissue plasminogen activator with a longer half-life that allows single-bolus administration rather than the hour-long infusion required for alteplase, has emerged as an increasingly attractive thrombolytic option for the transport setting specifically because of its logistic simplicity: a single intravenous push, given over five seconds, replaces an infusion pump, an hour of monitoring the infusion rate, and the risk of interruption or miscalculation that accompanies any continuous infusion during transport. Current evidence supports tenecteplase as non-inferior to alteplase for acute ischemic stroke, with comparable efficacy and safety profiles, and several national stroke guidelines have incorporated tenecteplase as an acceptable alternative. The transport clinician should know which agent their program carries and be prepared to administer it within the time window, recognizing that the simplicity of tenecteplase's bolus dosing is a genuine clinical advantage in the transport environment where infusion complexity is a liability.

### Mobile Stroke Unit Integration With Transport Medicine

Mobile stroke units--ambulances equipped with CT scanners, telemedicine capability, and thrombolytic medications--represent the intersection of stroke care and transport medicine, enabling prehospital imaging, diagnosis, and treatment initiation that can save thirty to sixty minutes compared to the traditional pathway of transport-to-hospital-to-imaging-to-treatment. Where available, mobile stroke unit deployment for stroke patients allows thrombolytic administration at the scene based on CT confirmation of ischemic stroke, transforming the transport from a pre-treatment conveyance into a post-treatment continuation-of-care transfer. The transport clinician operating within a mobile stroke unit system should understand the imaging and treatment protocols specific to that system, the telemedicine communication standards, and the integration of mobile stroke unit findings into the receiving facility's workflow.

## Stroke Mimics and the Differential Diagnosis During Transport

Not every patient transferred with a diagnosis of acute stroke actually has a stroke, and the transport clinician should maintain awareness of the common stroke mimics that can present with acute focal neurologic deficits: hypoglycemia (which should be excluded by point-of-care glucose in every patient with acute neurologic change), seizure with post-ictal Todd paralysis, complex migraine with aura, conversion disorder, intracranial mass lesion with acute decompensation, and drug intoxication or withdrawal. The transport clinician's role is not to definitively exclude these mimics during transport--that requires the imaging and laboratory resources of the receiving facility--but to ensure that easily reversible causes (hypoglycemia, opioid overdose) are identified and treated during transit and that the clinical trajectory is communicated to the receiving team so that their differential diagnosis is informed by the transport crew's observations.

## Acute Cerebral Venous Thrombosis in Transport

Cerebral venous sinus thrombosis presents with headache, seizures, focal neurologic deficits, and signs of elevated intracranial pressure that can mimic arterial stroke or subarachnoid hemorrhage, and is diagnosed definitively by CT venography or MR venography at the receiving facility. The transport management is anticoagulation with heparin (which may seem counterintuitive given that many patients with cerebral venous thrombosis also have associated hemorrhagic infarction, but anticoagulation has been shown to be safe and effective in this population) and management of elevated intracranial pressure using the principles from Chapter 11. The transport clinician should be aware that this diagnosis exists, that its management includes anticoagulation even in the presence of hemorrhage, and that the patient may require the same ICP monitoring and neuroprotective measures applied to other intracranial pathologies during transport.

## Blood Pressure Management Nuances Across Stroke Subtypes

Blood pressure management targets differ across stroke subtypes in ways that the transport clinician must actively reconcile rather than applying a single target to all stroke patients. Acute ischemic stroke without thrombolytic therapy: permissive hypertension up to 220/120 is generally acceptable, and aggressive lowering is avoided to maintain collateral perfusion to the ischemic penumbra. Acute ischemic stroke with thrombolytic therapy: the target drops to below 180/105 to reduce the risk of hemorrhagic transformation. Intracerebral hemorrhage: intensive lowering to systolic below 140 within the first hours reduces hematoma expansion. Subarachnoid hemorrhage with unsecured aneurysm: systolic below 160 to reduce rebleeding risk. The transport clinician should confirm the specific subtype and whether thrombolytics have been administered, then apply the correct target, since applying the permissive hypertension appropriate for untreated ischemic stroke to a patient who has received a thrombolytic exposes the patient to a hemorrhagic transformation risk that is directly preventable by tighter control.

## Additional Clinical Considerations for Transport Management

The management of patients in Chapter 10 requires attention to several additional transport-specific clinical factors that extend the principles established in the main body of the chapter. The transport clinician should be aware that the disease processes covered here interact with the transport environment in ways that are specific to the combination of the underlying pathophysiology and the particular environmental stressor encountered during a given mission, and that a management approach that is adequate for a short ground transport may be insufficient for a longer air transport at altitude, or vice versa. The serial reassessment protocol established in Chapter 2 provides the framework for detecting these interactions as they develop, and the Deterioration Signature introduced in this chapter names the most characteristic pattern by which they declare themselves.

Each patient transport is a unique combination of a specific patient's physiology, a specific set of ongoing therapies, a specific transport platform with its own environmental characteristics, and a specific mission profile with its own altitude, duration, and route constraints. The anticipatory approach to transport medicine that this text teaches is not a set of memorized responses to predetermined scenarios but a cognitive framework for analyzing the specific combination of variables present in any given transport and identifying, before departure, the most likely points of vulnerability where the transport environment will test the patient's physiologic reserve. This chapter's clinical content provides the disease-specific knowledge needed to apply that framework to the conditions covered here, while the Deterioration Signature provides the named pattern that makes the most characteristic transport-specific vulnerability explicit, recognizable, and actionable.

The receiving team's ability to continue the patient's care seamlessly after the transport crew departs depends entirely on the quality and completeness of the clinical information the transport crew provides, and for the conditions covered in this chapter, the specific information that matters most includes: the trajectory of the patient's primary condition during transport (improving, stable, or worsening, with specific details), any interventions performed during transport and their response, any new clinical findings identified by the transport crew that were not present at the sending facility, and any anticipated needs that the receiving team should prepare for based on the transport crew's clinical assessment. This information, communicated through the structured handoff format established in Chapter 2 and supplemented by the trajectory communication emphasis that is a recurring theme throughout this text, is the final clinical act of the transport and the one that determines whether the transport adds value to the patient's care continuum or merely moves the patient from one location to another without preserving the clinical narrative that only the transport crew was positioned to observe.

The clinical scenarios addressed in this chapter illustrate a principle that recurs throughout the text: the transport environment does not merely add logistic complexity to the management of critical illness--it introduces specific physiologic stressors that interact with the patient's underlying condition to produce clinical changes that would not occur at the bedside. The altitude-related gas expansion, preload shifts, oxygenation challenges, and monitoring degradation described in Chapter 1, combined with the pharmacologic and equipment considerations from Chapters 4 and 5, create a modified clinical environment in which every bedside management principle must be re-examined through the lens of transport-specific risk. The disease-specific management recommendations in this chapter have been written with this re-examination already performed, incorporating the transport modifications into the clinical recommendations rather than presenting bedside management followed by a separate list of transport considerations, because the integration of disease knowledge and transport awareness is the competency that this text is designed to develop.

Inter-professional collaboration during the management of the conditions in this chapter deserves specific emphasis, because the complexity of many transport patients exceeds the capability of any single clinician acting alone. The nurse-paramedic team, the nurse-physician team, or whatever crew configuration the program uses represents a collaborative unit whose combined clinical capability exceeds the sum of its individual members, provided that the communication, role allocation, and shared mental model practices described in Chapter 24 are actively maintained throughout the transport. A transport in which one crew member manages the airway while the other manages hemodynamics, with both monitoring different aspects of the same clinical picture and cross-checking each other's assessments, produces a more complete and reliable clinical picture than either clinician could achieve alone, and this collaborative advantage is greatest during the high-workload, high-stress scenarios that the conditions in this chapter frequently produce.

Quality improvement in the management of these conditions during transport depends on systematic outcome tracking that links transport-specific management decisions to patient outcomes at the receiving facility. Did the patient who received a specific intervention during transport have a better or worse outcome than comparable patients who did not? Did a specific monitoring strategy detect deterioration earlier and allow more effective intervention? Did advance communication with the receiving facility produce measurably faster time-to-treatment on arrival? These questions can only be answered by programs that collect and analyze outcome data systematically, and the transport clinician's contribution to this process is meticulous, contemporaneous documentation of every clinical decision, every intervention, and every trajectory observation during the transport, since this documentation is the raw material from which quality improvement insights are derived. A transport program that does not analyze its outcomes cannot improve them, and a transport clinician who does not document their clinical reasoning cannot contribute to the program's learning.

## THE IN-TRANSIT DETERIORATION SIGNATURE SYSTEM — Neurovascular Emergency Patterns

**Signature Introduced This Chapter:** Altitude-Potentiated Intracranial Pressure Elevation (new or worsening signs of elevated ICP temporally linked to ascent in a patient with acute intracranial pathology, driven by gas-expansion and transmural pressure changes at altitude).

**Neurovascular Pattern Logic:** This Signature connects the altitude-physiology foundation from Chapter 1 to the neurologic domain, extending the same gas-expansion principle that drove the Occult Pneumothorax Expansion Signature to intracranial air and pressure dynamics.

**Cross-Reference Forward:** Chapter 11 (Traumatic Brain Injury) extends the ICP management and altitude interaction principles to the trauma population; Chapter 12 (Status Epilepticus) addresses seizure-related neurologic deterioration during transport.

## Summary and Key Concepts

Large vessel occlusion screening using validated scales should be applied to every acute ischemic stroke transfer to ensure appropriate receiving facility selection.

Advance activation of the receiving neurointervention team is as clinically consequential as any medication administered during transit; every minute of delay translates into neural tissue loss.

Hemorrhagic stroke blood pressure management targets systolic below one hundred forty within the first hours; coagulopathy reversal should be initiated at the earliest opportunity.

Subarachnoid hemorrhage management during transport prioritizes rebleeding prevention through blood pressure control, with awareness that vasospasm requires the opposite hemodynamic strategy.

Serial neurologic reassessment at fixed intervals provides trajectory information that directly informs the receiving team's clinical decision-making and adds value beyond a single arrival examination.

Altitude-related gas expansion and pressure changes can potentiate intracranial pressure elevation in patients with acute intracranial pathology, making cabin altitude restriction a therapeutic intervention.

# CHAPTER 11: TRAUMATIC BRAIN INJURY AND INTRACRANIAL PRESSURE MANAGEMENT IN TRANSIT

**Learning Objectives**

1. Apply primary and secondary brain injury prevention principles adapted to the transport environment.
2. Interpret intracranial pressure monitoring data and waveform morphology during transit.
3. Administer hyperosmolar therapy and manage herniation syndromes en route.
4. Optimize ventilation strategies to maintain cerebral perfusion pressure targets during transport.
5. Coordinate cervical spine precautions with airway and positioning requirements in the multiply injured patient.

**Chapter Outline**

This chapter addresses the transport of patients with traumatic brain injury, extending the neuroprotective principles introduced in Chapter 10 to the specific pathophysiology and management challenges of traumatic intracranial injury. The transport clinician's central task is preventing secondary brain injury--the cascade of ischemia, edema, and metabolic failure that follows the primary mechanical insult--by maintaining cerebral perfusion pressure, avoiding hypoxemia and hypotension, and managing intracranial pressure through the physiologically hostile transit window.

## Primary and Secondary Brain Injury Prevention

### The Secondary Injury Cascade and Modifiable Transport Variables

Primary brain injury occurs at the moment of impact and is not modifiable by the transport clinician; what is modifiable is the secondary injury cascade--cerebral ischemia from hypotension, hypoxemia-driven neuronal injury, cerebral edema from hyperglycemia and hyperthermia, and excitotoxic damage amplified by seizure activity--each of which has a specific, evidence-based prevention strategy that the transport clinician must apply continuously throughout the transit window. A single episode of hypotension, defined as a systolic blood pressure below ninety millimeters of mercury in the adult, is independently associated with a doubling of mortality in moderate-to-severe traumatic brain injury, and the transport clinician's most impactful intervention may be nothing more sophisticated than maintaining adequate blood pressure throughout a thirty-minute flight--an intervention whose simplicity belies its outsized effect on outcome.

### Hypotension Avoidance and Blood Pressure Targets

Current guidelines for traumatic brain injury management recommend maintaining a systolic blood pressure at or above one hundred millimeters of mercury, and ideally above one hundred ten, throughout the acute phase, a target that directly conflicts with the altitude-related preload reduction and positional hemodynamic shifts described in Chapter 1. The transport clinician should establish continuous arterial pressure monitoring before departure for any patient with moderate-to-severe traumatic brain injury, and should have vasopressor therapy immediately available rather than deferred to a reactive deployment after hypotension has already occurred, since even a brief hypotensive episode during transit represents a potentially irreversible secondary insult to the injured brain.

### Hypoxemia Prevention and Oxygenation Targets

Hypoxemia is the second major modifiable secondary insult, and the transport clinician should target an oxygen saturation above ninety-four percent throughout transit, anticipating the altitude-related reduction in alveolar oxygen tension described in Chapter 1 and requesting a lower cabin altitude or increasing supplemental oxygen proactively rather than reactively. Hyperoxia, conversely, has been associated with worse outcomes in some traumatic brain injury populations through oxygen free radical-mediated injury, and the oxygenation target should aim for the normoxic range rather than supranormal values, a nuance that distinguishes evidence-based neuroprotective oxygen management from the reflexive maximal supplementation that is sometimes applied in the prehospital setting.

**KEY POINT:** A single episode of hypotension (systolic below 90 mmHg) in moderate-to-severe TBI is independently associated with doubled mortality; maintaining blood pressure above target throughout transport is one of the highest-impact interventions the transport clinician can deliver.

### Coagulopathy Assessment and Reversal in Traumatic Brain Injury

Traumatic brain injury releases tissue factor from damaged brain parenchyma, triggering a consumptive coagulopathy that can worsen intracranial hemorrhage and is present in up to a third of patients with severe traumatic brain injury at admission. The transport clinician should ascertain whether coagulation studies have been obtained at the sending facility and whether any reversal agents--fresh frozen plasma, prothrombin complex concentrate, tranexamic acid, or platelet transfusion--have been administered or are indicated. Tranexamic acid, an antifibrinolytic agent, has been studied in traumatic brain injury and is most likely beneficial when administered within three hours of injury, making the transport window a relevant treatment interval for patients being transferred early after injury. The drug's favorable safety profile and ease of administration by intravenous infusion make it a practical transport intervention when the clinical picture includes traumatic intracranial hemorrhage within the time window.

## External Ventricular Drain Transport Protocol

Transporting a patient with an external ventricular drain requires a specific, rehearsed protocol that addresses the drain at every transition point during the transport: clamping before any position change or movement, re-leveling to the tragus after every position change, confirming drainage height against the neurosurgical team's prescribed drainage level, and monitoring for signs of overdrainage (sudden headache, decreased consciousness, new subdural hemorrhage) or underdrainage (rising ICP, worsening neurologic examination). The drain collection system must be secured to prevent spillage, siphoning from height changes, or inadvertent disconnection, and the crew member responsible for drain management should be identified and assigned before departure as part of the same team role allocation described in Chapter 2.

## Pediatric Traumatic Brain Injury Transport Considerations

Children with traumatic brain injury present transport-specific management differences from adults: age-appropriate blood pressure targets are lower than adult targets but carry the same importance for secondary injury prevention, weight-based dosing for hyperosmolar therapy and sedation must be calculated precisely using the child's actual weight, and the immature brain's greater vulnerability to secondary insult amplifies the consequence of even brief hypotensive or hypoxemic episodes during transit. The Cushing response--hypertension with bradycardia as a late sign of herniation--may be less reliable in younger children, making serial pupillary assessment and GCS trending even more important as early herniation indicators in this population.

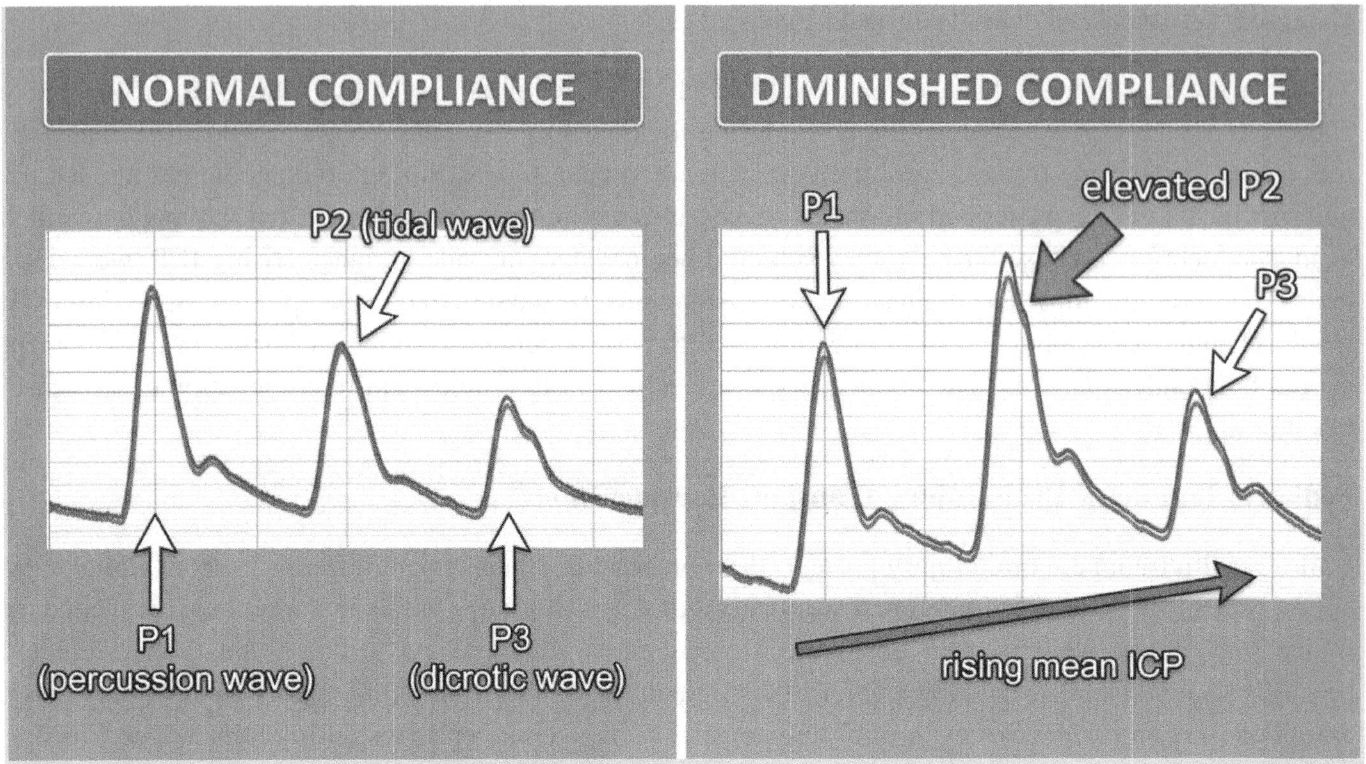


## Intracranial Pressure Monitoring and Waveform Interpretation

### ICP Monitor Types and Transport Compatibility

Patients transferred with intracranial pressure monitors in place typically have either an external ventricular drain, which provides both monitoring and therapeutic cerebrospinal fluid drainage, or a parenchymal fiberoptic or strain-gauge monitor, which provides monitoring only. The external ventricular drain requires particular attention during transport: it must be leveled to a consistent anatomic reference point (typically the tragus of the ear, approximating the foramen of Monro), clamped during loading and any position change that would alter the drain height relative to the patient's head, and reopened at the correct height once the patient is settled in transport position, since an improperly leveled drain can produce either overdrainage (risking ventricular collapse and subdural hemorrhage) or underdrainage (allowing intracranial pressure to rise unchecked).

### Waveform Morphology and Plateau Waves

The intracranial pressure waveform, where displayed on the transport monitor, provides information beyond the numeric value alone: a progressive loss of waveform compliance--flattening of the pulsatile morphology and elevation of the mean pressure--signals diminishing intracranial compensatory reserve, even when the absolute pressure remains within the target range. Plateau waves (Lundberg A waves), characterized by sustained elevations in intracranial pressure to forty to eighty millimeters of mercury lasting five to twenty minutes, represent a near-exhaustion of compensatory capacity and should trigger immediate intervention--cerebrospinal fluid drainage if an external ventricular drain is in place, hyperosmolar therapy, and re-verification of head positioning and ventilation targets--rather than watchful observation of whether the wave will spontaneously resolve.

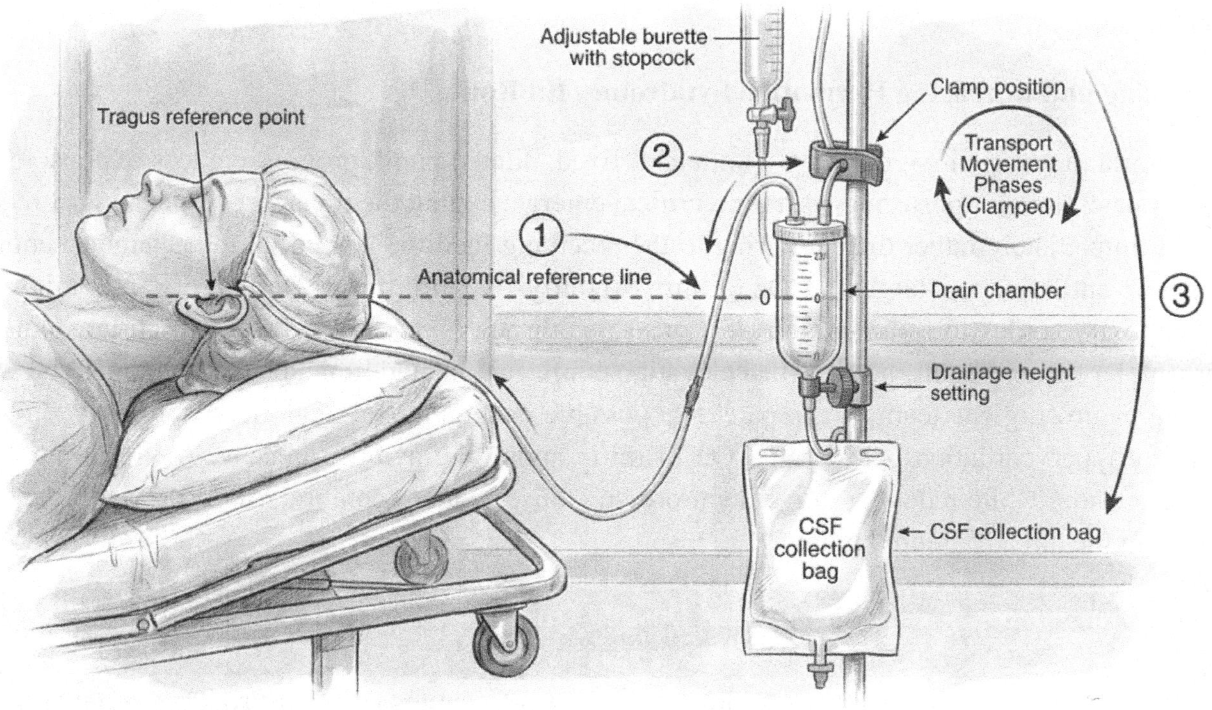


**Figure 11.2:** External Ventricular Drain Leveling and Clamping Protocol for Transport

### ICP Monitoring Troubleshooting During Transport

An ICP value that suddenly changes during transport should prompt a systematic check of the monitoring system before being accepted as a genuine physiologic event: for an external ventricular drain, the drain height relative to the tragus should be re-verified, the tubing should be inspected for kinking or air bubbles, and the transducer should be re-leveled and re-zeroed; for a parenchymal monitor, the cable connection and monitor display should be verified. A sudden, sustained ICP elevation that persists after system verification is a genuine clinical event requiring immediate treatment, while an abrupt, transient spike that coincides with a position change or a movement event and resolves spontaneously is more likely artifact or a brief, self-limited Lundberg B wave.

## Hyperosmolar Therapy and Herniation Management

### Mannitol and Hypertonic Saline: Selection and Administration

Hyperosmolar therapy with mannitol or hypertonic saline is the primary pharmacologic intervention for elevated intracranial pressure and impending herniation during transport. Mannitol, administered as an intravenous bolus, produces its osmotic effect within fifteen to thirty minutes and should be available in pre-measured doses for immediate administration; its principal transport-specific limitation is the osmotic diuresis it produces, which can exacerbate hypovolemia and hypotension in a patient who may already be volume-depleted from hemorrhage or inadequate resuscitation, making concurrent volume replacement and blood pressure monitoring essential. Hypertonic saline (typically three percent or twenty-three point four percent concentration) produces a comparable osmotic effect without the diuretic volume loss, making it the preferred agent in hypotensive patients or those in whom further volume depletion is unacceptable.

**Recognizing and Managing Herniation Syndromes En Route**

Transtentorial herniation--signaled by a unilateral fixed, dilated pupil, progressive loss of consciousness, and contralateral motor posturing--is a time-critical emergency that the transport clinician must recognize and treat immediately rather than deferring to the receiving facility. The initial management sequence is brief hyperventilation to a target PaCO2 of thirty to thirty-five millimeters of mercury (providing a rapid but temporary reduction in intracranial pressure through cerebral vasoconstriction), concurrent hyperosmolar therapy bolus, head-of-bed elevation confirmation, and immediate communication with the receiving neurosurgical team to prepare for possible emergent surgical decompression on arrival. Prolonged hyperventilation below a PaCO2 of thirty should be avoided because the resulting cerebral vasoconstriction, while reducing intracranial pressure, also reduces cerebral blood flow and can worsen ischemia in the already-injured brain.

| Hyperosmolar Agent | Typical Bolus Dose | Onset | Key Transport Consideration |
|---|---|---|---|
| Mannitol 20% | Confirm against current formulary | 15-30 minutes | Produces osmotic diuresis; monitor volume status and blood pressure closely |
| Hypertonic saline 3% | Confirm against current formulary | Minutes | No diuretic effect; preferred in hypotensive patients |
| Hypertonic saline 23.4% | Confirm against current formulary | Minutes | Requires central venous access for administration; potent osmotic effect |

**THE IN-TRANSIT DETERIORATION SIGNATURE SYSTEM — Position-Triggered Herniation Progression**

**The Signature:** Acute neurologic deterioration--new pupillary asymmetry, loss of previously present motor response, or a sudden drop in Glasgow Coma Scale score--that develops during or immediately after a positional change such as stretcher loading, head-down tilt during aircraft ascent, or repositioning for a procedural intervention during transport.

**Movement Trigger:** Positional changes that transiently increase intracranial venous pressure (head-down tilt), reduce cerebral perfusion pressure (systemic hypotension from the preload shifts described in Chapter

1), or mechanically shift intracranial contents (lateral or rotational head movement away from midline) can push a brain already operating at the limits of its compensatory capacity across the herniation threshold.

**Early Tell:** A subtle pupillary change--sluggish rather than absent reactivity, or a one-millimeter asymmetry--or a one-to-two-point decline in GCS motor score, noted by the serial neurologic reassessment protocol from Chapter 10, that appears temporally linked to a specific positional event rather than developing gradually over time.

**Trap Logic:** This pattern is frequently attributed to disease progression rather than recognized as a position-triggered event, because the clinical signs of herniation look identical regardless of the cause. The discriminating feature is the temporal link to a specific positional change, which is the cue to immediately reverse the position, re-confirm head-of-bed elevation and midline alignment, and deploy hyperosmolar therapy.

**Signature Anchor:** After any positional change in a patient with a known intracranial mass effect, perform an immediate focused neurologic reassessment--pupils and motor response at minimum--and treat any new asymmetry or decline as a position-triggered herniation event until the position has been corrected and the examination has been repeated.

## Ventilation Strategies to Optimize Cerebral Perfusion

### PaCO2 Targeting and the Danger of Inadvertent Hyperventilation

Carbon dioxide is a potent cerebral vasodilator, and its management during transport directly affects both intracranial pressure and cerebral blood flow. The target PaCO2 for most traumatic brain injury patients is thirty-five to forty millimeters of mercury--normocapnia--which maintains cerebral blood flow without exacerbating intracranial hypertension. Inadvertent hyperventilation, which is common during manual bag-valve ventilation and during the stress of a clinical deterioration, produces hypocapnia that reduces intracranial pressure through cerebral vasoconstriction but simultaneously reduces cerebral blood flow to potentially ischemic levels, producing a net worsening of secondary injury despite the apparent improvement in the intracranial pressure number. Continuous end-tidal capnography is the primary tool for preventing inadvertent hyperventilation during transport, though the clinician should be aware that end-tidal CO2 underestimates arterial PaCO2 by a variable margin that increases with dead space ventilation, making periodic correlation with arterial blood gas values important where point-of-care testing is available.

### Ventilator Settings for Neuroprotective Ventilation

Mechanical ventilation settings for the traumatic brain injury patient during transport should balance lung-protective targets (low tidal volume, appropriate PEEP) against the neuroprotective requirement for normocapnia, a balance that can be challenging when low tidal volume ventilation produces hypercapnia that elevates intracranial pressure. In practice, a modest increase in respiratory rate, rather than an increase in tidal volume, is the preferred method for maintaining normocapnia within a lung-protective tidal volume range, though excessive rate increases can produce auto-PEEP that raises intrathoracic pressure, impedes cerebral venous drainage, and paradoxically worsens intracranial pressure. The transport clinician should monitor for auto-PEEP through the ventilator waveform--specifically, the presence of flow at end-expiration on the flow-time curve--and reduce the respiratory rate if auto-PEEP develops rather than allowing it to persist.

## Cervical Spine Precautions and Multisystem Trauma Overlap

### Balancing Cervical Immobilization With Airway and ICP Management

Many patients with traumatic brain injury severe enough to require critical care transport also have confirmed or suspected cervical spine injuries, and the transport clinician must balance the competing requirements of cervical immobilization, airway access, and intracranial pressure management. A rigid cervical collar, while protecting the cervical spine, can impede jugular venous drainage and elevate intracranial pressure if applied too tightly or if the collar's anterior component compresses the internal jugular veins, and the transport clinician should verify that the collar is sized and applied appropriately, with adequate space for venous drainage, before departure.

### Prioritizing Competing Injuries During Transport

The multiply injured patient with both a traumatic brain injury and an extracranial hemorrhagic source presents a management tension that the transport clinician must navigate explicitly: traumatic brain injury management prioritizes maintaining a higher blood pressure target to preserve cerebral perfusion pressure, while hemorrhagic shock management focuses on damage control resuscitation with a lower, permissive hypotension target to reduce ongoing hemorrhage. In general, the brain injury target takes precedence, because the irreversible secondary brain injury produced by hypotension is less recoverable than the hemorrhagic insult, which can be addressed surgically at the receiving facility. This prioritization should be communicated to the receiving trauma team so that their resuscitation plan accounts for the higher pressure target and its implications for ongoing hemorrhage control.

### Seizure Prophylaxis and Management in TBI Transport

Early post-traumatic seizures occur in approximately ten to fifteen percent of patients with severe traumatic brain injury, and current evidence supports the use of a prophylactic anticonvulsant--typically levetiracetam, which has a favorable side effect profile and does not require serum level monitoring--during the first seven days after injury. The transport clinician should confirm whether seizure prophylaxis has been initiated at the sending facility and continue it without interruption during transport. If a seizure occurs during transport, the management follows the same principles described for stroke-related seizures in Chapter 10: first-line benzodiazepine therapy administered promptly, airway protection, and communication with the receiving team. A witnessed seizure in a patient with a known intracranial mass lesion should also trigger reassessment for herniation, since the metabolic stress and intracranial pressure elevation produced by seizure activity can push a marginally compensated brain across the herniation threshold.

## Temperature Management in Traumatic Brain Injury

Fever is associated with worse neurologic outcomes in traumatic brain injury through the same mechanisms described for stroke in Chapter 10--increased cerebral metabolic demand, enhanced excitotoxicity, and blood-brain barrier disruption--and should be treated aggressively during transport with antipyretic therapy and active cooling measures. Induced hypothermia as a targeted neuroprotective strategy in traumatic brain injury remains controversial, with the evidence from major randomized trials failing to demonstrate clear benefit and raising concerns about adverse effects including coagulopathy and cardiac arrhythmias, and it should generally not be initiated during transport unless specifically directed by the receiving neurosurgical team. Normothermia, maintained rigorously, is the evidence-based default target.

## Preparing the Receiving Team for Possible Decompressive Craniectomy

When the transport clinician observes a trajectory of rising intracranial pressure, worsening compliance on the ICP waveform, and neurologic deterioration despite maximal medical management during transit, communication with the receiving facility should explicitly raise the possibility of emergent decompressive craniectomy on arrival, so that the neurosurgical team, operating room, and anesthesia resources can be mobilized before the patient's arrival rather than after. This advance communication is the neurosurgical equivalent of the catheterization laboratory activation described for STEMI in Chapter 6 and the neurointervention activation described for stroke in Chapter 10, and it can convert a receiving facility's response from reactive to proactive, saving minutes that directly affect outcome in a patient whose remaining compensatory capacity is measured in those same minutes.

Consider a twenty-three-year-old man with a severe traumatic brain injury from a motorcycle collision, GCS of six at the sending facility with a right-sided fixed and dilated pupil, and a CT showing a large left-sided epidural hematoma with significant midline shift. The sending facility has intubated the patient and placed an external ventricular drain, and the patient is being transferred to a Level I trauma center for emergent craniotomy. During the stretcher loading sequence for a rotor-wing transport, the crew notes that the previously reactive left pupil has become sluggish, and the ICP, which had been fifteen millimeters of mercury, has risen to twenty-eight, temporally coinciding with the brief head-down tilt that occurred during litter loading. Recognizing the Position-Triggered Herniation Progression Signature, the crew immediately returns the patient to a head-up position, confirms midline alignment, drains ten milliliters of cerebrospinal fluid through the external ventricular drain, and administers a hypertonic saline bolus. The ICP returns to sixteen within three minutes, and the left pupil reactivity returns. The crew delays departure by four minutes to confirm hemodynamic and neurologic stability before proceeding, a decision that prioritizes patient safety over transport speed and prevents the crew from beginning a flight with an actively herniating patient whose intervention options in the air would be more limited.

**CLINICAL PEARL:** A four-minute delay at the helipad to stabilize a herniating patient is always preferable to departing with an actively deteriorating patient whose management options narrow once the aircraft is airborne.

## Advanced TBI Management During Transport

### Cerebral Perfusion Pressure Optimization: The CPP Equation

Cerebral perfusion pressure equals mean arterial pressure minus intracranial pressure, and the transport clinician managing a patient with ICP monitoring can directly calculate and target CPP as a more physiologically meaningful goal than either MAP or ICP alone. A CPP target of sixty to seventy millimeters of mercury is generally recommended for adult traumatic brain injury, though the optimal target may be individualized based on the patient's autoregulatory status (a concept discussed further below). Maintaining CPP requires simultaneous attention to both components of the equation: MAP must be kept above the threshold that produces adequate CPP, and ICP must be kept below the threshold that degrades CPP, and changes in either component require adjustment of the other. A falling CPP can result from a falling MAP (managed with volume and vasopressors) or a rising ICP (managed with CSF drainage, hyperosmolar therapy, and positioning), and the transport clinician must identify which component is driving the change to apply the correct intervention.

### Cerebrovascular Autoregulation and Its Relevance to Transport

In the healthy brain, cerebrovascular autoregulation maintains relatively constant cerebral blood flow across a wide range of mean arterial pressures (approximately fifty to one hundred fifty millimeters of mercury in a normotensive individual) by adjusting cerebrovascular resistance in response to pressure changes. In traumatic brain injury, autoregulation is frequently impaired in the injured hemisphere, meaning that cerebral blood flow becomes directly pressure-dependent: when MAP falls, cerebral blood flow falls proportionally rather than being maintained by autoregulatory vasodilation, and when MAP rises, cerebral blood flow and volume rise proportionally, potentially worsening cerebral edema and ICP. This autoregulatory impairment has direct transport implications: the altitude-related preload reduction, positional hemodynamic shifts, and acceleration forces described in Chapter 1 produce MAP fluctuations that, in a patient with impaired autoregulation, translate directly into cerebral blood flow fluctuations--a mechanism that converts the routine hemodynamic variability of transport into a direct threat to the injured brain.

### The Concept of Optimal CPP and Pressure Reactivity

Research into individualized CPP targeting has identified the concept of optimal CPP--the specific mean arterial pressure at which a given patient's pressure reactivity index (a measure of how ICP responds to changes in MAP) indicates the best preserved autoregulation. While continuous pressure reactivity monitoring is typically available only in specialized neurocritical care units and not during transport, the transport clinician should understand the concept because it informs the management philosophy: the optimal CPP target for a specific patient may differ from the population-based target of sixty to seventy, and the receiving neurocritical care team may adjust the target based on individualized monitoring data after arrival. During transport, the population-based target provides a reasonable default, but the transport clinician should communicate any observed relationship between MAP changes and ICP responses (e.g., "when the MAP dropped during loading, the ICP rose disproportionately") to the receiving team, as this observation provides informal autoregulation data that the receiving team can use.

### Decompressive Craniectomy: What the Transport Clinician Should Know

Decompressive craniectomy, the surgical removal of a portion of the skull to allow the swelling brain to expand without being constrained by the fixed cranial vault, may be performed at the sending facility before transport or may be the specific intervention the patient is being transferred to receive. The transport clinician managing a post-craniectomy patient should be aware that the surgically created cranial defect is a direct vulnerability during transport: the unprotected brain beneath the defect is susceptible to direct trauma from contact with the stretcher or equipment, atmospheric pressure changes at altitude can alter the transdefect pressure gradient and produce brain herniation through the craniectomy site, and the patient's neurologic examination may be affected by the altered intracranial dynamics in ways that differ from a patient with an intact skull. A protective helmet or padded headrest should be used for any post-craniectomy patient during transport, and the crew should be aware that cabin pressurization changes can produce visible changes in the scalp flap tension that may correlate with intracranial pressure shifts.

### Prognostication Discipline: What NOT to Communicate During Transport

The transport clinician frequently encounters families who ask about prognosis during the emotionally charged period surrounding an acute traumatic brain injury, and the appropriate response is to acknowledge the severity of the situation while explicitly deferring prognostic statements to the receiving neurosurgical team, who will have access to imaging, monitoring, and examination data over time that the transport clinician does not possess. Premature prognostication during transport--whether optimistic ("he's going to be fine") or pessimistic ("this doesn't look good")--is both clinically irresponsible (because the data is insufficient) and potentially harmful (because it anchors the family's expectations in a direction that the subsequent clinical course may not support). The transport clinician's communication with the family should focus on what is being done right now to protect the patient's brain, where the patient is being taken and why, and what the family can expect to happen in the first hours after arrival.

### Additional Clinical Considerations for Transport Management

The management of patients in Chapter 11 requires attention to several additional transport-specific clinical factors that extend the principles established in the main body of the chapter. The transport clinician should be aware that the disease processes covered here interact with the transport environment in ways that are specific to the combination of the underlying pathophysiology and the particular environmental stressor encountered during a given mission, and that a management approach that is adequate for a short ground transport may be insufficient for a longer air transport at altitude, or vice versa. The serial reassessment protocol established in Chapter 2 provides the framework for detecting these interactions as they develop, and the Deterioration Signature introduced in this chapter names the most characteristic pattern by which they declare themselves.

Each patient transport is a unique combination of a specific patient's physiology, a specific set of ongoing therapies, a specific transport platform with its own environmental characteristics, and a specific mission profile with its own altitude, duration, and route constraints. The anticipatory approach to transport medicine that this text teaches is not a set of memorized responses to predetermined scenarios but a cognitive framework for analyzing the specific combination of variables present in any given transport and identifying, before departure, the most likely points of vulnerability where the transport environment will test the patient's physiologic reserve. This chapter's clinical content provides the disease-specific knowledge needed to apply that framework to the conditions covered here, while the Deterioration Signature provides the named pattern that makes the most characteristic transport-specific vulnerability explicit, recognizable, and actionable.

The receiving team's ability to continue the patient's care seamlessly after the transport crew departs depends entirely on the quality and completeness of the clinical information the transport crew provides, and for the conditions covered in this chapter, the specific information that matters most includes: the trajectory of the patient's primary condition during transport (improving, stable, or worsening, with specific details), any interventions performed during transport and their response, any new clinical findings identified by the transport crew that were not present at the sending facility, and any anticipated needs that the receiving team should prepare for based on the transport crew's clinical assessment. This information, communicated through the structured handoff format established in Chapter 2 and supplemented by the trajectory communication emphasis that is a recurring theme throughout this text, is the final clinical act of the transport and the one that determines whether the transport adds value to the patient's care continuum or merely moves the patient from one location to another without preserving the clinical narrative that only the transport crew was positioned to observe.

The clinical scenarios addressed in this chapter illustrate a principle that recurs throughout the text: the transport environment does not merely add logistic complexity to the management of critical illness--it introduces specific physiologic stressors that interact with the patient's underlying condition to produce clinical changes that would not occur at the bedside. The altitude-related gas expansion, preload shifts, oxygenation challenges, and monitoring degradation described in Chapter 1, combined with the pharmacologic and equipment considerations from Chapters 4 and 5, create a modified clinical environment in which every bedside management principle must be re-examined through the lens of transport-specific risk. The disease-specific management recommendations in this chapter have been written with this re-examination already performed, incorporating the transport modifications into the clinical recommendations rather than presenting bedside management followed by a separate list of transport considerations, because the integration of disease knowledge and transport awareness is the competency that this text is designed to develop.

Inter-professional collaboration during the management of the conditions in this chapter deserves specific emphasis, because the complexity of many transport patients exceeds the capability of any single clinician acting alone. The nurse-paramedic team, the nurse-physician team, or whatever crew configuration the program uses represents a collaborative unit whose combined clinical capability exceeds the sum of its individual members, provided that the communication, role allocation, and shared mental model practices described in Chapter 24 are actively maintained throughout the transport. A transport in which one crew member manages the airway while the other manages hemodynamics, with both monitoring different aspects of the same clinical picture and cross-checking each other's assessments, produces a more complete and reliable clinical picture than either clinician could achieve alone, and this collaborative advantage is greatest during the high-workload, high-stress scenarios that the conditions in this chapter frequently produce.

Quality improvement in the management of these conditions during transport depends on systematic outcome tracking that links transport-specific management decisions to patient outcomes at the receiving facility. Did the patient who received a specific intervention during transport have a better or worse outcome than comparable patients who did not? Did a specific monitoring strategy detect deterioration earlier and allow more effective intervention? Did advance communication with the receiving facility produce measurably faster time-to-treatment on arrival? These questions can only be answered by programs that collect and analyze outcome data systematically, and the transport clinician's contribution to this process is meticulous, contemporaneous documentation of every clinical decision, every intervention, and every trajectory observation during the transport, since this documentation is the raw material from which quality improvement insights are derived. A transport program that does not analyze its outcomes cannot improve them, and a transport clinician who does not document their clinical reasoning cannot contribute to the program's learning.

**THE IN-TRANSIT DETERIORATION SIGNATURE SYSTEM — Traumatic Brain Injury Movement Patterns**

**Signature Introduced This Chapter:** Position-Triggered Herniation Progression (acute neurologic deterioration temporally linked to a positional change that transiently worsens intracranial dynamics in a patient with marginal compensatory reserve).

**TBI Pattern Logic:** This Signature extends the altitude-potentiated ICP Signature from Chapter 10 to the positional domain, recognizing that any movement event--not just altitude change--can push a brain at the limits of its compensatory capacity across the herniation threshold if the crew does not perform an immediate neurologic reassessment after the event.

**Cross-Reference Forward:** Chapter 13 (Multisystem Trauma) addresses the management tension between traumatic brain injury targets and hemorrhagic shock targets in the multiply injured patient; Chapter 15 (Sepsis) extends the cerebral perfusion pressure optimization framework to sepsis-associated encephalopathy.

## Summary and Key Concepts

Preventing secondary brain injury through continuous hypotension avoidance and hypoxemia prevention is the transport clinician's highest-impact intervention in traumatic brain injury.

Intracranial pressure waveform morphology, not just the numeric value, provides information about remaining compensatory reserve; a progressive loss of compliance signals impending decompensation.

Hyperosmolar therapy with mannitol or hypertonic saline should be immediately available for herniation management; hypertonic saline is preferred in hypotensive patients because it avoids the osmotic diuresis that mannitol produces.

Normocapnia ($PaCO_2$ 35-40 mmHg) is the ventilation target for most TBI patients; inadvertent hyperventilation reduces cerebral blood flow and worsens secondary injury despite the apparent improvement in ICP.

Positional changes during loading and transit can precipitate herniation in a patient with marginal compensatory reserve; immediate neurologic reassessment after every position change is mandatory.

In the multiply injured patient with both TBI and hemorrhagic shock, the brain injury blood pressure target generally takes precedence because hypotension-mediated secondary brain injury is less recoverable than surgically addressable hemorrhage.

# CHAPTER 12: STATUS EPILEPTICUS AND NEUROMUSCULAR EMERGENCIES IN TRANSIT

**Learning Objectives**

1. Recognize convulsive and nonconvulsive status epilepticus and initiate staged pharmacologic management during transport.
2. Manage refractory status epilepticus with continuous infusion therapy in the transport environment.
3. Identify neuromuscular weakness syndromes presenting with ventilatory failure requiring transport for definitive management.
4. Titrate sedation and paralytic agents with awareness of their interactions with underlying neuromuscular pathology.
5. Perform structured post-ictal and altered mental status assessment during transit.

**Chapter Outline**

This chapter addresses two categories of neurologic emergency that the transport clinician encounters with distinct frequency and management urgency: status epilepticus, which requires time-sensitive staged pharmacologic intervention that must proceed during transit without access to electroencephalography or neurologic consultation, and acute neuromuscular weakness syndromes, which present as ventilatory failure requiring intubation and transport to a facility capable of definitive diagnosis and treatment. Both conditions share the common transport challenge that the neurologic examination is the primary clinical tool, and that sedation and paralysis--often necessary for airway and ventilator management--ablate the very examination findings the clinician depends on to assess treatment response and detect progression.

## Seizure Recognition and First-Line Management

### Convulsive Status Epilepticus: Definition and Time-Sensitive Staging

Convulsive status epilepticus is defined as continuous seizure activity lasting five or more minutes, or two or more discrete seizures without return to baseline consciousness between them, and it represents a genuine neurologic emergency in which the duration of seizure activity directly correlates with the difficulty of termination and the severity of neurologic injury. The first-line treatment is a benzodiazepine--midazolam intramuscularly or intravenously, or lorazepam intravenously--administered as rapidly as possible once status epilepticus is recognized, and the transport clinician should not delay treatment to obtain vascular access if intramuscular midazolam is available, since the time to treatment is more important than the route of delivery at this stage.

## Second-Line Anticonvulsant Loading During Transport

If benzodiazepine therapy does not terminate seizure activity within five to ten minutes, second-line treatment with an intravenous anticonvulsant loading dose is indicated. Levetiracetam, fosphenytoin, and valproic acid are all acceptable second-line agents, each with specific transport considerations: levetiracetam has the most favorable hemodynamic profile and does not require cardiac monitoring during infusion, making it the most transport-friendly option; fosphenytoin requires cardiac monitoring during infusion due to the risk of hypotension and arrhythmia, a manageable but attention-consuming requirement; and valproic acid is effective but carries hepatotoxicity risk and is contraindicated in pregnancy and mitochondrial disorders, which may not be fully screened in a transport patient with an incomplete history.

## Recognizing Nonconvulsive Status Epilepticus Without EEG

Nonconvulsive status epilepticus--ongoing seizure activity without overt convulsive movements, presenting instead as fluctuating consciousness, subtle repetitive behaviors, or unexplained unresponsiveness--is the most diagnostically challenging seizure presentation in the transport environment, because definitive diagnosis requires electroencephalography that is unavailable during transit. The transport clinician's role is suspicion rather than diagnosis: any patient with an unexplained alteration in consciousness, particularly one with a known seizure history or acute brain injury, who is not improving as expected should be considered a possible nonconvulsive status epilepticus case, and this suspicion should be communicated to the receiving team so that emergent electroencephalography can be prioritized on arrival. A therapeutic trial of a benzodiazepine in a patient with suspected nonconvulsive status epilepticus may produce visible clinical improvement that supports the suspicion, though the absence of improvement does not exclude the diagnosis.

| Treatment Stage | Agent | Timing | Key Transport Consideration |
|---|---|---|---|
| First-line | Midazolam IM or lorazepam IV | Immediate on recognition | Do not delay for IV access if IM available |
| Second-line | Levetiracetam, fosphenytoin, or valproic acid IV | If seizure persists after 5-10 min | Levetiracetam most transport-friendly (no cardiac monitoring needed) |
| Refractory (third-line) | Midazolam or propofol continuous infusion | If seizure persists after second-line agent | Requires intubation, continuous monitoring, vasopressor readiness |
| Super-refractory | Pentobarbital or ketamine infusion | If seizure persists despite third-line | Typically initiated at receiving facility; transport role is to arrive safely |

## Refractory Status Epilepticus and Continuous Infusion Therapy

### Initiating Continuous Infusion Anticonvulsant Therapy in Transit

Refractory status epilepticus--seizure activity that persists despite adequate first- and second-line therapy--requires continuous infusion of a sedating anticonvulsant, typically midazolam or propofol, at doses sufficient to suppress seizure activity, which in practice means intubation, mechanical ventilation, and continuous hemodynamic monitoring, all of which should already be in place or rapidly established. The transport-specific challenge is that the clinician cannot confirm seizure suppression without electroencephalography, and must instead titrate the infusion to clinical endpoints: cessation of any visible motor activity, hemodynamic stability, and a level of sedation deep enough to suppress the seizure without producing refractory hypotension from the sedative infusion itself.

### Hemodynamic Consequences of Deep Sedation for Seizure Suppression

The deep sedation required for continuous infusion seizure suppression produces the same pharmacologically mediated hemodynamic vulnerability described in the Masked Hemodynamic Collapse Signature from Chapter 4: blood pressure declines gradually without compensatory tachycardia, and the sedated patient cannot communicate distress or discomfort that would otherwise alert the crew to a developing problem. The transport clinician should have vasopressor therapy running or immediately available for any patient receiving continuous infusion seizure suppression, and should monitor blood pressure trends at frequent intervals through the continuous arterial line that should already be in place for this acuity level.

### THE IN-TRANSIT DETERIORATION SIGNATURE SYSTEM — Sedation-Masked Seizure Recurrence

**The Signature:** Recurrence of seizure activity in a deeply sedated and possibly paralyzed patient during transport, detectable only through subtle indirect signs--unexplained tachycardia, rising end-tidal CO2, new hemodynamic instability, or a pupillary change--because the motor manifestations of the seizure are pharmacologically suppressed.

**Movement Trigger:** The infusion rate of the continuous anticonvulsant may become subtherapeutic during transport due to pump interruption during a line transition, cold-induced flow slowing, or vibration-induced delivery irregularities described in Chapter 4, allowing seizure activity to resume beneath the surface of pharmacologic suppression.

**Early Tell:** An unexplained rise in heart rate, blood pressure, or end-tidal CO2 in a deeply sedated patient, without any corresponding change in sedation dose or ventilator settings, suggesting increased metabolic demand from subclinical seizure activity that the paralyzed or deeply sedated patient cannot manifest as visible convulsions.

**Trap Logic:** These hemodynamic and metabolic changes are easily attributed to pain, inadequate sedation depth, or a primary hemodynamic event rather than recognized as the indirect signature of ongoing seizure activity. The discriminating feature is the pattern: seizure-driven metabolic stress produces a concordant rise in heart rate, blood pressure, temperature, and $CO_2$ production that is difficult to explain by any single alternative mechanism.

**Signature Anchor:** In any deeply sedated or paralyzed patient being treated for status epilepticus, treat an unexplained, concordant rise in heart rate, blood pressure, and end-tidal $CO_2$ as possible seizure recurrence, verify the anticonvulsant infusion rate and line integrity, and administer a benzodiazepine bolus while communicating the concern to the receiving team for urgent EEG on arrival.

## Neuromuscular Weakness and Ventilatory Failure

### Guillain-Barre Syndrome and Myasthenic Crisis in Transport

Acute neuromuscular weakness syndromes--most commonly Guillain-Barre syndrome (acute inflammatory demyelinating polyneuropathy) and myasthenic crisis--present in the transport setting as patients with progressive ascending weakness and ventilatory failure who require intubation and transfer to a facility with neuromuscular expertise. The transport clinician's primary concerns are airway management, ventilator support, and autonomic instability monitoring, since both conditions can produce unpredictable swings in heart rate and blood pressure from autonomic dysfunction that are distinct from the hemodynamic changes seen in other transport populations and may not respond predictably to standard vasoactive agents.

### Ventilatory Monitoring and Forced Vital Capacity Assessment

In the patient with neuromuscular weakness who has not yet been intubated, serial assessment of ventilatory adequacy--including negative inspiratory force and forced vital capacity measurements where available, supplemented by clinical assessment of respiratory effort, accessory muscle use, and the ability to count to twenty in a single breath--should be performed at frequent intervals to detect the trajectory toward ventilatory failure before it becomes a respiratory arrest. The threshold for pre-departure intubation should be low in any patient with a progressive neuromuscular weakness trajectory, since intubation in a moving vehicle during an acute respiratory decompensation from neuromuscular failure is substantially more dangerous than a controlled, elective intubation at the sending bedside.

Figure 12.1: Clinical Assessment of Progressive Neuromuscular Ventilatory Failure

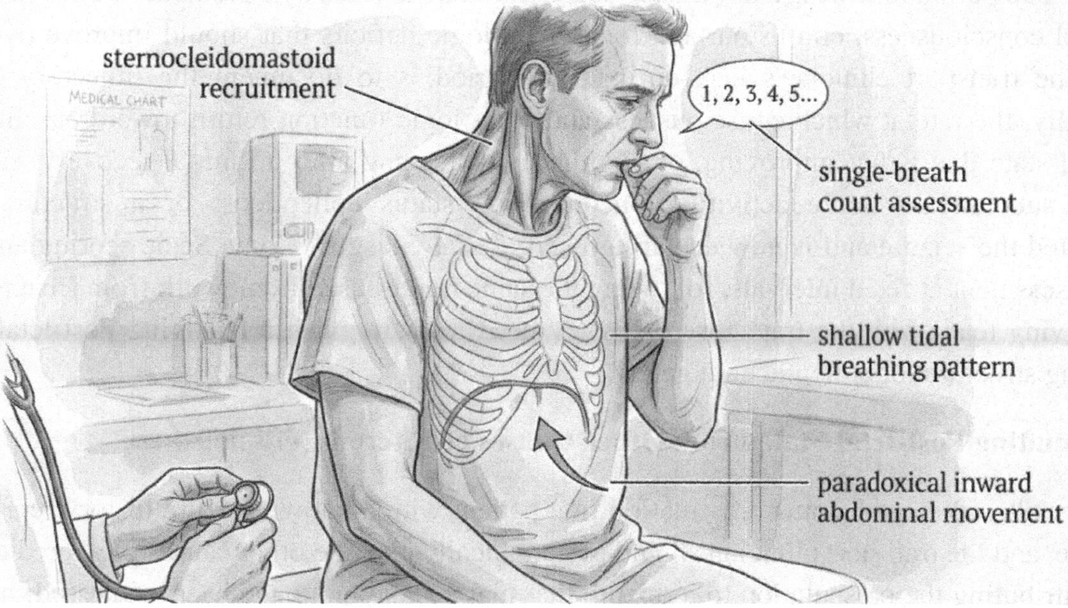


## Sedation and Paralytic Considerations During Transport

### Avoiding Exacerbating Agents in Neuromuscular Disease

Certain medications commonly used in the transport setting carry specific risks in patients with neuromuscular disease: succinylcholine is absolutely contraindicated in Guillain-Barre syndrome and many other denervation conditions due to the risk of fatal hyperkalemia from upregulated acetylcholine receptor proliferation, and non-depolarizing neuromuscular blocking agents (rocuronium, vecuronium) produce prolonged, unpredictable blockade in myasthenic patients whose neuromuscular junction is already impaired. The transport clinician must screen for these conditions before administering any paralytic agent, and should default to rocuronium (with sugammadex availability confirmed for reversal if needed) for intubation in any patient with a known or suspected neuromuscular disorder, avoiding succinylcholine entirely.

### Autonomic Instability Monitoring and Management

Both Guillain-Barre syndrome and myasthenic crisis can produce autonomic instability characterized by alternating episodes of tachycardia and bradycardia, hypertension and hypotension, and excessive secretions that are unpredictable and may not respond to standard interventions in the expected manner. The transport clinician should anticipate these swings and manage them conservatively, since overreacting to a transient hypertensive episode with aggressive antihypertensive therapy can produce profound rebound hypotension that is harder to correct than the original hypertension, and similarly, treating a transient bradycardia aggressively can provoke a rebound tachycardia that destabilizes the patient further.

## Post-Ictal and Altered Mental Status Assessment

### Structured Post-Ictal Assessment During Transport

The post-ictal period following a terminated seizure is characterized by a predictable but variable sequence of altered consciousness, confusion, and focal neurologic deficits that should improve over minutes to hours. The transport clinician's task during this period is to document the trajectory of recovery--specifically, the rate at which consciousness and neurologic function return toward baseline--because a post-ictal state that is not improving, or one that is worsening after an initial recovery, suggests either ongoing subclinical seizure activity (nonconvulsive status epilepticus) or a structural lesion that precipitated the seizure and is now declaring itself. Serial Glasgow Coma Scale scoring and lateralizing motor assessment at fixed intervals, following the same trend-based framework from Chapter 2, provides the receiving team with the trajectory data they need to distinguish a resolving post-ictal state from a worsening structural or epileptic emergency.

### Differentiating Post-Ictal State From Other Causes of Altered Consciousness

Not every altered mental status presentation in a patient with a known seizure history represents a post-ictal state, and the transport clinician should systematically exclude other causes of altered consciousness before attributing the presentation to a seizure that may or may not have been witnessed: hypoglycemia, which can both cause seizures and mimic a post-ictal state, should be excluded by point-of-care glucose measurement; drug intoxication or withdrawal, which can also cause both seizures and altered consciousness, should be considered in the clinical context; and a new structural lesion such as an intracranial hemorrhage should remain in the differential until the receiving facility can obtain imaging.

Consider a fifty-two-year-old woman with a known seizure disorder, found unresponsive after a witnessed generalized seizure at a skilled nursing facility, transferred by ground critical care ambulance for further evaluation after the sending facility's CT scan was equivocal. During transport, the crew performs serial neurologic assessments every ten minutes. At the first assessment, the patient's GCS is eight with no lateralizing motor deficit. By the twenty-minute mark, the GCS has improved to eleven with purposeful withdrawal bilaterally. However, at the forty-minute assessment, the crew notes that the GCS has declined back to nine and a new right-sided facial droop has appeared that was not present at the previous assessment. Rather than attributing this decline to normal fluctuation in the post-ictal period, the crew recognizes the non-improving trajectory as a red flag for either nonconvulsive seizure recurrence or a structural lesion declaring itself, administers a benzodiazepine bolus empirically for possible nonconvulsive status, and communicates the trajectory to the receiving facility, which prioritizes emergent EEG and repeat imaging on arrival. The imaging ultimately reveals a small acute subdural hematoma that was not visible on the initial equivocal CT and that had expanded during the transport window, producing the new focal deficit. The crew's serial assessment and trajectory communication allowed the receiving team to identify the surgical lesion minutes earlier than they would have from a single arrival examination.

## Additional Clinical Considerations for Transport Management

The management of patients in Chapter 12 requires attention to several additional transport-specific clinical factors that extend the principles established in the main body of the chapter. The transport clinician should be aware that the disease processes covered here interact with the transport environment in ways that are specific to the combination of the underlying pathophysiology and the particular environmental stressor encountered during a given mission, and that a management approach that is adequate for a short ground transport may be insufficient for a longer air transport at altitude, or vice versa. The serial reassessment protocol established in Chapter 2 provides the framework for detecting these interactions as they develop, and the Deterioration Signature introduced in this chapter names the most characteristic pattern by which they declare themselves.

Each patient transport is a unique combination of a specific patient's physiology, a specific set of ongoing therapies, a specific transport platform with its own environmental characteristics, and a specific mission profile with its own altitude, duration, and route constraints. The anticipatory approach to transport medicine that this text teaches is not a set of memorized responses to predetermined scenarios but a cognitive framework for analyzing the specific combination of variables present in any given transport and identifying, before departure, the most likely points of vulnerability where the transport environment will test the patient's physiologic reserve. This chapter's clinical content provides the disease-specific knowledge needed to apply that framework to the conditions covered here, while the Deterioration Signature provides the named pattern that makes the most characteristic transport-specific vulnerability explicit, recognizable, and actionable.

The receiving team's ability to continue the patient's care seamlessly after the transport crew departs depends entirely on the quality and completeness of the clinical information the transport crew provides, and for the conditions covered in this chapter, the specific information that matters most includes: the trajectory of the patient's primary condition during transport (improving, stable, or worsening, with specific details), any interventions performed during transport and their response, any new clinical findings identified by the transport crew that were not present at the sending facility, and any anticipated needs that the receiving team should prepare for based on the transport crew's clinical assessment. This information, communicated through the structured handoff format established in Chapter 2 and supplemented by the trajectory communication emphasis that is a recurring theme throughout this text, is the final clinical act of the transport and the one that determines whether the transport adds value to the patient's care continuum or merely moves the patient from one location to another without preserving the clinical narrative that only the transport crew was positioned to observe.

The transport clinician managing the conditions addressed in this chapter should develop a systematic pre-departure assessment that specifically identifies the highest-risk transport-environment interaction for each patient's specific disease process, the monitoring parameters that will detect that interaction earliest, and the intervention that will address it most effectively. This pre-departure risk analysis, adapted from the general pre-mission physiologic risk profile introduced in Chapter 1, should be specific enough to generate a concrete prediction: what is the single most likely way this specific patient's condition will interact with the specific transport environment of this specific mission? Answering that question before departure, rather than discovering the answer during transit, is the practical application of the anticipatory transport medicine framework that this entire text is designed to develop.

Clinical case presentations embedded throughout this chapter illustrate the principle that transport-specific deterioration patterns are predictable rather than random, recognizable rather than mysterious, and preventable rather than inevitable, provided the clinician applies the systematic assessment, continuous monitoring, and named-pattern recognition framework that the Deterioration Signature System codifies. Each case demonstrates the same three-part sequence: a patient with a specific disease process encounters a specific transport-environment stressor, produces a specific clinical change that could be attributed to either the disease or the environment, and is correctly managed because the transport clinician recognized the specific named Signature and applied the correct transport-specific intervention rather than the generic disease-specific response that would have been appropriate at the bedside but is insufficient or incorrect in the transport context.

The evidence base for transport-specific management of the conditions in this chapter continues to evolve, with ongoing research into optimal monitoring strategies, transport-adapted treatment protocols, and outcome data that will refine the recommendations presented here. The transport clinician should maintain awareness of emerging evidence through continuing education, program-sponsored journal clubs, and the quality improvement processes described in Chapter 24, since the standard of care for transport medicine is not static and the recommendations in any textbook represent a snapshot of evidence at the time of writing rather than a permanent standard. The principles, however, are durable: anticipate rather than react, monitor trends rather than thresholds, communicate trajectories rather than snapshots, and recognize that the transport environment is a clinical variable that acts on every patient's physiology, not a neutral conduit between two points of care.

Finally, the transport clinician should recognize that the clinical expertise required to manage these conditions during transport represents a distinct competency that builds on but extends beyond the bedside critical care training that most transport clinicians bring to their role. A clinician who is expert in managing these conditions in the intensive care unit is not automatically expert in managing them during transport, because the environmental, equipment, monitoring, and resource constraints of transport introduce variables that bedside practice never encounters. Conversely, a transport clinician who has mastered the anticipatory, environment-aware management approach described in this text brings a perspective to patient care that the bedside clinician lacks: the ability to see the patient's physiology not as a fixed state being managed in a controlled environment, but as a dynamic process interacting continuously with an environment that is itself changing throughout the transport. This dual awareness--of the disease and of the environment acting on it--is the defining competency of transport critical care medicine, and it is what this text, from its first chapter through its last, is designed to develop.

**THE IN-TRANSIT DETERIORATION SIGNATURE SYSTEM — Seizure and Neuromuscular Emergency Patterns**

**Signature Introduced This Chapter:** Sedation-Masked Seizure Recurrence (seizure activity beneath pharmacologic suppression, detectable only through indirect metabolic and hemodynamic signs in a paralyzed or deeply sedated patient).

**Seizure Pattern Logic:** This Signature extends the Masked Hemodynamic Collapse Signature from Chapter 4 to the neurologic domain: deep sedation suppresses not only compensatory hemodynamic responses but also the motor manifestations of seizure activity, requiring the clinician to rely on indirect metabolic indicators (heart rate, CO2 production, temperature) to detect a process that would ordinarily be clinically obvious.

**Cross-Reference Forward:** Chapter 20 (Toxicologic Emergencies) addresses seizures from toxic ingestion, where the underlying cause requires specific antidotal therapy in addition to anticonvulsant management; Chapter 23 (Pediatric Critical Care) addresses pediatric status epilepticus dosing and management differences.

## Summary and Key Concepts

Status epilepticus is a time-critical emergency in which first-line benzodiazepine therapy should not be delayed for vascular access; intramuscular midazolam is an acceptable initial route.

Refractory status epilepticus requiring continuous infusion therapy during transport necessitates intubation, continuous monitoring, and vasopressor readiness for sedation-mediated hemodynamic compromise.

Nonconvulsive status epilepticus cannot be definitively diagnosed during transport without EEG, but clinical suspicion should be communicated to the receiving team for emergent EEG prioritization.

Succinylcholine is absolutely contraindicated in Guillain-Barre syndrome and other denervation conditions; the transport clinician must screen for neuromuscular disease before administering any depolarizing agent.

Post-ictal trajectory, not a single snapshot, distinguishes a resolving seizure from nonconvulsive recurrence or a structural lesion declaring itself; serial assessment at fixed intervals is mandatory.

# CHAPTER 13: ACUTE RESPIRATORY FAILURE AND ARDS MANAGEMENT IN TRANSIT

**Learning Objectives**

1. Differentiate hypoxemic from hypercapnic respiratory failure and apply the distinction to ventilator strategy selection during transport.
2. Implement lung-protective ventilation and driving-pressure optimization for ARDS patients in the transport environment.
3. Apply prone positioning and rescue oxygenation strategies adapted to the constraints of a moving vehicle or aircraft.
4. Select and manage high-flow nasal cannula and noninvasive ventilation during transport.
5. Recognize transport-specific triggers for respiratory deterioration including altitude-mediated hypoxemia and equipment-related ventilation failure.

**Chapter Outline**

This chapter addresses the transport of patients with acute respiratory failure and acute respiratory distress syndrome, extending the ventilator management framework from Chapter 3 and the altitude physiology from Chapter 1 into the specific clinical challenges of maintaining gas exchange in a patient whose lungs are the primary failing organ. The transport clinician managing an ARDS patient operates under a fundamental tension: the lung-protective ventilation strategy that preserves long-term lung function may produce short-term gas exchange that is barely adequate at sea level and becomes inadequate at altitude, forcing a continuous recalibration of ventilator settings against the specific oxygen environment of the transport.

## Hypoxemic and Hypercapnic Respiratory Failure Differentiation

### Mechanisms and Transport Implications of Each Phenotype

Hypoxemic respiratory failure, characterized by a $PaO_2/FiO_2$ ratio that falls despite increasing supplemental oxygen, results from shunt physiology (perfused but unventilated lung units) or severe ventilation-perfusion mismatch, and is the hallmark of ARDS, pneumonia, pulmonary edema, and massive atelectasis. Hypercapnic respiratory failure results from inadequate alveolar ventilation--either from reduced respiratory drive, neuromuscular weakness, or severe airflow obstruction--and presents with a rising $PaCO_2$ and respiratory acidosis. The distinction matters for transport because the primary therapeutic intervention differs: hypoxemic failure is managed primarily through oxygenation strategies ($FiO_2$, PEEP, positioning), while hypercapnic failure is managed primarily through ventilation strategies (minute ventilation optimization), and misidentifying the predominant mechanism leads to the wrong therapeutic emphasis.

### Mixed Respiratory Failure and the Overlap Population

Many transport patients present with mixed hypoxemic and hypercapnic failure--the COPD patient with a superimposed pneumonia, the obese patient with ARDS, or the neuromuscular patient with atelectasis--and the transport clinician must address both mechanisms simultaneously, titrating PEEP and FiO2 for oxygenation while adjusting respiratory rate and tidal volume for ventilation, a dual-target optimization that is more complex than managing either mechanism alone and that must be sustained continuously across the transport window.

## ARDS Ventilator Strategies for Transport

### Lung-Protective Tidal Volume and Plateau Pressure Targets

Lung-protective ventilation with a tidal volume of six to eight milliliters per kilogram of predicted body weight, a plateau pressure below thirty centimeters of water, and the lowest driving pressure achievable is the evidence-based standard for ARDS management and must be maintained without interruption during transport, applying the same equipment-transition verification described in Chapter 3's Silent Lung-Protection Lapse Signature. The transport ventilator's ability to display plateau pressure, either directly or through an inspiratory hold maneuver, should be confirmed before departure, since monitoring plateau pressure is the primary tool for detecting a compliance change that could signal worsening edema, developing pneumothorax, or progressive atelectasis.

### PEEP Titration and Recruitment at Altitude

Positive end-expiratory pressure titration in ARDS aims to maintain alveolar recruitment while avoiding overdistention, and the optimal PEEP level may need adjustment during transport as altitude-related changes in ambient pressure alter the effective transpulmonary pressure. A PEEP level that was appropriately set at sea level may provide relatively less alveolar distending pressure at a higher cabin altitude where ambient pressure is lower, potentially allowing recruited alveoli to de-recruit; conversely, the same nominal PEEP represents a higher fraction of the reduced ambient pressure, which may increase the risk of barotrauma. The practical approach is to monitor oxygenation and compliance trends continuously and adjust PEEP in response to the patient's gas exchange at the actual operating altitude rather than assuming that a ground-level PEEP setting remains optimal throughout a flight.

### Permissive Hypercapnia and Acidosis Tolerance

Accepting a PaCO2 above the normal range in exchange for maintaining low tidal volumes and plateau pressures is a standard component of lung-protective ventilation for ARDS, and the transport clinician should communicate the acceptable PaCO2 range and pH floor to the receiving team so that the receiving team does not reflexively correct a respiratory acidosis that was deliberately tolerated as part of a lung-protective strategy. An arterial pH below 7.20, however, carries increasing risk of hemodynamic compromise and cardiac arrhythmia, and most clinicians treat the acidosis at this threshold with either a modest ventilator adjustment or, in severe cases, sodium bicarbonate infusion, recognizing that the bicarbonate itself generates CO2 that must be ventilated.

| ARDS Severity | PaO2/FiO2 Ratio | Mortality Range | Transport Monitoring Priority |
|---|---|---|---|
| Mild | 201-300 | 27% | Trend oxygenation; may tolerate noninvasive support |
| Moderate | 101-200 | 32% | Invasive ventilation with lung-protective settings; continuous SpO2 and ETCO2 |
| Severe | ≤100 | 45% | Maximum ventilatory support; prone positioning consideration; vasopressor readiness |

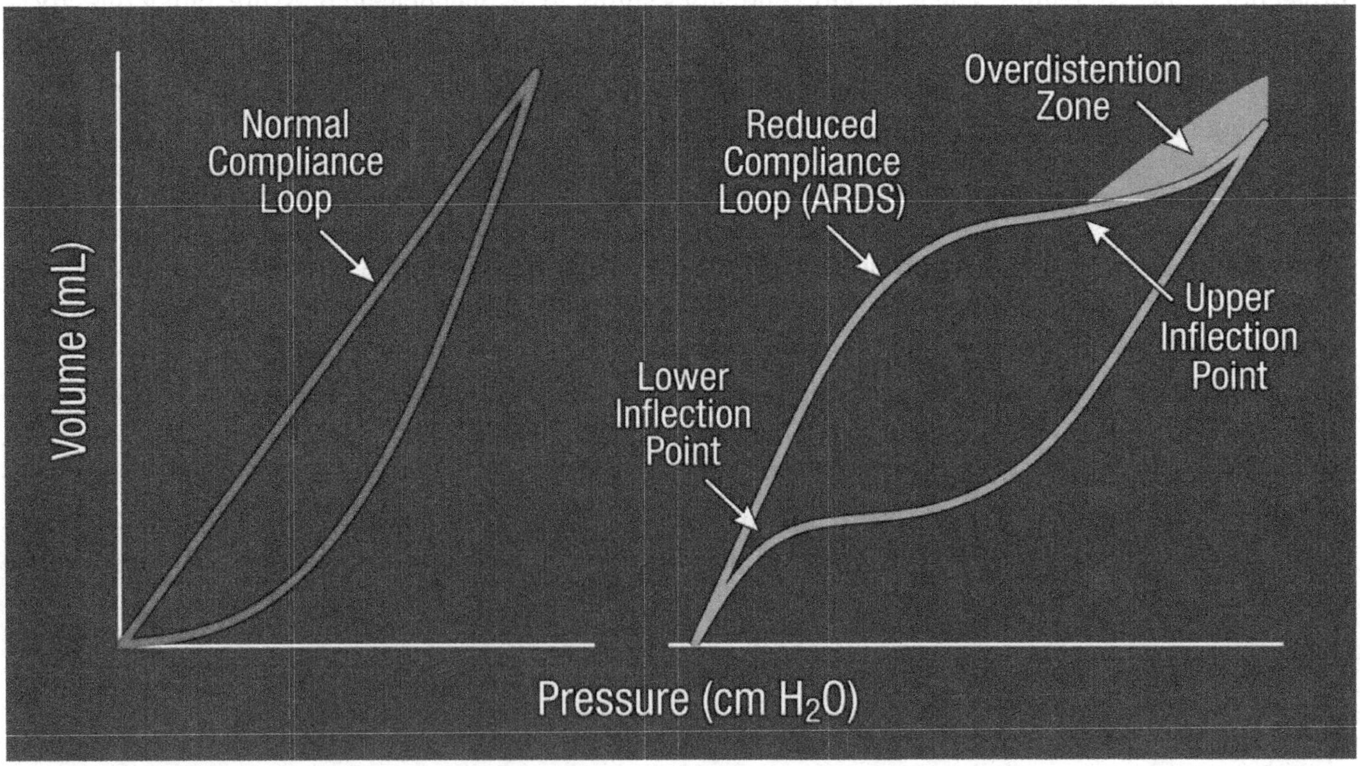

## Prone Positioning and Rescue Oxygenation Therapies

### Prone Positioning Feasibility and Safety in Transport

Prone positioning improves oxygenation in moderate-to-severe ARDS by redistributing ventilation to dorsal lung regions that are better perfused, and its mortality benefit has been demonstrated in prolonged prone sessions in the ICU setting. Proning a patient during transport is logistically challenging but not impossible, and some specialized transport programs perform prone transports routinely for severe ARDS patients. The transport-specific considerations include: securing all lines, tubes, and monitoring cables against the mechanical stress of the turn and the prone position; ensuring that the airway remains accessible and the endotracheal tube is not compressed or kinked; and maintaining continuous monitoring throughout, since a prone patient's face-down position makes direct clinical assessment substantially more difficult than in the supine position.

### Inhaled Pulmonary Vasodilators and Other Rescue Therapies

Inhaled nitric oxide and inhaled epoprostenol, introduced in Chapter 7 for right ventricular failure, also serve as rescue oxygenation therapies in severe ARDS by selectively vasodilating ventilated lung units and improving ventilation-perfusion matching. Their transport logistics are identical to those described in Chapter 7, including the risk of rebound hypoxemia if delivery is interrupted. Neuromuscular blockade, which has been shown to improve oxygenation and reduce ventilator-induced lung injury in early severe ARDS, may be initiated or continued during transport with the same monitoring requirements described in Chapters 4 and 12.

### THE IN-TRANSIT DETERIORATION SIGNATURE SYSTEM — Altitude-Driven ARDS Oxygenation Collapse

**The Signature:** A progressive, disproportionate decline in oxygen saturation during ascent or at altitude in an ARDS patient whose ventilator settings have not changed, exceeding what would be predicted by the Dalton's law reduction in alveolar oxygen tension alone and suggesting active alveolar de-recruitment superimposed on the altitude effect.

**Movement Trigger:** The combination of reduced ambient pressure at altitude (lowering effective transpulmonary distending pressure and promoting alveolar collapse) with the vibration-induced positional shifts that redistribute perfusion away from recruited lung regions produces a synergistic oxygenation decline that is greater than either mechanism alone.

**Early Tell:** A fall in oxygen saturation that begins during climb and continues to worsen after level flight is reached, rather than stabilizing once the altitude effect plateaus, suggesting that ongoing de-recruitment is compounding the initial altitude-mediated hypoxemia.

**Trap Logic:** The initial oxygenation decline is correctly attributed to altitude, but the continued worsening after reaching cruise altitude is the signal that a second mechanism--alveolar de-recruitment--is now operating, and this second mechanism requires a different intervention (PEEP adjustment or recruitment maneuver) than the altitude effect alone (which would respond to increased FiO2 or cabin altitude restriction).

**Signature Anchor:** In any ARDS patient whose oxygenation continues to worsen after reaching cruise altitude despite FiO2 optimization, consider alveolar de-recruitment as the additional mechanism and respond with a PEEP increase or a cautious recruitment maneuver, in addition to requesting a lower cabin altitude if feasible.

## High-Flow and Noninvasive Ventilation En Route

### High-Flow Nasal Cannula in the Transport Environment

High-flow nasal cannula provides humidified, heated oxygen at flow rates up to sixty liters per minute, generating a modest positive airway pressure effect and washing out nasopharyngeal dead space, which can delay or prevent intubation in patients with hypoxemic respiratory failure who retain adequate respiratory drive and airway protective reflexes. The transport-specific limitations include gas consumption (high-flow devices consume oxygen at rates that can rapidly exhaust portable cylinder supplies), device compatibility with transport oxygen systems, and the need for a reliable power source for the heating and humidification unit. The crew should calculate oxygen supply duration at the planned flow rate before departure and have a contingency plan for transitioning to a conventional delivery system if the supply runs low.

### Noninvasive Ventilation Continuation and Failure Recognition

Noninvasive positive pressure ventilation, whether CPAP or BiPAP, can be continued during transport for patients in whom it was effective at the sending facility, but the transport clinician must define clear failure criteria before departure: a rising oxygen requirement, worsening respiratory rate or accessory muscle use, inability to maintain the mask seal, or hemodynamic instability should each trigger reassessment and consideration of intubation rather than prolonged persistence with a failing noninvasive strategy. Intubation during transport is categorically more difficult than at a stationary bedside, which argues for a lower threshold for elective intubation before departure in a patient whose noninvasive ventilation trajectory is borderline rather than clearly improving.

**Figure 13.2: Pressure-Volume Loop Interpretation for PEEP Optimization**

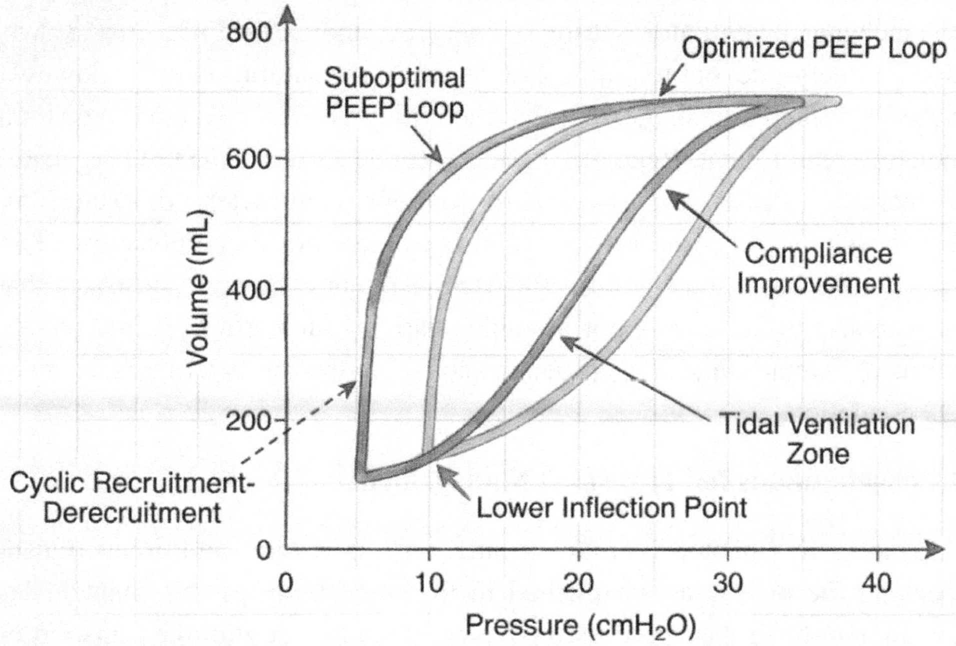


## Weaning and Extubation Readiness Considerations

### Assessing Extubation Readiness Before Transport

A patient who is being considered for extubation at the sending facility should generally be extubated before transport if they meet standard readiness criteria, since reintubation in a moving vehicle is substantially more dangerous than at a stationary bedside, and a patient who fails extubation mid-transport creates a genuine airway emergency in a confined space. Conversely, a patient who is improving but has not yet met readiness criteria should remain intubated for the duration of transport, with extubation deferred to the receiving facility, since the transport environment--with its altitude-related oxygenation challenges, vibration, and limited backup--is not an appropriate setting for a marginal extubation trial.

### Transport-Specific Extubation Contraindications

Beyond the standard extubation readiness criteria, the transport environment imposes additional relative contraindications: any patient with a known or suspected difficult airway, a recent difficult intubation, or significant upper airway edema should not be extubated before transport even if ventilatory parameters appear favorable, because the consequences of a failed reintubation in transit are disproportionately severe compared to the bedside setting. The transport clinician should apply a conservative threshold for extubation that accounts for the reduced rescue capability of the transport environment, not merely the patient's current ventilatory performance.

Consider a forty-four-year-old woman with moderate ARDS from community-acquired pneumonia, ventilated with lung-protective settings at a community hospital and transferred by fixed-wing aircraft to a tertiary ARDS referral center. Her pre-departure PaO2/FiO2 ratio is 145 on a PEEP of twelve and FiO2 of 0.6. During climb to a cabin altitude of six thousand feet, her SpO2 drops from ninety-four to eighty-eight percent despite unchanged ventilator settings. The crew increases FiO2 to 0.8, which briefly stabilizes the saturation at ninety-one, but ten minutes into cruise the saturation drifts downward again to eighty-seven despite the FiO2 increase, suggesting that the initial altitude-mediated hypoxemia has been compounded by alveolar de-recruitment. Recognizing the Altitude-Driven ARDS Oxygenation Collapse Signature, the crew increases PEEP from twelve to fourteen centimeters of water, monitors for hemodynamic consequences, and requests a lower cabin altitude from the flight crew. The saturation stabilizes at ninety-two within five minutes of the PEEP adjustment. The case illustrates that an ARDS patient's oxygenation response to altitude is not a single, static event but a dynamic process in which altitude and de-recruitment interact, and the correct response addresses both mechanisms rather than relying solely on FiO2 escalation.

**Additional Clinical Considerations for Transport Management**

The management of patients in Chapter 13 requires attention to several additional transport-specific clinical factors that extend the principles established in the main body of the chapter. The transport clinician should be aware that the disease processes covered here interact with the transport environment in ways that are specific to the combination of the underlying pathophysiology and the particular environmental stressor encountered during a given mission, and that a management approach that is adequate for a short ground transport may be insufficient for a longer air transport at altitude, or vice versa. The serial reassessment protocol established in Chapter 2 provides the framework for detecting these interactions as they develop, and the Deterioration Signature introduced in this chapter names the most characteristic pattern by which they declare themselves.

Each patient transport is a unique combination of a specific patient's physiology, a specific set of ongoing therapies, a specific transport platform with its own environmental characteristics, and a specific mission profile with its own altitude, duration, and route constraints. The anticipatory approach to transport medicine that this text teaches is not a set of memorized responses to predetermined scenarios but a cognitive framework for analyzing the specific combination of variables present in any given transport and identifying, before departure, the most likely points of vulnerability where the transport environment will test the patient's physiologic reserve. This chapter's clinical content provides the disease-specific knowledge needed to apply that framework to the conditions covered here, while the Deterioration Signature provides the named pattern that makes the most characteristic transport-specific vulnerability explicit, recognizable, and actionable.

The receiving team's ability to continue the patient's care seamlessly after the transport crew departs depends entirely on the quality and completeness of the clinical information the transport crew provides, and for the conditions covered in this chapter, the specific information that matters most includes: the trajectory of the patient's primary condition during transport (improving, stable, or worsening, with specific details), any interventions performed during transport and their response, any new clinical findings identified by the transport crew that were not present at the sending facility, and any anticipated needs that the receiving team should prepare for based on the transport crew's clinical assessment. This information, communicated through the structured handoff format established in Chapter 2 and supplemented by the trajectory communication emphasis that is a recurring theme throughout this text, is the final clinical act of the transport and the one that determines whether the transport adds value to the patient's care continuum or merely moves the patient from one location to another without preserving the clinical narrative that only the transport crew was positioned to observe.

The transport clinician managing the conditions addressed in this chapter should develop a systematic pre-departure assessment that specifically identifies the highest-risk transport-environment interaction for each patient's specific disease process, the monitoring parameters that will detect that interaction earliest, and the intervention that will address it most effectively. This pre-departure risk analysis, adapted from the general pre-mission physiologic risk profile introduced in Chapter 1, should be specific enough to generate a concrete prediction: what is the single most likely way this specific patient's condition will interact with the specific transport environment of this specific mission? Answering that question before departure, rather than discovering the answer during transit, is the practical application of the anticipatory transport medicine framework that this entire text is designed to develop.

Clinical case presentations embedded throughout this chapter illustrate the principle that transport-specific deterioration patterns are predictable rather than random, recognizable rather than mysterious, and preventable rather than inevitable, provided the clinician applies the systematic assessment, continuous monitoring, and named-pattern recognition framework that the Deterioration Signature System codifies. Each case demonstrates the same three-part sequence: a patient with a specific disease process encounters a specific transport-environment stressor, produces a specific clinical change that could be attributed to either the disease or the environment, and is correctly managed because the transport clinician recognized the specific named Signature and applied the correct transport-specific intervention rather than the generic disease-specific response that would have been appropriate at the bedside but is insufficient or incorrect in the transport context.

The evidence base for transport-specific management of the conditions in this chapter continues to evolve, with ongoing research into optimal monitoring strategies, transport-adapted treatment protocols, and outcome data that will refine the recommendations presented here. The transport clinician should maintain awareness of emerging evidence through continuing education, program-sponsored journal clubs, and the quality improvement processes described in Chapter 24, since the standard of care for transport medicine is not static and the recommendations in any textbook represent a snapshot of evidence at the time of writing rather than a permanent standard. The principles, however, are durable: anticipate rather than react, monitor trends rather than thresholds, communicate trajectories rather than snapshots, and recognize that the transport environment is a clinical variable that acts on every patient's physiology, not a neutral conduit between two points of care.

Finally, the transport clinician should recognize that the clinical expertise required to manage these conditions during transport represents a distinct competency that builds on but extends beyond the bedside critical care training that most transport clinicians bring to their role. A clinician who is expert in managing these conditions in the intensive care unit is not automatically expert in managing them during transport, because the environmental, equipment, monitoring, and resource constraints of transport introduce variables that bedside practice never encounters. Conversely, a transport clinician who has mastered the anticipatory, environment-aware management approach described in this text brings a perspective to patient care that the bedside clinician lacks: the ability to see the patient's physiology not as a fixed state being managed in a controlled environment, but as a dynamic process interacting continuously with an environment that is itself changing throughout the transport. This dual awareness--of the disease and of the environment acting on it--is the defining competency of transport critical care medicine, and it is what this text, from its first chapter through its last, is designed to develop.

**THE IN-TRANSIT DETERIORATION SIGNATURE SYSTEM — Respiratory Failure Transport Patterns**

**Signature Introduced This Chapter:** Altitude-Driven ARDS Oxygenation Collapse (progressive oxygenation decline from combined altitude-mediated hypoxemia and vibration/position-induced alveolar de-recruitment, producing a synergistic decline that exceeds either mechanism alone).

**Respiratory Pattern Logic:** This Signature combines two previously introduced mechanisms--Dalton's law altitude hypoxemia from Chapter 1 and positional hemodynamic shifts from Chapter 7--into a respiratory-specific pattern where both operate simultaneously on a lung with minimal reserve, producing a decline steeper than either would explain individually.

**Cross-Reference Forward:** Chapter 14 (Pneumothorax and Thoracic Emergencies) addresses the thoracic trauma overlap with ARDS; Chapter 15 (Multisystem Trauma) addresses the trauma-ARDS interface with hemorrhagic shock management.

## Summary and Key Concepts

Hypoxemic and hypercapnic respiratory failure require different primary interventions; misidentifying the predominant mechanism leads to the wrong therapeutic emphasis.

Lung-protective ventilation targets must be maintained without interruption during transport, with equipment-transition verification at every ventilator change.

PEEP optimization may require real-time adjustment at altitude as reduced ambient pressure alters effective transpulmonary distending pressure.

High-flow nasal cannula and noninvasive ventilation can be continued during transport but require clear failure criteria and a low threshold for pre-departure intubation in borderline patients.

An ARDS patient whose oxygenation continues to worsen after reaching cruise altitude despite $FiO_2$ optimization should be assessed for alveolar de-recruitment as an additional mechanism requiring PEEP adjustment.

# CHAPTER 14: PNEUMOTHORAX, CHEST TRAUMA, AND THORACIC EMERGENCIES IN TRANSIT

**Learning Objectives**

1. Recognize tension pneumothorax in the transport environment and perform needle or finger thoracostomy under transit conditions.
2. Manage chest tube drainage systems during air and ground transport.
3. Identify and manage hemothorax, flail chest, and massive hemoptysis during transit.
4. Recognize pulmonary embolism and initiate risk-stratified management during interfacility transport.
5. Anticipate altitude-related worsening of thoracic injuries using the gas-law framework from Chapter 1.

**Chapter Outline**

This chapter extends the Occult Pneumothorax Expansion at Altitude Signature introduced in Chapter 1 to the full spectrum of thoracic emergencies encountered in critical care transport, including traumatic pneumothorax, hemothorax, flail chest, and pulmonary embolism. These conditions share a common transport vulnerability: the thoracic cavity is a gas-containing, pressure-sensitive space that is directly affected by the altitude-related pressure changes and the mechanical forces of the transport environment, making thoracic pathology uniquely susceptible to transport-triggered deterioration.

## Tension Pneumothorax Recognition and Needle/Finger Thoracostomy

### Clinical Recognition Under Transport Monitoring Constraints

Tension pneumothorax during transport presents with the classic combination of hypotension, hypoxemia, absent breath sounds on the affected side, and tracheal deviation, but the transport environment degrades the clinician's ability to detect these findings: auscultation is unreliable in a noisy cabin, tracheal deviation is a late and unreliable sign, and the hypotension and desaturation may initially be attributed to equipment artifact or altitude-related changes rather than recognized as a thoracic emergency. The most reliable early indicators in the transport environment are a sudden, sustained rise in peak airway pressures on the ventilator (in a mechanically ventilated patient), a concordant fall in oxygen saturation and blood pressure, and a loss of chest wall movement symmetry visible on direct inspection--a combination that should trigger immediate decompression rather than further diagnostic workup.

### Needle Versus Finger Thoracostomy in the Transport Environment

Needle decompression using a large-bore needle or angiocatheter at the second intercostal space, midclavicular line, or the fifth intercostal space, anterior axillary line, provides immediate but temporary relief of tension physiology and can be performed with minimal equipment and space--advantages that make it feasible in the confined cabin of a moving vehicle or aircraft. Its principal limitation is the high failure rate from needle length inadequacy in patients with significant chest wall thickness, needle kinking, and reaccumulation of air, all of which may necessitate a repeat attempt or conversion to a finger thoracostomy. Finger thoracostomy--a small incision through the chest wall with digital confirmation of pleural entry and placement of a gloved finger into the pleural space to release trapped air--provides more definitive decompression and is increasingly taught as the primary transport decompression technique for clinicians trained in the procedure.

### Performing Thoracic Procedures in a Moving Vehicle

Both procedures are substantially more difficult to perform in a moving vehicle than at a stationary bedside: patient positioning may be constrained by stretcher restraints, the procedural field moves with vehicle vibration, sterile technique is compromised by the confined and non-sterile cabin environment, and the clinician performing the procedure cannot simultaneously monitor the patient or manage other aspects of the clinical picture. The decision to perform a thoracic procedure during active transport versus requesting a stop should weigh the urgency of the decompression against the brief delay of stopping, recognizing that for true tension physiology, the urgency is absolute and the procedure must proceed without delay, while for a suspected but non-tension pneumothorax, a brief stop may produce a better procedural outcome than an attempt during active turbulence.

**KEY POINT:** In the transport environment, a sudden concordant rise in peak airway pressures plus a fall in $SpO_2$ and blood pressure should trigger immediate thoracic decompression rather than further diagnostic workup; tension pneumothorax is treated on clinical suspicion, not confirmed by imaging.

Figure 14.1: Needle and Finger Thoracostomy Anatomic Landmarks

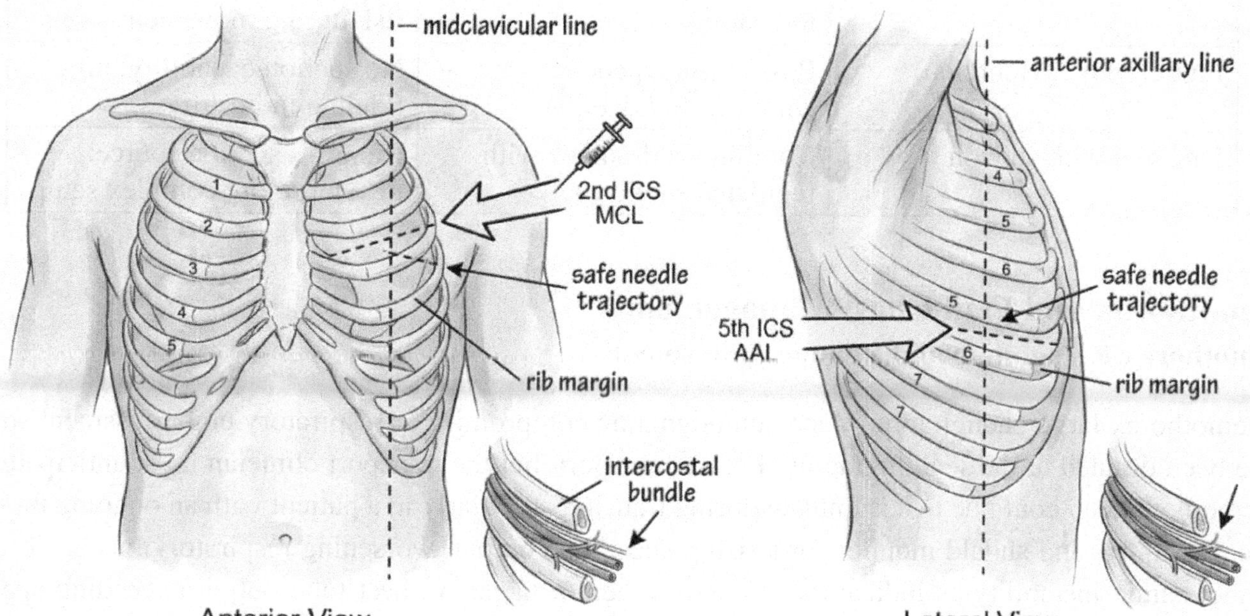


## Chest Tube Management During Transport

### Drainage System Types and Transport Compatibility

Chest tubes placed before transport may be connected to a water-seal drainage system, a one-way flutter valve (Heimlich valve), or a dry-seal system, each with different transport handling requirements. Water-seal systems must remain upright to function correctly and are vulnerable to spillage during the tilting and movement of transport, making them less transport-friendly than flutter valves, which allow drainage in any position and do not require a water column. For patients with ongoing air leaks or significant pleural fluid output, a drainage system that provides continuous suction through a regulated source is ideal but may not be available on all transport platforms, in which case a flutter valve with a collection bag provides adequate drainage without suction for the transport duration.

### Monitoring Drainage Output and Detecting Complications

The chest tube drainage output should be monitored at fixed intervals during transport, both for total volume and for the character of the output (serous, sanguineous, or purulent), since a sudden increase in sanguineous drainage may indicate active hemorrhage that requires escalation, while a sudden cessation of drainage in a patient who was previously draining may indicate tube occlusion, kinking, or malposition rather than resolution of the pleural process. The tube itself should be visually inspected at each reassessment for kinking at the skin exit site or where it traverses the stretcher edge, and the connections between tube, drainage system, and any suction source should be checked for security, since a disconnection during transport produces an immediate open pneumothorax through the chest wall defect around the tube.

| Drainage System | Transport Advantage | Transport Limitation |
|---|---|---|
| Water-seal | Familiar; provides tidaling indicator | Must remain upright; spillage risk during movement |
| Flutter valve (Heimlich) | Position-independent; compact; lightweight | No suction capability; no tidaling indicator |
| Dry-seal with suction | Continuous drainage with regulated suction | Requires suction source; heavier; more complex setup |

## Hemothorax and Flail Chest Management

### Hemothorax Recognition and Volume Assessment

A hemothorax large enough to produce hemodynamic compromise or respiratory embarrassment should have been drained at the sending facility before transport, but the transport clinician must anticipate that a hemothorax can continue to accumulate during transit, particularly in a patient with an ongoing thoracic vascular injury, and should monitor for a rising chest tube output, worsening respiratory mechanics, and hemodynamic instability as indicators of ongoing hemorrhage. A chest tube output exceeding specific volume thresholds over a defined time period (typically cited as initial output exceeding one thousand milliliters or ongoing output exceeding two hundred milliliters per hour) suggests a surgical hemorrhage that the receiving facility should be alerted to in advance so that thoracic surgical resources are mobilized before the patient's arrival.

### Flail Chest and Pulmonary Contusion Management

Flail chest--a segment of chest wall with fractures in two or more ribs at two sites each, producing paradoxical motion--compromises ventilatory mechanics through the flail segment's paradoxical inward movement during inspiration, but the more important clinical concern is typically the underlying pulmonary contusion, which produces progressive hypoxemia over hours as the contusion matures and edema accumulates. The transport clinician managing a flail chest patient should anticipate worsening oxygenation during a transport that falls within the twelve-to-forty-eight-hour window after injury, when contusion-related edema is typically increasing, and should have ventilator support ready for escalation even if the patient is currently managing on supplemental oxygen alone.

### Pain Management for Chest Wall Injury During Transport

Adequate analgesia for thoracic wall injuries is both a humanitarian and a physiologic priority during transport: undertreated chest wall pain produces splinting, hypoventilation, atelectasis, and progressive hypoxemia that can convert a stable patient into one requiring intubation and mechanical ventilation. The multimodal analgesic approach from Chapter 4 applies directly, with fentanyl as the primary agent and ketamine at sub-dissociative doses as an adjunct. Regional anesthesia techniques such as intercostal nerve blocks or serratus anterior plane blocks, if performed at the sending facility before transport, provide superior analgesia to systemic opioids alone and should be continued and monitored during transit.

## Massive Hemoptysis and Airway Protection

### Airway Management in Active Hemorrhage

Massive hemoptysis--typically defined as more than one hundred milliliters in twenty-four hours or any amount sufficient to produce airway compromise--represents one of the most dangerous airway emergencies in the transport setting because blood in the airway simultaneously threatens both oxygenation (by flooding alveolar gas exchange surfaces) and ventilation (by obstructing the endotracheal tube or tracheobronchial tree). Airway protection with a large-bore endotracheal tube that allows passage of a suction catheter is the first priority, and positioning the patient with the bleeding side down (if identified) uses gravity to protect the non-bleeding lung from contamination. Continuous suction capability, verified as described in Chapter 5, is essential for the duration of the transport, since recurrent airway bleeding can obstruct the tube or circuit at any time.

## Pulmonary Embolism Recognition and Management in Transit

### Risk Stratification and Treatment Decisions During Transport

Pulmonary embolism encountered during transport ranges from hemodynamically stable presentations managed with anticoagulation alone to massive, hemodynamically compromising events that may require thrombolytic therapy or catheter-directed intervention at the receiving facility. The transport clinician's primary tasks are risk stratification--using clinical findings, right ventricular strain markers on ECG, and point-of-care echocardiography where available to classify the patient as low, submassive, or massive--and initiation of systemic anticoagulation with heparin unless contraindicated, since the time to therapeutic anticoagulation directly affects the risk of clot propagation and hemodynamic deterioration during the transport window.

### Right Ventricular Failure Management in Massive PE

Massive pulmonary embolism producing right ventricular failure requires the same right-heart-specific management approach described in Chapter 7: avoidance of excessive volume loading that worsens right ventricular distention, norepinephrine as the first-line vasopressor to maintain coronary perfusion pressure to the failing right ventricle, and generous oxygenation to minimize hypoxic pulmonary vasoconstriction that adds to the right ventricular afterload burden. The altitude-related increase in pulmonary vascular resistance described in Chapter 7 applies with particular force to the PE patient, and the transport clinician should proactively request a lower cabin altitude or maximize oxygenation for any PE patient with evidence of right ventricular strain.

### THE IN-TRANSIT DETERIORATION SIGNATURE SYSTEM — Chest Tube Obstruction Masquerading as Primary Pulmonary Deterioration

---

**The Signature:** Progressive respiratory distress, rising peak airway pressures, and hemodynamic instability in a patient with a chest tube in place, initially attributed to a primary pulmonary process such as worsening ARDS or contusion maturation, but actually caused by chest tube occlusion or kinking that has allowed a recurrent pneumothorax or hemothorax to re-accumulate undetected.

**Movement Trigger:** The mechanical stresses of transport--stretcher repositioning, loading tilt, vibration, and patient movement during clinical care--can kink, displace, or occlude a chest tube at the skin exit site, at the point where it crosses the stretcher edge, or at the connection to the drainage system, producing a functional loss of drainage that is not visible on the external portion of the tube.

**Early Tell:** A cessation of previously present drainage output, loss of the respiratory swing or tidaling in the drainage system, or a change in the tube's position relative to the patient's skin exit site, any of which should prompt inspection of the tube and drainage system before attributing the respiratory change to a primary pulmonary process.

**Trap Logic:** This pattern is particularly dangerous because the chest tube's presence creates a false sense of security that the pleural space is being drained when in fact it is not, and the respiratory and hemodynamic changes produced by a recurrent pneumothorax or hemothorax are identical to those produced by primary pulmonary deterioration, directing the clinician's attention toward the lungs rather than toward the tube.

**Signature Anchor:** In any patient with a chest tube who develops new respiratory distress or hemodynamic instability during transport, inspect the tube and drainage system for patency, position, and drainage output before initiating treatment for a primary pulmonary process; a kinked or occluded tube is immediately correctable, while the recurrent collection it has allowed to accumulate is the actual clinical problem.

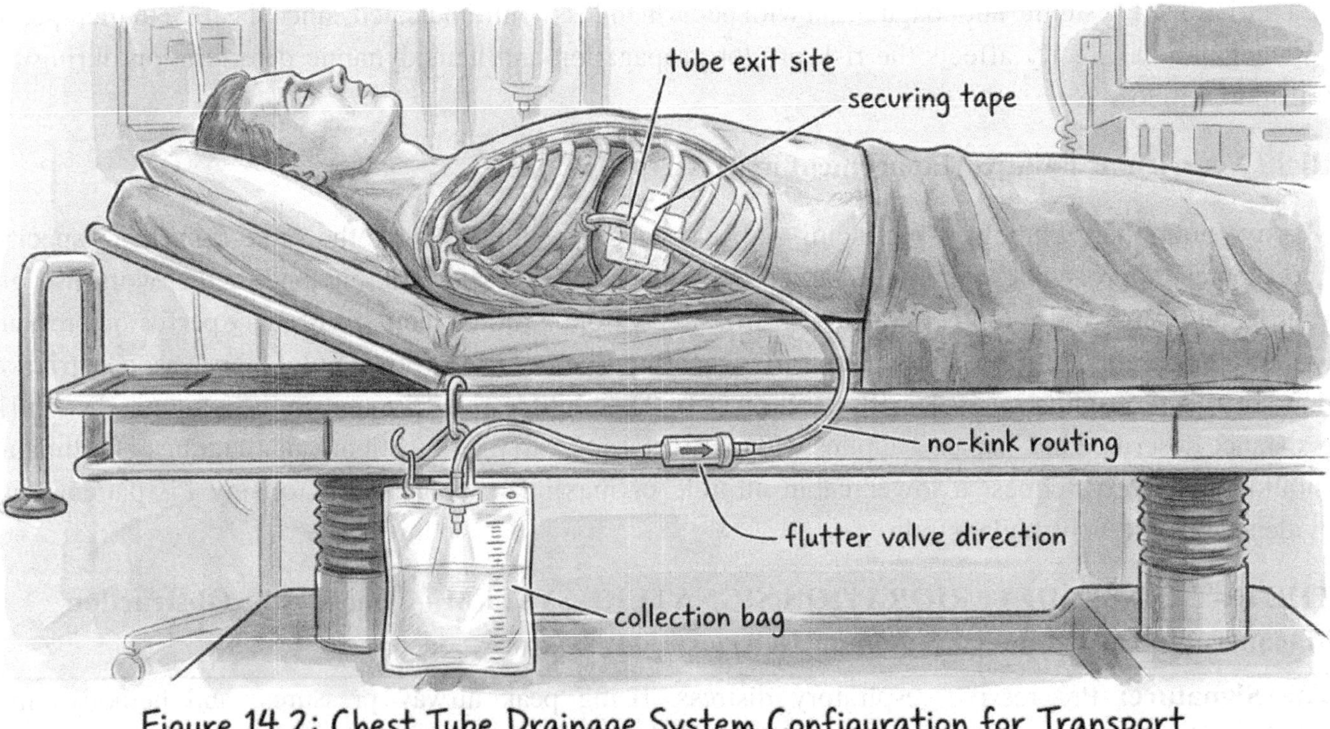


Figure 14.2: Chest Tube Drainage System Configuration for Transport

Consider a thirty-six-year-old man with a traumatic pneumothorax and two rib fractures, chest tube placed at the sending facility with good initial drainage and lung re-expansion confirmed on post-placement radiograph, transported by ground critical care ambulance. Twenty minutes into transport, the crew notes a gradual rise in peak airway pressures and a subtle decline in oxygen saturation. The initial assessment focuses on the ventilator circuit and airway--ruling out tube migration, mucus plugging, and bronchospasm. However, a crew member inspecting the chest tube notes that the tube has kinked at the point where it crosses the stretcher rail, and the flutter valve has stopped oscillating with respiration. Unkinking the tube produces an immediate rush of air and a small amount of sanguineous fluid into the collection bag, and the peak airway pressures and saturation normalize within two minutes. The case illustrates the Chest Tube Obstruction Signature: the chest tube's presence created a false assumption that the pleural space was being managed, when in fact the tube had been functionally non-draining since the kink occurred during the loading process, allowing a recurrent pneumothorax to accumulate gradually.

**Additional Clinical Considerations for Transport Management**

The management of patients in Chapter 14 requires attention to several additional transport-specific clinical factors that extend the principles established in the main body of the chapter. The transport clinician should be aware that the disease processes covered here interact with the transport environment in ways that are specific to the combination of the underlying pathophysiology and the particular environmental stressor encountered during a given mission, and that a management approach that is adequate for a short ground transport may be insufficient for a longer air transport at altitude, or vice versa. The serial reassessment protocol established in Chapter 2 provides the framework for detecting these interactions as they develop, and the Deterioration Signature introduced in this chapter names the most characteristic pattern by which they declare themselves.

Each patient transport is a unique combination of a specific patient's physiology, a specific set of ongoing therapies, a specific transport platform with its own environmental characteristics, and a specific mission profile with its own altitude, duration, and route constraints. The anticipatory approach to transport medicine that this text teaches is not a set of memorized responses to predetermined scenarios but a cognitive framework for analyzing the specific combination of variables present in any given transport and identifying, before departure, the most likely points of vulnerability where the transport environment will test the patient's physiologic reserve. This chapter's clinical content provides the disease-specific knowledge needed to apply that framework to the conditions covered here, while the Deterioration Signature provides the named pattern that makes the most characteristic transport-specific vulnerability explicit, recognizable, and actionable.

The receiving team's ability to continue the patient's care seamlessly after the transport crew departs depends entirely on the quality and completeness of the clinical information the transport crew provides, and for the conditions covered in this chapter, the specific information that matters most includes: the trajectory of the patient's primary condition during transport (improving, stable, or worsening, with specific details), any interventions performed during transport and their response, any new clinical findings identified by the transport crew that were not present at the sending facility, and any anticipated needs that the receiving team should prepare for based on the transport crew's clinical assessment. This information, communicated through the structured handoff format established in Chapter 2 and supplemented by the trajectory communication emphasis that is a recurring theme throughout this text, is the final clinical act of the transport and the one that determines whether the transport adds value to the patient's care continuum or merely moves the patient from one location to another without preserving the clinical narrative that only the transport crew was positioned to observe.

The transport clinician managing the conditions addressed in this chapter should develop a systematic pre-departure assessment that specifically identifies the highest-risk transport-environment interaction for each patient's specific disease process, the monitoring parameters that will detect that interaction earliest, and the intervention that will address it most effectively. This pre-departure risk analysis, adapted from the general pre-mission physiologic risk profile introduced in Chapter 1, should be specific enough to generate a concrete prediction: what is the single most likely way this specific patient's condition will interact with the specific transport environment of this specific mission? Answering that question before departure, rather than discovering the answer during transit, is the practical application of the anticipatory transport medicine framework that this entire text is designed to develop.

Clinical case presentations embedded throughout this chapter illustrate the principle that transport-specific deterioration patterns are predictable rather than random, recognizable rather than mysterious, and preventable rather than inevitable, provided the clinician applies the systematic assessment, continuous monitoring, and named-pattern recognition framework that the Deterioration Signature System codifies. Each case demonstrates the same three-part sequence: a patient with a specific disease process encounters a specific transport-environment stressor, produces a specific clinical change that could be attributed to either the disease or the environment, and is correctly managed because the transport clinician recognized the specific named Signature and applied the correct transport-specific intervention rather than the generic disease-specific response that would have been appropriate at the bedside but is insufficient or incorrect in the transport context.

The evidence base for transport-specific management of the conditions in this chapter continues to evolve, with ongoing research into optimal monitoring strategies, transport-adapted treatment protocols, and outcome data that will refine the recommendations presented here. The transport clinician should maintain awareness of emerging evidence through continuing education, program-sponsored journal clubs, and the quality improvement processes described in Chapter 24, since the standard of care for transport medicine is not static and the recommendations in any textbook represent a snapshot of evidence at the time of writing rather than a permanent standard. The principles, however, are durable: anticipate rather than react, monitor trends rather than thresholds, communicate trajectories rather than snapshots, and recognize that the transport environment is a clinical variable that acts on every patient's physiology, not a neutral conduit between two points of care.

Finally, the transport clinician should recognize that the clinical expertise required to manage these conditions during transport represents a distinct competency that builds on but extends beyond the bedside critical care training that most transport clinicians bring to their role. A clinician who is expert in managing these conditions in the intensive care unit is not automatically expert in managing them during transport, because the environmental, equipment, monitoring, and resource constraints of transport introduce variables that bedside practice never encounters. Conversely, a transport clinician who has mastered the anticipatory, environment-aware management approach described in this text brings a perspective to patient care that the bedside clinician lacks: the ability to see the patient's physiology not as a fixed state being managed in a controlled environment, but as a dynamic process interacting continuously with an environment that is itself changing throughout the transport. This dual awareness--of the disease and of the environment acting on it--is the defining competency of transport critical care medicine, and it is what this text, from its first chapter through its last, is designed to develop.

**THE IN-TRANSIT DETERIORATION SIGNATURE SYSTEM — Thoracic Emergency Transport Patterns**

**Signature Introduced This Chapter:** Chest Tube Obstruction Masquerading as Primary Pulmonary Deterioration (functional loss of chest tube drainage from transport-related mechanical occlusion, allowing recurrent pneumothorax or hemothorax to re-accumulate undetected).

**Thoracic Pattern Logic:** This Signature completes the thoracic arc begun in Chapter 1 with the Occult Pneumothorax Expansion Signature: Chapter 1 addressed the patient who arrives without a chest tube and whose occult pneumothorax expands at altitude, while this chapter addresses the patient who has a chest tube that fails mechanically during transport, allowing a previously drained pneumothorax to recur.

**Cross-Reference Forward:** Chapter 15 (Multisystem Trauma) addresses the interaction between thoracic injuries, hemorrhagic shock, and traumatic brain injury in the multiply injured patient; Chapter 16 (Burns) addresses inhalation injury overlap with thoracic management.

## Summary and Key Concepts

Tension pneumothorax in transit should be treated on clinical suspicion--concordant rise in airway pressures plus hemodynamic compromise--without waiting for imaging confirmation.

Chest tube drainage systems must be compatible with the transport environment; flutter valves are more transport-friendly than water-seal systems but provide no suction.

A sudden cessation of chest tube drainage during transport should prompt immediate tube and drainage system inspection before attributing respiratory changes to a primary pulmonary process.

Massive hemoptysis requires large-bore endotracheal tube placement, affected-side-down positioning, and continuous suction capability throughout transport.

Pulmonary embolism risk stratification and early anticoagulation are the primary transport management tasks; altitude-related pulmonary vasoconstriction worsens right ventricular afterload in massive PE.

# CHAPTER 15: MULTISYSTEM TRAUMA AND HEMORRHAGIC SHOCK IN TRANSIT

**Learning Objectives**

1. Perform a structured primary and secondary trauma survey adapted to the transport environment.
2. Implement massive transfusion protocol principles during interfacility transport.
3. Apply damage control resuscitation strategies including permissive hypotension, hemostatic resuscitation, and hypothermia prevention.
4. Manage pelvic and extremity hemorrhage control during transit.
5. Coordinate communication with receiving trauma centers for advance activation of surgical resources.

**Chapter Outline**

This chapter addresses the transport of the multiply injured patient in hemorrhagic shock, one of the most time-critical and physiologically demanding transport scenarios in critical care medicine. The transport clinician managing a hemorrhagic shock patient must simultaneously manage active hemorrhage control, volume resuscitation, hemodynamic support, and secondary injury prevention while moving toward a surgical facility that can provide the definitive hemorrhage control that resuscitation alone cannot achieve.

## Primary and Secondary Trauma Survey in the Transport Setting

### Rapid Assessment and Injury Prioritization

The primary trauma survey in the transport setting follows the same airway-breathing-circulation-disability-exposure sequence used at the scene, but the transport clinician performs it with a different purpose: not as a first assessment of an unknown patient, but as an independent verification of the sending facility's assessment and a baseline against which subsequent changes during transit will be measured. Injuries missed by the sending team's evaluation are not uncommon, particularly soft-tissue injuries, posterior wounds, and subtle musculoskeletal injuries that were lower priority during the sending facility's resuscitation-focused evaluation, and the transport crew's independent secondary survey frequently identifies findings that change the receiving facility's surgical planning.

### Reassessment Intervals for the Trauma Patient

The multiply injured patient requires more frequent reassessment during transport than most other patient populations, because the trajectory of hemorrhagic shock can change rapidly, and a patient who appears hemodynamically stable at departure may deteriorate within minutes if an initially tamponaded hemorrhage source re-opens with the positional and mechanical stresses of transport. Reassessment intervals of every five to ten minutes, rather than the fifteen-to-twenty-minute intervals adequate for most medical patients, should be the standard for any trauma patient with hemodynamic instability or a significant mechanism of injury.

## Massive Transfusion Protocol Adaptation for Transport

### Blood Product Logistics in the Transport Environment

Massive transfusion during transport requires advance planning that begins before the crew arrives at the sending facility: the type and quantity of blood products available, the cooler and storage capability of the transport platform, the ABO compatibility status of the patient, and the availability of emergency release uncrossmatched blood (typically O-negative packed red blood cells and AB plasma) must all be confirmed before departure. Many transport programs carry a limited supply of emergency-release blood products on the transport platform itself, while others rely on products prepared by the sending facility's blood bank, and the crew must know which arrangement applies to their specific program and mission.

### Balanced Resuscitation: Red Cells, Plasma, and Platelets

Damage control resuscitation emphasizes a balanced ratio of red blood cells, plasma, and platelets--typically approaching a one-to-one-to-one ratio by unit--to replace not only oxygen-carrying capacity but also clotting factors and platelet function that are consumed and diluted during hemorrhagic shock. The transport clinician should administer blood products in this balanced fashion rather than defaulting to crystalloid-heavy resuscitation, since excessive crystalloid dilutes the remaining clotting factors, worsens hypothermia from unwarmed fluid, and contributes to the coagulopathy that is already the primary threat to the hemorrhaging patient.

### Tranexamic Acid Administration

Tranexamic acid, an antifibrinolytic agent, reduces mortality in hemorrhagic trauma when administered within three hours of injury, and the transport window frequently falls within this treatment interval. A loading dose followed by a maintenance infusion should be initiated as early as possible in any patient with significant traumatic hemorrhage, ideally at the sending facility before departure or during the early phase of transport. The drug's benefit diminishes sharply after three hours, and there is evidence that late administration beyond three hours may be harmful, making accurate documentation of injury time and early drug administration a transport-specific priority.

| Resuscitation Component | Transport Priority | Key Consideration |
|---|---|---|
| Packed red blood cells | Highest -- oxygen carrying capacity | O-negative emergency release if crossmatch unavailable |
| Fresh frozen plasma | High -- clotting factor replacement | Thaw time required; coordinate with sending blood bank before departure |

| | | |
|---|---|---|
| Platelets | Moderate -- maintain platelet function | Storage and availability limited in many community hospitals |
| Tranexamic acid | High -- antifibrinolytic benefit within 3-hour window | Administer as early as possible; document injury time |
| Crystalloid | Low -- use only as bridge until blood products available | Excessive crystalloid worsens coagulopathy, hypothermia, and acidosis |

**Figure 15.1: Damage Control Resuscitation Components and Timing**

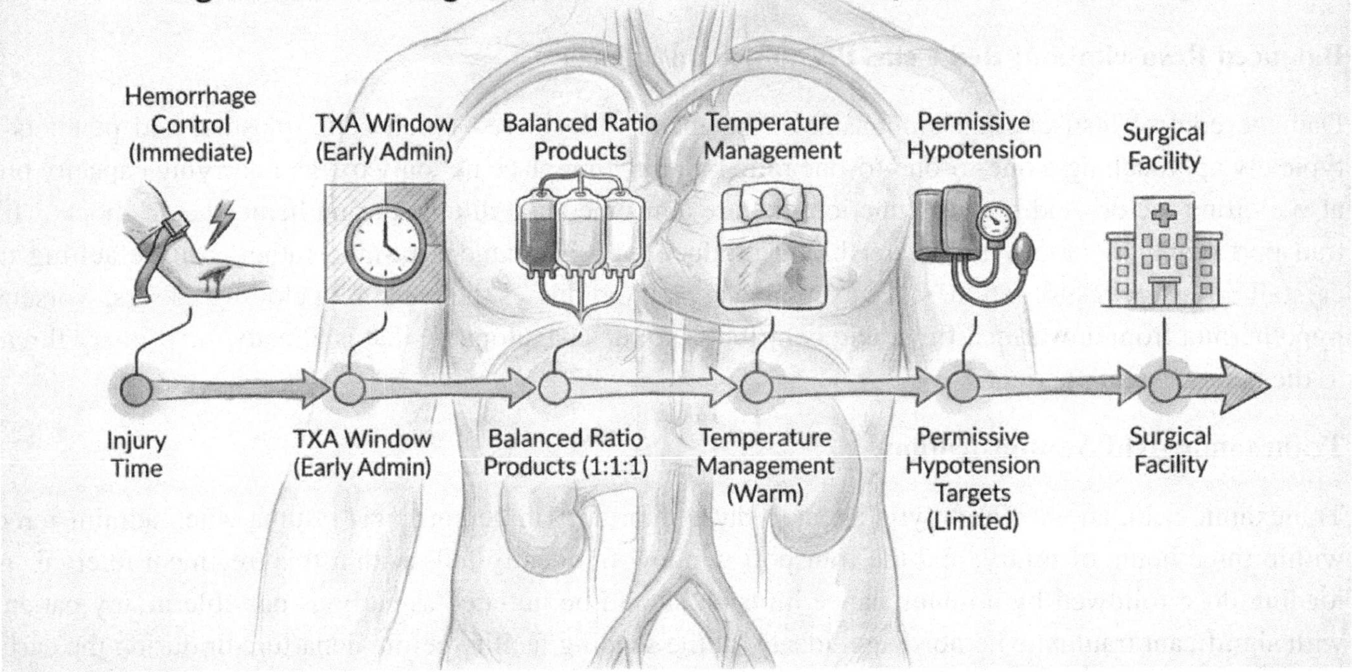


## Damage Control Resuscitation Principles

### Permissive Hypotension: Rationale and Limits

Permissive hypotension--accepting a systolic blood pressure lower than the normal target, typically sixty to eighty millimeters of mercury in the absence of traumatic brain injury--reduces the driving pressure behind active hemorrhage and allows clot formation at injured vascular sites to proceed without being disrupted by higher flow rates. This strategy is specifically contraindicated in the presence of traumatic brain injury, where the cerebral perfusion pressure implications of systemic hypotension produce irreversible secondary brain injury, as discussed in Chapter 11. The transport clinician must identify the presence or absence of traumatic brain injury early in the assessment, since it determines which blood pressure target applies for the duration of the transport.

### Hypothermia Prevention: The Lethal Triad

Hypothermia, acidosis, and coagulopathy form the lethal triad that drives mortality in hemorrhagic trauma, and each component worsens the others in a self-reinforcing cycle. Hypothermia prevention during transport follows the principles from Chapter 1: active warming with forced-air blankets, warmed intravenous fluids administered through in-line warmers where available, and passive insulation to minimize radiant and convective heat loss. The transport environment is particularly hostile to temperature maintenance because the combination of vehicle or aircraft exposure, unwarmed blood products and fluids, and the patient's impaired thermoregulatory capacity from hemorrhagic shock produces a temperature decline that is faster and more difficult to reverse than in a controlled hospital environment.

## Pelvic and Extremity Hemorrhage Control

### Pelvic Binder Application and Monitoring

Pelvic fractures with hemodynamic instability require circumferential pelvic compression with a commercial pelvic binder or a bedsheet wrap applied at the level of the greater trochanters to reduce pelvic volume and promote clot formation. The binder should be applied at the sending facility before transport and should remain in place for the duration of transport without removal, since releasing pelvic compression can disrupt clots and re-initiate hemorrhage. The transport clinician should verify binder position at each reassessment interval, since stretcher movement can shift the binder superiorly or inferiorly from its intended position, reducing its effectiveness.

### Tourniquet Management and Extremity Hemorrhage

Tourniquets applied for life-threatening extremity hemorrhage should remain in place during transport and should not be loosened or removed in transit, since the transport environment is not the appropriate setting for reassessing tourniquet necessity--that decision belongs to the receiving trauma team. The time of tourniquet application should be clearly documented on the tourniquet itself and in the transport record, since prolonged tourniquet time carries ischemic limb consequences that the receiving team must factor into their surgical planning.

### THE IN-TRANSIT DETERIORATION SIGNATURE SYSTEM — Rebleeding After Position-Disrupted Tamponade

**The Signature:** A sudden, disproportionate hemodynamic deterioration in a previously stable or stabilizing trauma patient that occurs during or immediately after a positional change such as stretcher loading, aircraft ascent, or patient repositioning for a procedure.

**Movement Trigger:** Positional changes, acceleration forces, and the mechanical jarring of loading and movement can disrupt a tamponaded hemorrhage source--a retroperitoneal hematoma stabilized by intra-abdominal pressure, a pelvic fracture stabilized by a binder, or a hepatic laceration stabilized by surrounding tissue--re-initiating hemorrhage that had been controlled by the patient's immobility.

**Early Tell:** A rising heart rate or falling blood pressure that appears abruptly rather than gradually, temporally linked to a specific movement event, and out of proportion to the expected hemodynamic effect of the position change itself.

**Trap Logic:** This pattern is frequently attributed to the expected hemodynamic effects of position change (the preload shifts described in Chapter 1) rather than recognized as a rebleeding event, particularly because the patient was previously stable and the hemodynamic change coincides with a known position-related stressor. The discriminating feature is the magnitude and persistence of the change: a preload-mediated position effect is typically mild and self-limited, while a rebleeding event produces a sustained, progressive decline that does not stabilize despite positioning correction.

**Signature Anchor:** In any trauma patient who develops a sudden, disproportionate hemodynamic deterioration during or after a positional change, treat the event as possible rebleeding until proven otherwise, initiate volume resuscitation and blood product administration, reassess hemorrhage control measures (binder position, tourniquet integrity), and communicate the trajectory to the receiving trauma team as a possible surgical hemorrhage re-activation.

## Abdominal and Solid Organ Injury Considerations

### Nonoperative Management Patients Requiring Transfer

Many patients with solid organ injuries--hepatic lacerations, splenic injuries, and renal injuries--are managed nonoperatively at the sending facility based on hemodynamic stability and imaging findings, and are transferred to a trauma center for continued observation and the availability of surgical backup if nonoperative management fails. The transport clinician's task for these patients is vigilant hemodynamic monitoring with a specific awareness that nonoperative management can fail at any time, and that the transition from stable nonoperative patient to one requiring emergent surgery may be signaled by nothing more than a subtle, sustained downward trend in hemoglobin or blood pressure that the crew is positioned to detect only if trending rather than snapshot monitoring is in place.

### Damage Control Surgery Patients in Transport

Patients transported after damage control surgery--abbreviated laparotomy with temporary abdominal closure, packing for hemorrhage control, and planned return to the operating room for definitive repair--present specific transport challenges: the temporary abdominal closure must be monitored for integrity, intra-abdominal packing can shift with transport movement potentially releasing a tamponaded hemorrhage source, and the patient typically has ongoing massive transfusion requirements, hypothermia, and coagulopathy that must be managed aggressively throughout the transport. These patients are among the most critically ill in interfacility transport, and the transport clinician should anticipate a trajectory of ongoing physiologic instability rather than expecting the stability typically associated with a postoperative patient.

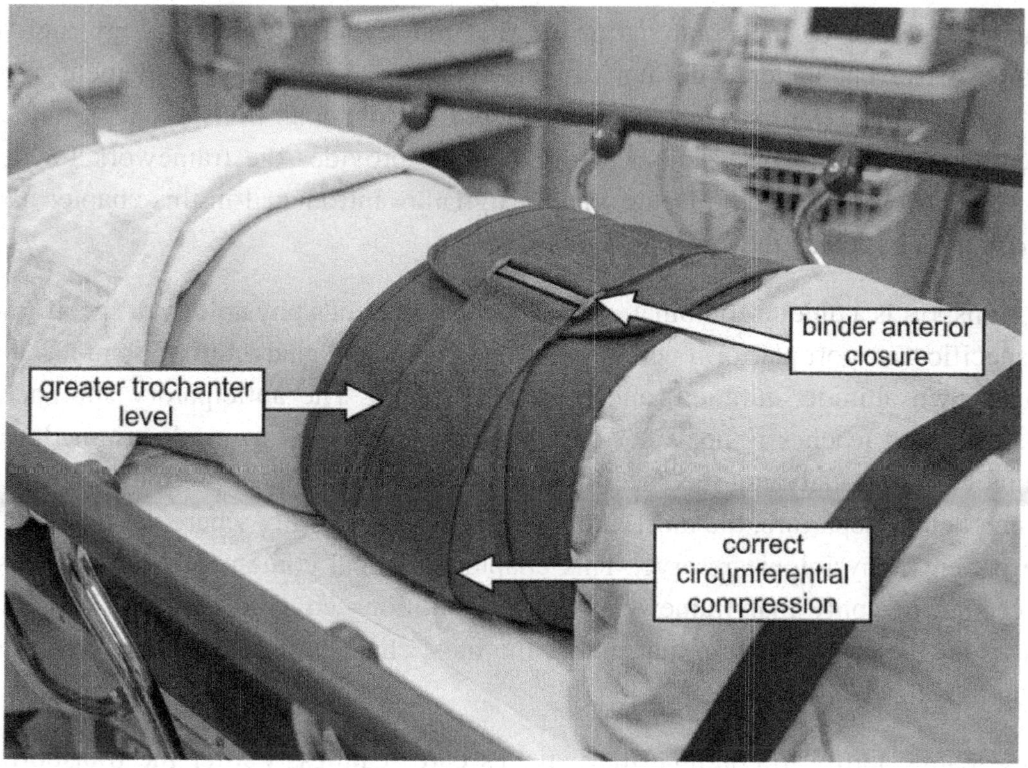


Consider a twenty-nine-year-old man with a high-speed motorcycle collision, hemodynamically stabilized at a Level III trauma center with two units of packed red blood cells and a pelvic binder for an open-book pelvic fracture, transferred by rotor-wing to a Level I trauma center for angioembolization. His blood pressure is ninety-eight systolic and heart rate is one hundred twelve at the time of departure, trending stable over the preceding thirty minutes. During the loading process for the helicopter, as the stretcher tilts head-up during litter rail insertion, the crew notes an abrupt drop in blood pressure to seventy-two systolic with a simultaneous rise in heart rate to one hundred thirty-eight. Rather than attributing this solely to the expected preload-related hemodynamic shift of the tilt, the crew recognizes the magnitude and persistence of the change as disproportionate and immediately initiates a second blood product transfusion, verifies the pelvic binder position (which has shifted superiorly during the loading movement), repositions the binder to the greater trochanter level, and communicates the trajectory change to the receiving trauma team. The blood pressure stabilizes at eighty-six systolic with ongoing transfusion, and the patient arrives at the receiving facility with the interventional radiology team already mobilized based on the crew's en-route communication. The case illustrates the Rebleeding After Position-Disrupted Tamponade Signature: the loading-related positional change likely disrupted the tamponaded retroperitoneal hematoma, and the binder shift reduced the circumferential compression, together re-initiating a hemorrhage that had been controlled by immobility and compression.

**Additional Clinical Considerations for Transport Management**

The management of patients in Chapter 15 requires attention to several additional transport-specific clinical factors that extend the principles established in the main body of the chapter. The transport clinician should be aware that the disease processes covered here interact with the transport environment

in ways that are specific to the combination of the underlying pathophysiology and the particular environmental stressor encountered during a given mission, and that a management approach that is adequate for a short ground transport may be insufficient for a longer air transport at altitude, or vice versa. The serial reassessment protocol established in Chapter 2 provides the framework for detecting these interactions as they develop, and the Deterioration Signature introduced in this chapter names the most characteristic pattern by which they declare themselves.

Each patient transport is a unique combination of a specific patient's physiology, a specific set of ongoing therapies, a specific transport platform with its own environmental characteristics, and a specific mission profile with its own altitude, duration, and route constraints. The anticipatory approach to transport medicine that this text teaches is not a set of memorized responses to predetermined scenarios but a cognitive framework for analyzing the specific combination of variables present in any given transport and identifying, before departure, the most likely points of vulnerability where the transport environment will test the patient's physiologic reserve. This chapter's clinical content provides the disease-specific knowledge needed to apply that framework to the conditions covered here, while the Deterioration Signature provides the named pattern that makes the most characteristic transport-specific vulnerability explicit, recognizable, and actionable.

The receiving team's ability to continue the patient's care seamlessly after the transport crew departs depends entirely on the quality and completeness of the clinical information the transport crew provides, and for the conditions covered in this chapter, the specific information that matters most includes: the trajectory of the patient's primary condition during transport (improving, stable, or worsening, with specific details), any interventions performed during transport and their response, any new clinical findings identified by the transport crew that were not present at the sending facility, and any anticipated needs that the receiving team should prepare for based on the transport crew's clinical assessment. This information, communicated through the structured handoff format established in Chapter 2 and supplemented by the trajectory communication emphasis that is a recurring theme throughout this text, is the final clinical act of the transport and the one that determines whether the transport adds value to the patient's care continuum or merely moves the patient from one location to another without preserving the clinical narrative that only the transport crew was positioned to observe.

The transport clinician managing the conditions addressed in this chapter should develop a systematic pre-departure assessment that specifically identifies the highest-risk transport-environment interaction for each patient's specific disease process, the monitoring parameters that will detect that interaction earliest, and the intervention that will address it most effectively. This pre-departure risk analysis, adapted from the general pre-mission physiologic risk profile introduced in Chapter 1, should be specific enough to generate a concrete prediction: what is the single most likely way this specific patient's condition will interact with the specific transport environment of this specific mission? Answering that question before departure, rather than discovering the answer during transit, is the practical application of the anticipatory transport medicine framework that this entire text is designed to develop.

Clinical case presentations embedded throughout this chapter illustrate the principle that transport-specific deterioration patterns are predictable rather than random, recognizable rather than mysterious, and preventable rather than inevitable, provided the clinician applies the systematic assessment, continuous monitoring, and named-pattern recognition framework that the Deterioration Signature System codifies. Each case demonstrates the same three-part sequence: a patient with a specific disease process encounters a specific transport-environment stressor, produces a specific clinical change that could be attributed to either the disease or the environment, and is correctly managed because the transport clinician recognized the specific named Signature and applied the correct transport-specific intervention rather than the generic disease-specific response that would have been appropriate at the bedside but is insufficient or incorrect in the transport context.

The evidence base for transport-specific management of the conditions in this chapter continues to evolve, with ongoing research into optimal monitoring strategies, transport-adapted treatment protocols, and outcome data that will refine the recommendations presented here. The transport clinician should maintain awareness of emerging evidence through continuing education, program-sponsored journal clubs, and the quality improvement processes described in Chapter 24, since the standard of care for transport medicine is not static and the recommendations in any textbook represent a snapshot of evidence at the time of writing rather than a permanent standard. The principles, however, are durable: anticipate rather than react, monitor trends rather than thresholds, communicate trajectories rather than snapshots, and recognize that the transport environment is a clinical variable that acts on every patient's physiology, not a neutral conduit between two points of care.

Finally, the transport clinician should recognize that the clinical expertise required to manage these conditions during transport represents a distinct competency that builds on but extends beyond the bedside critical care training that most transport clinicians bring to their role. A clinician who is expert in managing these conditions in the intensive care unit is not automatically expert in managing them during transport, because the environmental, equipment, monitoring, and resource constraints of transport introduce variables that bedside practice never encounters. Conversely, a transport clinician who has mastered the anticipatory, environment-aware management approach described in this text brings a perspective to patient care that the bedside clinician lacks: the ability to see the patient's physiology not as a fixed state being managed in a controlled environment, but as a dynamic process interacting continuously with an environment that is itself changing throughout the transport. This dual awareness--of the disease and of the environment acting on it--is the defining competency of transport critical care medicine, and it is what this text, from its first chapter through its last, is designed to develop.

### THE IN-TRANSIT DETERIORATION SIGNATURE SYSTEM — Hemorrhagic Trauma Transport Patterns

---

**Signature Introduced This Chapter:** Rebleeding After Position-Disrupted Tamponade (sudden hemodynamic deterioration from re-initiation of a tamponaded hemorrhage source disrupted by transport-related positional changes).

**Trauma Pattern Logic:** This Signature connects the positional hemodynamic shifts from Chapter 1 to the specific vulnerability of the trauma patient: where Chapter 1 described a predictable, physiologic preload reduction with ascent, this chapter describes a catastrophic, pathologic hemorrhage re-activation triggered by the same positional forces, and the discriminating feature is the magnitude and persistence of the change.

**Cross-Reference Forward:** Chapter 16 (Burn Injury) extends the resuscitation and hypothermia prevention framework to the burn-specific population; Chapter 11 (TBI) addresses the blood pressure target tension between traumatic brain injury and hemorrhagic shock in the multiply injured patient.

## Summary and Key Concepts

The transport crew's independent secondary survey frequently identifies injuries missed during the sending facility's resuscitation-focused evaluation.

Massive transfusion during transport requires pre-departure coordination with the sending blood bank for product availability, type, and cooler logistics.

Damage control resuscitation emphasizes balanced blood product ratios rather than crystalloid-heavy resuscitation, since excessive crystalloid worsens the lethal triad.

Permissive hypotension is specifically contraindicated in the presence of traumatic brain injury, where cerebral perfusion pressure preservation takes priority.

Pelvic binder position should be verified at each reassessment interval, since transport movement can shift the binder from its effective position at the greater trochanters.

A sudden, disproportionate hemodynamic deterioration during a positional change in a trauma patient should be treated as possible rebleeding rather than attributed solely to the expected hemodynamic effects of position change.

# CHAPTER 16: BURN INJURY MANAGEMENT IN TRANSIT

**Learning Objectives**

1. Assess burn depth and calculate total body surface area using standardized methods adapted to the transport environment.
2. Apply the Parkland formula and modified resuscitation endpoints for fluid management during burn transport.
3. Recognize inhalation injury and secure the airway proactively before transport when upper airway edema is anticipated.
4. Manage pain and sedation in burn patients with attention to the pharmacokinetic alterations produced by burn pathophysiology.
5. Identify electrical and chemical burn presentations requiring specialty-specific transport considerations.

**Chapter Outline**

This chapter addresses the transport of patients with burn injuries, one of the most resource-intensive and physiologically complex critical care transport populations. Burn patients present a unique convergence of challenges: massive fluid shifts requiring continuous resuscitation titration, airway vulnerability from inhalation injury that may worsen progressively during the transport window, pain management demands that exceed those of most other transport populations, and thermoregulatory failure from loss of the skin's barrier function that is compounded by the environmental exposures of transport described in Chapter 1.

## Burn Depth and Total Body Surface Area Assessment

### Burn Depth Classification and Its Transport Implications

Burn depth is classified as superficial (epidermal only), superficial partial-thickness (into the papillary dermis), deep partial-thickness (into the reticular dermis), and full-thickness (through the entire dermis into subcutaneous tissue), and the distinction between these depths has direct transport management implications beyond wound care. Superficial and superficial partial-thickness burns are painful because sensory nerve endings are intact, requiring aggressive analgesia during transport, while full-thickness burns are characteristically insensate at the wound surface because the nerve endings have been destroyed, a distinction that can paradoxically cause the transport clinician to underestimate pain management needs if they assess pain solely at the wound surface rather than at the wound margins and surrounding partial-thickness zones where sensation is preserved and intense.

### Circumferential Burns and Compartment Syndrome Risk

Circumferential full-thickness burns of the extremities, chest, or abdomen carry a specific transport-related risk: the inelastic eschar formed by the burned tissue acts as a constricting band that, as underlying tissue edema develops during resuscitation, can produce compartment syndrome in the extremities or restrict chest wall excursion and ventilation. The transport clinician should monitor distal pulses, capillary refill, and sensation in any extremity with circumferential burns at each reassessment interval, and should be aware that escharotomy--incision through the eschar to release the constriction--may be necessary as an emergent procedure during transport if compartment syndrome develops, though the procedure is typically deferred to the receiving burn center unless limb-threatening ischemia is progressing during transit.

### Total Body Surface Area Calculation for Resuscitation Planning

Accurate total body surface area calculation is essential because it drives the fluid resuscitation calculation that will govern the patient's hemodynamic management throughout the transport window. The rule of nines provides a rapid estimation suitable for the transport setting: each upper extremity represents nine percent, each lower extremity eighteen percent, the anterior and posterior trunk each eighteen percent, the head nine percent, and the perineum one percent. The transport clinician should perform their own independent TBSA assessment rather than relying solely on the sending facility's estimate, since TBSA estimates are notoriously variable between assessors and even a modest over- or underestimation produces a clinically significant error in the resuscitation volume calculation.

**Figure 16.1: Rule of Nines for Total Body Surface Area Estimation**

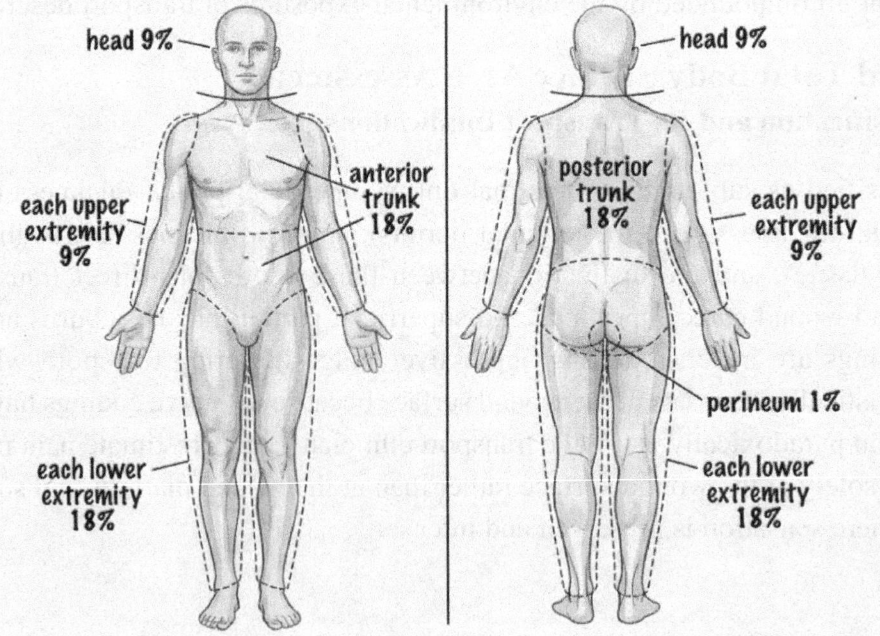

## Fluid Resuscitation Formulas and Titration En Route

### Parkland Formula and Resuscitation Initiation

The Parkland formula estimates the total crystalloid resuscitation volume for the first twenty-four hours as four milliliters per kilogram of body weight per percent total body surface area burned, with half of the calculated volume administered in the first eight hours from the time of injury and the remaining half over the subsequent sixteen hours. The transport clinician must calculate the resuscitation rate based on the specific time that has elapsed since injury, not since the start of transport, since a patient who arrives at the sending facility two hours after injury and spends another hour before transport departs has already consumed three of the eight first-phase hours, and the remaining fluid volume must be distributed across the remaining five hours rather than restarted from the beginning of a new eight-hour clock.

### Resuscitation Endpoint Titration During Transport

The Parkland formula provides a starting point, not a fixed prescription, and the transport clinician should titrate the resuscitation rate against clinical endpoints rather than adhering rigidly to the calculated rate. The primary resuscitation endpoint is urine output, targeting 0.5 to 1 milliliter per kilogram per hour in adults, monitored through an indwelling urinary catheter that should be confirmed in place and functioning before departure. Over-resuscitation is as dangerous as under-resuscitation in the burn population: excessive fluid administration drives tissue edema, compartment syndrome, abdominal compartment syndrome, and pulmonary edema, all of which are harder to reverse than the hypovolemia they were intended to prevent. The transport clinician who monitors urine output and adjusts the infusion rate accordingly provides more effective resuscitation than one who adheres to the Parkland number without adjustment.

| Resuscitation Parameter | Target | Transport Monitoring Method |
|---|---|---|
| Urine output (adult) | 0.5-1 mL/kg/hr | Hourly catheter output measurement |
| Urine output (pediatric) | 1-1.5 mL/kg/hr | Hourly catheter output measurement |
| Mean arterial pressure | Patient-specific baseline per Chapter 2 | Continuous arterial line monitoring |
| Lactate trend | Declining toward normal | Point-of-care testing where available |
| Base deficit | Improving | Serial blood gas analysis |

## Airway Management in Inhalation Injury

### Recognizing Inhalation Injury Before Airway Compromise Develops

Inhalation injury is the most immediately life-threatening component of burn injury during transport, because the upper airway edema it produces is progressive and time-dependent: a patient who has an adequate airway at the time of the transport crew's arrival at the sending facility may develop critical airway narrowing during the transport window as edema continues to develop over the first twelve to twenty-four hours after exposure. The clinical indicators of inhalation injury--facial burns, singed nasal hair, carbonaceous sputum, hoarseness or voice change, stridor, and a history of exposure in an enclosed space--should trigger a proactive decision to intubate before departure rather than a watchful waiting approach that risks managing a lost airway in a moving vehicle.

### Intubation Considerations for the Burn Airway

When inhalation injury is suspected or confirmed, intubation should be performed with the largest endotracheal tube that will pass through the edematous glottis, since the progressive nature of the edema means that a tube placed now will need to accommodate continued swelling, and a tube that is marginal at the time of placement may become effectively obstructed as the tissue swells around it during transport. Video laryngoscopy is strongly preferred for the burn airway because it provides the visual confirmation of tube passage through an edematous and potentially distorted glottis that direct laryngoscopy cannot reliably offer, and because it allows the clinician to assess the degree of supraglottic and glottic edema as a prognostic indicator of how rapidly the airway situation is evolving.

### THE IN-TRANSIT DETERIORATION SIGNATURE SYSTEM — Inhalation-Masked Airway Compromise

**The Signature:** Progressive upper airway edema from thermal or chemical inhalation that develops insidiously during transport and becomes a critical airway emergency only after the edema has progressed beyond the point where a controlled intubation is easily achievable.

**Movement Trigger:** The time-dependent progression of inhalation-induced upper airway edema coincides with the transport window, and the transport environment's limited airway resources make a late, emergency intubation through a severely edematous glottis substantially more dangerous than a proactive, early intubation at the sending bedside.

**Early Tell:** Progressive voice change from normal to hoarse to muffled, increasing difficulty handling secretions, subtle inspiratory stridor audible only on close auscultation over the anterior neck, and visible facial or lip swelling that is worsening compared to the initial assessment.

**Trap Logic:** This pattern is frequently missed because the airway appeared adequate at the initial assessment, and the progressive changes are gradual enough to be normalized by a crew that is focused on the more visually dramatic burn wounds rather than monitoring the airway trajectory. The discriminating feature is the trajectory: any worsening of voice, stridor, or secretion handling over the transport window, however subtle, indicates continuing edema progression and warrants immediate airway intervention rather than continued observation.

**Signature Anchor:** In any patient with suspected inhalation injury, secure the airway proactively before departure if any clinical indicator of upper airway involvement is present, and if the patient departs with an unsecured airway, treat any progression of voice change, stridor, or facial edema during transport as an indication for immediate intubation rather than continued monitoring.

**CAUTION:** The window for controlled intubation in inhalation injury is time-limited and closes progressively during transport; a patient whose airway appears adequate at departure may become unintubatable by conventional means within thirty to sixty minutes as edema progresses.

## Electrical and Chemical Burn Considerations

### Electrical Injury: Hidden Tissue Destruction and Cardiac Risk

Electrical burns produce tissue destruction that extends far deeper than the visible skin injury suggests, because electrical current follows the path of least resistance through deep tissues--nerves, blood vessels, and muscle--causing rhabdomyolysis, compartment syndrome, and internal organ injury that may not be apparent on surface examination. The transport clinician should monitor for signs of rhabdomyolysis (dark urine, rising creatine kinase where point-of-care testing allows, and renal function decline) and should ensure aggressive fluid resuscitation sufficient to maintain a high urine output to prevent myoglobin-induced acute kidney injury. Cardiac arrhythmias, including ventricular fibrillation, can occur acutely or in a delayed fashion following electrical injury, and continuous cardiac monitoring should be maintained throughout transport for any patient with a significant electrical exposure.

### Chemical Burns: Decontamination and Ongoing Injury Prevention

Chemical burns differ from thermal burns in that the injurious agent may continue to cause tissue destruction until it is removed, making decontamination a higher priority than it is for thermal injuries. The sending facility should have completed copious water irrigation before the transport crew's arrival, but the transport clinician should confirm that decontamination was performed, verify that no residual chemical agent remains on the patient or their clothing, and be aware that certain chemicals--hydrofluoric acid, phenol, and alkali agents--require specific antidotal treatment beyond water irrigation. Hydrofluoric acid burns in particular can produce life-threatening hypocalcemia and hypomagnesemia through fluoride ion chelation of calcium and magnesium, requiring calcium gluconate gel application to the burn site and potentially intravenous calcium supplementation, a clinical scenario that connects directly to the electrolyte management principles from Chapter 19.

## Pain and Sedation Management for Burn Patients

### Pharmacokinetic Alterations in Major Burns

Major burns produce significant pharmacokinetic alterations that affect drug dosing during transport: the massive capillary leak and third-spacing of fluid increase the volume of distribution for water-soluble medications, requiring higher-than-expected doses to achieve therapeutic effect; hepatic and renal blood flow changes alter drug metabolism and clearance; and protein binding is reduced due to hypoalbuminemia, increasing the free fraction of protein-bound drugs and potentially producing toxicity at doses that would be safe in an unburned patient. The transport clinician should anticipate that standard dosing may be inadequate for analgesia and sedation in the major burn patient and should titrate to clinical effect rather than relying on weight-based calculations derived from non-burn populations.

### Multimodal Analgesia in the Transport Setting

Burn pain during transport is among the most severe pain encountered in any transport population, and inadequate pain management is both inhumane and physiologically counterproductive, driving tachycardia, hypertension, increased metabolic demand, and catecholamine release that worsen the already-stressed cardiovascular system. The multimodal approach from Chapter 4 applies with particular force: fentanyl as the primary opioid for its rapid onset and hemodynamic stability, ketamine at sub-dissociative or dissociative doses for its potent analgesic and sedative properties without respiratory depression, and consideration of anxiolytic therapy with midazolam for the psychological distress that accompanies severe burn injury. The transport clinician should not underdose analgesia out of concern for hemodynamic effects, since the hemodynamic consequences of undertreated pain are typically worse than the hemodynamic effects of appropriately dosed analgesia.

Figure 16.2: Burn Depth Classification and Tissue Layer Involvement

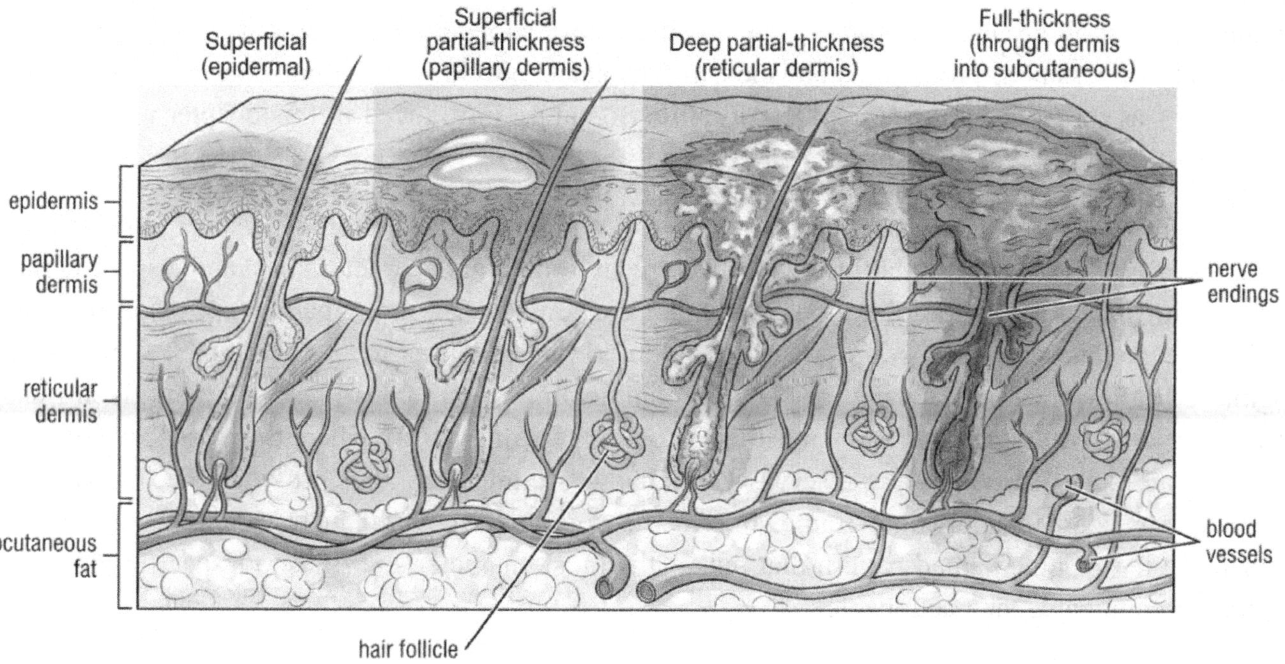


Consider a thirty-two-year-old man rescued from a house fire with forty percent total body surface area burns including circumferential full-thickness burns to both upper extremities, facial burns with singed nasal hair, and carbonaceous sputum. The sending emergency department has initiated Parkland-based crystalloid resuscitation and placed a urinary catheter but has not intubated the patient, who is currently speaking in a hoarse but audible voice. The transport crew, recognizing the multiple indicators of inhalation injury and the time-dependent nature of upper airway edema, elects to intubate before departure using video laryngoscopy, successfully passing a 7.5 endotracheal tube through a moderately edematous glottis that they note would likely have been significantly more difficult to navigate an hour later. During the sixty-minute ground transport to the regional burn center, the crew monitors urine output at fifteen-minute intervals, adjusting the resuscitation rate twice to maintain the target range, and performs neurovascular checks on both upper extremities at each assessment, noting progressive swelling but maintained distal pulses throughout. The crew communicates the TBSA estimate, the airway findings, and the resuscitation trajectory to the receiving burn team, who have the burn intensive care unit bed and the surgical team for potential escharotomy assessment ready on arrival. This case illustrates the chapter's central management triad: proactive airway protection before edema progression closes the window, continuous resuscitation titration against endpoints rather than formula adherence, and structured neurovascular surveillance for compartment syndrome in circumferential injuries.

## Additional Clinical Considerations for Transport Management

The management of patients in Chapter 16 requires attention to several additional transport-specific clinical factors that extend the principles established in the main body of the chapter. The transport clinician should be aware that the disease processes covered here interact with the transport environment

in ways that are specific to the combination of the underlying pathophysiology and the particular environmental stressor encountered during a given mission, and that a management approach that is adequate for a short ground transport may be insufficient for a longer air transport at altitude, or vice versa. The serial reassessment protocol established in Chapter 2 provides the framework for detecting these interactions as they develop, and the Deterioration Signature introduced in this chapter names the most characteristic pattern by which they declare themselves.

Each patient transport is a unique combination of a specific patient's physiology, a specific set of ongoing therapies, a specific transport platform with its own environmental characteristics, and a specific mission profile with its own altitude, duration, and route constraints. The anticipatory approach to transport medicine that this text teaches is not a set of memorized responses to predetermined scenarios but a cognitive framework for analyzing the specific combination of variables present in any given transport and identifying, before departure, the most likely points of vulnerability where the transport environment will test the patient's physiologic reserve. This chapter's clinical content provides the disease-specific knowledge needed to apply that framework to the conditions covered here, while the Deterioration Signature provides the named pattern that makes the most characteristic transport-specific vulnerability explicit, recognizable, and actionable.

The receiving team's ability to continue the patient's care seamlessly after the transport crew departs depends entirely on the quality and completeness of the clinical information the transport crew provides, and for the conditions covered in this chapter, the specific information that matters most includes: the trajectory of the patient's primary condition during transport (improving, stable, or worsening, with specific details), any interventions performed during transport and their response, any new clinical findings identified by the transport crew that were not present at the sending facility, and any anticipated needs that the receiving team should prepare for based on the transport crew's clinical assessment. This information, communicated through the structured handoff format established in Chapter 2 and supplemented by the trajectory communication emphasis that is a recurring theme throughout this text, is the final clinical act of the transport and the one that determines whether the transport adds value to the patient's care continuum or merely moves the patient from one location to another without preserving the clinical narrative that only the transport crew was positioned to observe.

The transport clinician managing the conditions addressed in this chapter should develop a systematic pre-departure assessment that specifically identifies the highest-risk transport-environment interaction for each patient's specific disease process, the monitoring parameters that will detect that interaction earliest, and the intervention that will address it most effectively. This pre-departure risk analysis, adapted from the general pre-mission physiologic risk profile introduced in Chapter 1, should be specific enough to generate a concrete prediction: what is the single most likely way this specific patient's condition will interact with the specific transport environment of this specific mission? Answering that question before departure, rather than discovering the answer during transit, is the practical application of the anticipatory transport medicine framework that this entire text is designed to develop.

Clinical case presentations embedded throughout this chapter illustrate the principle that transport-specific deterioration patterns are predictable rather than random, recognizable rather than mysterious, and preventable rather than inevitable, provided the clinician applies the systematic assessment, continuous monitoring, and named-pattern recognition framework that the Deterioration Signature System codifies. Each case demonstrates the same three-part sequence: a patient with a specific disease process encounters a specific transport-environment stressor, produces a specific clinical change that could be attributed to either the disease or the environment, and is correctly managed because the transport clinician recognized the specific named Signature and applied the correct transport-specific intervention rather than the generic disease-specific response that would have been appropriate at the bedside but is insufficient or incorrect in the transport context.

The evidence base for transport-specific management of the conditions in this chapter continues to evolve, with ongoing research into optimal monitoring strategies, transport-adapted treatment protocols, and outcome data that will refine the recommendations presented here. The transport clinician should maintain awareness of emerging evidence through continuing education, program-sponsored journal clubs, and the quality improvement processes described in Chapter 24, since the standard of care for transport medicine is not static and the recommendations in any textbook represent a snapshot of evidence at the time of writing rather than a permanent standard. The principles, however, are durable: anticipate rather than react, monitor trends rather than thresholds, communicate trajectories rather than snapshots, and recognize that the transport environment is a clinical variable that acts on every patient's physiology, not a neutral conduit between two points of care.

Finally, the transport clinician should recognize that the clinical expertise required to manage these conditions during transport represents a distinct competency that builds on but extends beyond the bedside critical care training that most transport clinicians bring to their role. A clinician who is expert in managing these conditions in the intensive care unit is not automatically expert in managing them during transport, because the environmental, equipment, monitoring, and resource constraints of transport introduce variables that bedside practice never encounters. Conversely, a transport clinician who has mastered the anticipatory, environment-aware management approach described in this text brings a perspective to patient care that the bedside clinician lacks: the ability to see the patient's physiology not as a fixed state being managed in a controlled environment, but as a dynamic process interacting continuously with an environment that is itself changing throughout the transport. This dual awareness--of the disease and of the environment acting on it--is the defining competency of transport critical care medicine, and it is what this text, from its first chapter through its last, is designed to develop.

**THE IN-TRANSIT DETERIORATION SIGNATURE SYSTEM — Inhalation-Masked Airway Compromise Patterns**

**Signature Introduced This Chapter:** Inhalation-Masked Airway Compromise -- a transport-specific deterioration pattern unique to burn depth assessment.

**Pattern Logic:** This Signature extends the foundational transport-physiology principles from Chapter 1 and the assessment framework from Chapter 2 into this disease domain.

**Cross-Reference Forward:** This Signature is indexed in the Anchor Section's Master Signature Atlas by organ system and clinical category.

## Summary and Key Concepts

The transport environment modifies the management of burn depth assessment, total body surface area calculation, fluid resuscitation, and inhalation injury management in specific, predictable ways beyond what bedside training addresses.

Trend-based monitoring at fixed intervals is the primary tool for detecting the disease-specific deterioration patterns described in this chapter's Signature.

Pharmacologic management follows the Chapter 4 framework with disease-specific modifications; infusion continuity requires particular attention.

Anticipatory contingency planning for the most likely complications is more effective than reactive management in the resource-constrained transport environment.

Advance communication with the receiving facility, including trajectory updates, is a direct clinical intervention improving care on arrival.

# CHAPTER 17: SEPSIS AND SEPTIC SHOCK IN TRANSIT

**Learning Objectives**

1. Recognize sepsis and septic shock using current diagnostic criteria adapted to the transport assessment framework.
2. Initiate and titrate fluid resuscitation and vasopressor therapy for septic shock during interfacility transport.
3. Apply antimicrobial timing principles and source control considerations specific to the transport window.
4. Recognize septic cardiomyopathy and distinguish it from primary cardiac dysfunction in the septic patient.
5. Monitor for multi-organ dysfunction progression during transit using trend-based perfusion assessment.

**Chapter Outline**

This chapter addresses the transport of patients with sepsis and septic shock, one of the most common indications for critical care interfacility transfer. The septic patient in transport presents a dynamic clinical challenge: the hemodynamic picture evolves continuously, fluid responsiveness changes over hours as resuscitation progresses, and the adequacy of tissue perfusion cannot be assessed from vital signs alone but requires the trend-based, multi-parameter monitoring framework established in Chapter 2.

## Sepsis Recognition and Source Control Considerations

### Current Diagnostic Criteria and Their Transport Application

Sepsis is defined as life-threatening organ dysfunction caused by a dysregulated host response to infection, operationalized clinically as a suspected or confirmed infection with an acute increase in the Sequential Organ Failure Assessment score of two or more points. In the transport setting, formal SOFA scoring may not be feasible, and the transport clinician should use the clinical surrogates embedded in the qSOFA criteria--altered mentation, systolic blood pressure at or below one hundred millimeters of mercury, and respiratory rate at or above twenty-two breaths per minute--as a rapid screening framework, recognizing that these criteria were designed for bedside identification of patients at risk for poor outcomes rather than as a diagnostic standard. The presence of two or more qSOFA criteria in a patient with suspected infection should heighten the transport clinician's vigilance for hemodynamic deterioration and should lower the threshold for establishing invasive monitoring, initiating vasopressor therapy, and communicating the trajectory proactively to the receiving facility.

### Source Control Assessment Before Transport

Source control--the identification and treatment of the anatomic source of infection through drainage, debridement, or removal of an infected device--is a primary determinant of outcome in sepsis, and the transport clinician should assess whether source control has been achieved, attempted, or is the specific reason for the transfer. A patient transferred for surgical drainage of an intra-abdominal abscess has a fundamentally different transport management posture than one transferred for medical management of a pneumonia-driven sepsis where source control is antimicrobial therapy alone: the former may deteriorate rapidly if the undrained source continues to drive the septic response during transport, while the latter's trajectory is more likely to be influenced by the adequacy of antimicrobial coverage and hemodynamic support.

### The One-Hour Sepsis Bundle and Transport Timing

Current sepsis guidelines emphasize completion of a resuscitation bundle within the first hour of sepsis recognition, including blood cultures, broad-spectrum antimicrobial administration, fluid resuscitation initiation, and vasopressor therapy if shock is present after initial fluid resuscitation. The transport clinician should confirm which bundle elements have been completed at the sending facility before departure, since any element not yet completed becomes the transport crew's responsibility to initiate during transit. Antimicrobial administration in particular should not be delayed for the sake of expediting departure; the mortality benefit of early antibiotics is well established, and a fifteen-minute delay in departure to ensure that the first antimicrobial dose has been administered and is infusing is a clinically superior choice to departing immediately with antibiotics still pending.

**KEY POINT:** Antimicrobial administration should never be delayed for transport departure; the mortality benefit of early antibiotics outweighs any time saved by departing before the first dose is infusing.

## Fluid Resuscitation and Vasopressor Titration

### Initial Resuscitation Volume and Reassessment

An initial crystalloid bolus of thirty milliliters per kilogram is the standard starting point for sepsis-related hypotension or hypoperfusion, though this volume should be administered with attention to the patient's cardiac function and volume tolerance rather than as a reflexive, unmonitored bolus. The transport clinician inheriting a patient who has already received the initial resuscitation volume should assess the response to that volume using the dynamic fluid responsiveness tools from Chapter 7--pulse pressure variation, passive leg raise, or ultrasound-guided IVC assessment--before administering further fluid, since excessive crystalloid administration beyond the point of fluid responsiveness produces tissue edema, pulmonary congestion, and increased extravascular lung water without further hemodynamic benefit.

### Vasopressor Selection and Titration Strategy

Norepinephrine is the first-line vasopressor for septic shock, applied through the vasoactive framework from Chapter 4. In the transport setting, the crew should have a norepinephrine infusion prepared and primed before departure for any patient with hemodynamic instability or a trajectory suggesting evolving shock, rather than deferring vasopressor initiation to a reactive decision after hypotension has already developed during transit. Vasopressin as a fixed-dose adjunct is typically added when the norepinephrine requirement is escalating toward moderate-to-high doses, and its non-catecholamine mechanism provides an independent vasoconstrictive pathway that may reduce the norepinephrine dose required to maintain the target pressure.

### Steroid Consideration in Refractory Septic Shock

Hydrocortisone administration for refractory septic shock--defined as shock requiring escalating vasopressor doses despite adequate volume resuscitation--may be initiated at the sending facility or during transport, and the transport clinician should confirm whether stress-dose steroids have been given and, if not, whether the current vasopressor trajectory suggests they are indicated. The decision to initiate steroids during transport should be made in consultation with the receiving critical care team where communication allows, since the evidence base remains debated and the receiving team may have a specific preference based on the patient's full clinical picture.

| Sepsis Bundle Element | Sending Facility Responsibility | Transport Crew Responsibility |
|---|---|---|
| Blood cultures | Obtain before antibiotics if possible | Confirm obtained; not a transport intervention |
| Broad-spectrum antimicrobials | Administer within 1 hour of recognition | Confirm infusing; complete if not yet given |
| Initial crystalloid bolus (30 mL/kg) | Initiate | Reassess response; administer remainder if indicated |
| Vasopressor therapy (if MAP <65 after fluids) | Initiate norepinephrine | Titrate continuously during transport; add vasopressin if escalating |
| Lactate measurement | Obtain initial value | Repeat at midpoint if point-of-care available; trend is more valuable than a single number |

**Figure 17.1: Septic Shock Hemodynamic Assessment Using Point-of-Care Ultrasound**

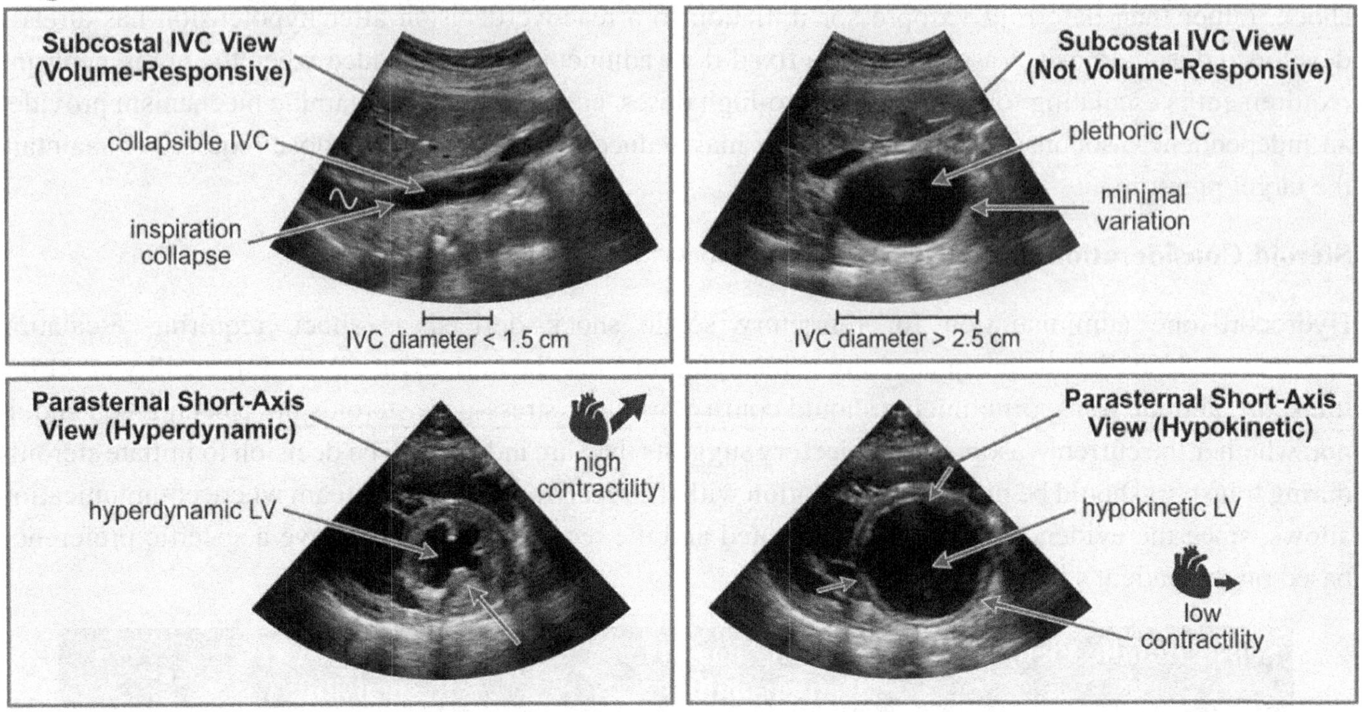


## Antimicrobial Timing and Selection in the Transport Setting

### First-Dose Timing and the Transport Decision

The relationship between antimicrobial timing and mortality in septic shock is steep and well documented: each hour of delay in appropriate antimicrobial administration is associated with a measurable increase in mortality, and this relationship does not pause during transport. The transport clinician should verify that the first dose of a broad-spectrum antimicrobial has been administered before departure and should confirm the specific agent, dose, and time of administration for communication to the receiving team, since the receiving team's subsequent antimicrobial decisions depend on knowing what was given, when, and whether it was an appropriate empiric choice for the suspected source.

### Antimicrobial Infusion Management During Transport

Certain antimicrobials require extended infusion times or specific infusion rates that the transport clinician must manage during transit: vancomycin infusions must be administered slowly to avoid red man syndrome, beta-lactam extended infusions are increasingly used for pharmacokinetic optimization in sepsis, and amphotericin B formulations carry infusion-related toxicities that require monitoring. The infusion pump management and battery considerations from Chapter 4 apply directly, and the crew should verify that the infusion pump is programmed for the correct rate and concentration and that sufficient battery reserve exists for the full infusion duration.

## Septic Cardiomyopathy Recognition

### Distinguishing Sepsis-Induced Cardiac Dysfunction From Primary Cardiac Disease

Septic cardiomyopathy--a reversible, cytokine-mediated depression of myocardial contractility that occurs in approximately forty percent of patients with septic shock--can produce a hemodynamic picture indistinguishable from primary cardiogenic shock if the clinician does not consider the septic context. The point-of-care ultrasound assessment described in Chapters 2 and 6 is the transport clinician's primary tool for identifying this complication: a patient in septic shock whose ultrasound shows a hyperdynamic, well-contracting ventricle requires a different vasoactive strategy (primarily vasopressor) than one whose ultrasound shows a dilated, hypokinetic ventricle (requiring inotropic support in addition to vasopressor therapy), and this distinction cannot be made from blood pressure and heart rate alone.

### Inotropic Augmentation in Sepsis-Induced Cardiac Dysfunction

When septic cardiomyopathy is suspected or confirmed by bedside ultrasound, dobutamine or low-dose epinephrine provides inotropic augmentation that addresses the contractile component of shock that vasopressor therapy alone cannot correct. The transport clinician should initiate inotropic support if the hemodynamic picture suggests combined distributive and cardiogenic shock, with continuous monitoring for the arrhythmogenic effects of both agents, and should communicate the ultrasound findings and the inotropic support decision to the receiving team so that their initial echocardiographic assessment accounts for the transport crew's bedside findings.

## Multi-Organ Dysfunction Monitoring En Route

### Perfusion Assessment Beyond Blood Pressure

Blood pressure is a necessary but grossly insufficient marker of perfusion adequacy in septic shock, because the septic vasculature can maintain a numerically acceptable blood pressure through compensatory tachycardia and vasoconstriction while tissue-level perfusion is critically inadequate. The transport clinician must assess perfusion through multiple converging indicators: mentation as a surrogate for cerebral perfusion, urine output as a surrogate for renal perfusion, lactate trend as a global marker of anaerobic metabolism, capillary refill time as a peripheral perfusion indicator, and skin mottling pattern and extent as an increasingly validated bedside marker of microcirculatory dysfunction in septic shock.

### THE IN-TRANSIT DETERIORATION SIGNATURE SYSTEM — Cryptic Hypoperfusion Behind Normalizing Vitals

---

**The Signature:** A patient whose vital signs appear to be improving or stabilizing during transport--blood pressure normalizing on a stable vasopressor dose, heart rate trending downward--but whose tissue perfusion markers are worsening: lactate continuing to rise, mottling extending, capillary refill prolonging, or urine output declining, indicating that the hemodynamic improvement is compensatory and not a reflection of genuine tissue-level clinical improvement.

**Movement Trigger:** The transport environment contributes by limiting the clinician's ability to perform a comprehensive perfusion assessment: noise and lighting constraints impair skin and mottling assessment, vibration degrades capillary refill assessment reliability, and point-of-care lactate measurement may not be available, leaving blood pressure and heart rate as the only easily monitored parameters and creating a false sense of hemodynamic improvement.

**Early Tell:** A discordance between improving macro-hemodynamic parameters (blood pressure, heart rate trending toward normal) and worsening micro-perfusion indicators (extending mottling, prolonging capillary refill, declining urine output, or a lactate that is not clearing despite hemodynamic improvement), detectable only when the clinician actively assesses perfusion markers rather than relying solely on the monitor display.

**Trap Logic:** This pattern is particularly dangerous because the normalizing vital signs provide exactly the reassurance that the clinician is looking for, and the effort required to assess perfusion markers beyond the monitor display is substantial enough that it can be skipped under workload pressure, particularly when the displayed numbers are trending in the right direction.

**Signature Anchor:** In every septic shock patient during transport, perform a deliberate perfusion assessment--including at minimum capillary refill, skin mottling, and urine output check--at each scheduled reassessment interval, independent of and in addition to the monitored vital signs, and treat any discordance between improving vitals and worsening perfusion markers as a signal that the current resuscitation strategy is insufficient despite its apparent hemodynamic success.

### Lactate Trending and Its Transport Application

Serial lactate measurement, where point-of-care testing is available, provides the most objective single marker of resuscitation adequacy: a declining lactate indicates improving tissue perfusion, while a stable or rising lactate despite normalized blood pressure indicates ongoing tissue hypoperfusion that requires further resuscitation intensity. The transport clinician should obtain a lactate measurement at departure and, for transports exceeding thirty minutes, repeat it at the midpoint to generate a two-point trend that the receiving team can use to assess the trajectory of resuscitation response, a contribution that a single arrival lactate cannot provide.

**Figure 17.2: Skin Mottling Score Assessment for Perfusion Monitoring**

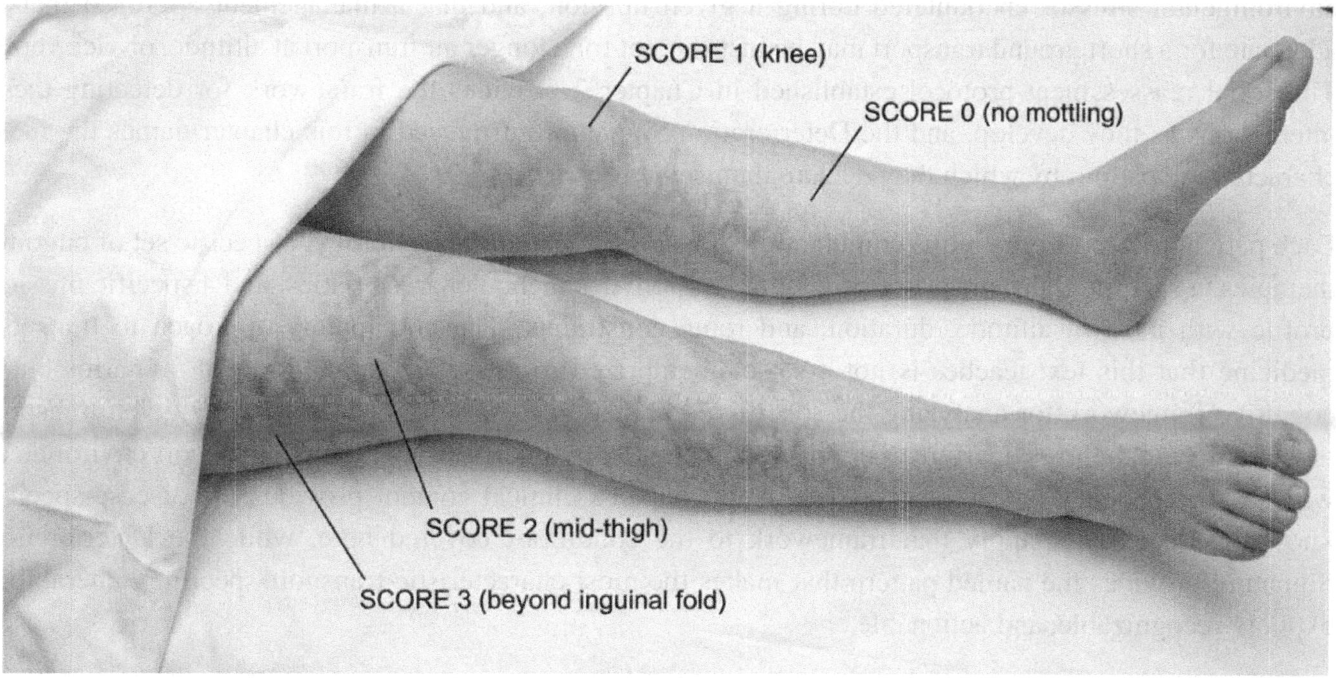


Consider a fifty-nine-year-old woman with urosepsis and septic shock, receiving norepinephrine at a moderate dose, transferred by ground critical care ambulance for surgical drainage of a perinephric abscess. Her blood pressure has stabilized at a mean arterial pressure of sixty-seven on the current norepinephrine dose, and her heart rate has trended down from one hundred thirty-two to one hundred fourteen over the preceding hour, findings that the sending team characterizes as improving. The transport crew's independent perfusion assessment, however, notes that capillary refill remains four seconds, skin mottling extends to the mid-thigh bilaterally, and the most recent urine output over the preceding hour is only fifteen milliliters, all of which indicate persistent tissue hypoperfusion despite the numerically acceptable blood pressure. Recognizing the Cryptic Hypoperfusion Signature, the crew assesses fluid responsiveness with a passive leg raise (positive, with a transient rise in pulse pressure), administers an additional five-hundred-milliliter crystalloid bolus, and increases the norepinephrine rate modestly. A repeat lactate at the transport midpoint shows a decline from 5.8 to 4.2, confirming that the resuscitation escalation is producing genuine perfusion improvement that the initial vital-sign trend alone had falsely suggested was already underway. This case illustrates the chapter's central argument: in septic shock, vital signs are the beginning of the assessment, not its completion, and the transport clinician who stops at improving blood pressure and heart rate without checking perfusion markers risks delivering a falsely reassuring picture to the receiving team.

### Additional Clinical Considerations for Transport Management

The management of patients in Chapter 17 requires attention to several additional transport-specific clinical factors that extend the principles established in the main body of the chapter. The transport clinician should be aware that the disease processes covered here interact with the transport environment

in ways that are specific to the combination of the underlying pathophysiology and the particular environmental stressor encountered during a given mission, and that a management approach that is adequate for a short ground transport may be insufficient for a longer air transport at altitude, or vice versa. The serial reassessment protocol established in Chapter 2 provides the framework for detecting these interactions as they develop, and the Deterioration Signature introduced in this chapter names the most characteristic pattern by which they declare themselves.

Each patient transport is a unique combination of a specific patient's physiology, a specific set of ongoing therapies, a specific transport platform with its own environmental characteristics, and a specific mission profile with its own altitude, duration, and route constraints. The anticipatory approach to transport medicine that this text teaches is not a set of memorized responses to predetermined scenarios but a cognitive framework for analyzing the specific combination of variables present in any given transport and identifying, before departure, the most likely points of vulnerability where the transport environment will test the patient's physiologic reserve. This chapter's clinical content provides the disease-specific knowledge needed to apply that framework to the conditions covered here, while the Deterioration Signature provides the named pattern that makes the most characteristic transport-specific vulnerability explicit, recognizable, and actionable.

The receiving team's ability to continue the patient's care seamlessly after the transport crew departs depends entirely on the quality and completeness of the clinical information the transport crew provides, and for the conditions covered in this chapter, the specific information that matters most includes: the trajectory of the patient's primary condition during transport (improving, stable, or worsening, with specific details), any interventions performed during transport and their response, any new clinical findings identified by the transport crew that were not present at the sending facility, and any anticipated needs that the receiving team should prepare for based on the transport crew's clinical assessment. This information, communicated through the structured handoff format established in Chapter 2 and supplemented by the trajectory communication emphasis that is a recurring theme throughout this text, is the final clinical act of the transport and the one that determines whether the transport adds value to the patient's care continuum or merely moves the patient from one location to another without preserving the clinical narrative that only the transport crew was positioned to observe.

The transport clinician managing the conditions addressed in this chapter should develop a systematic pre-departure assessment that specifically identifies the highest-risk transport-environment interaction for each patient's specific disease process, the monitoring parameters that will detect that interaction earliest, and the intervention that will address it most effectively. This pre-departure risk analysis, adapted from the general pre-mission physiologic risk profile introduced in Chapter 1, should be specific enough to generate a concrete prediction: what is the single most likely way this specific patient's condition will interact with the specific transport environment of this specific mission? Answering that question before departure, rather than discovering the answer during transit, is the practical application of the anticipatory transport medicine framework that this entire text is designed to develop.

Clinical case presentations embedded throughout this chapter illustrate the principle that transport-specific deterioration patterns are predictable rather than random, recognizable rather than mysterious, and preventable rather than inevitable, provided the clinician applies the systematic assessment, continuous monitoring, and named-pattern recognition framework that the Deterioration Signature System codifies. Each case demonstrates the same three-part sequence: a patient with a specific disease process encounters a specific transport-environment stressor, produces a specific clinical change that could be attributed to either the disease or the environment, and is correctly managed because the transport clinician recognized the specific named Signature and applied the correct transport-specific intervention rather than the generic disease-specific response that would have been appropriate at the bedside but is insufficient or incorrect in the transport context.

The evidence base for transport-specific management of the conditions in this chapter continues to evolve, with ongoing research into optimal monitoring strategies, transport-adapted treatment protocols, and outcome data that will refine the recommendations presented here. The transport clinician should maintain awareness of emerging evidence through continuing education, program-sponsored journal clubs, and the quality improvement processes described in Chapter 24, since the standard of care for transport medicine is not static and the recommendations in any textbook represent a snapshot of evidence at the time of writing rather than a permanent standard. The principles, however, are durable: anticipate rather than react, monitor trends rather than thresholds, communicate trajectories rather than snapshots, and recognize that the transport environment is a clinical variable that acts on every patient's physiology, not a neutral conduit between two points of care.

Finally, the transport clinician should recognize that the clinical expertise required to manage these conditions during transport represents a distinct competency that builds on but extends beyond the bedside critical care training that most transport clinicians bring to their role. A clinician who is expert in managing these conditions in the intensive care unit is not automatically expert in managing them during transport, because the environmental, equipment, monitoring, and resource constraints of transport introduce variables that bedside practice never encounters. Conversely, a transport clinician who has mastered the anticipatory, environment-aware management approach described in this text brings a perspective to patient care that the bedside clinician lacks: the ability to see the patient's physiology not as a fixed state being managed in a controlled environment, but as a dynamic process interacting continuously with an environment that is itself changing throughout the transport. This dual awareness--of the disease and of the environment acting on it--is the defining competency of transport critical care medicine, and it is what this text, from its first chapter through its last, is designed to develop.

**THE IN-TRANSIT DETERIORATION SIGNATURE SYSTEM — Cryptic Hypoperfusion Behind Normalizing Vitals Patterns**

**Signature Introduced This Chapter:** Cryptic Hypoperfusion Behind Normalizing Vitals -- a transport-specific deterioration pattern unique to sepsis recognition.

**Pattern Logic:** This Signature extends the foundational transport-physiology principles from Chapter 1 and the assessment framework from Chapter 2 into this disease domain.

**Cross-Reference Forward:** This Signature is indexed in the Anchor Section's Master Signature Atlas by organ system and clinical category.

## Summary and Key Concepts

The transport environment modifies the management of sepsis recognition, source control considerations, vasopressor titration, fluid resuscitation, and antimicrobial timing in specific, predictable ways beyond what bedside training addresses.

Trend-based monitoring at fixed intervals is the primary tool for detecting the disease-specific deterioration patterns described in this chapter's Signature.

Pharmacologic management follows the Chapter 4 framework with disease-specific modifications; infusion continuity requires particular attention.

Anticipatory contingency planning for the most likely complications is more effective than reactive management in the resource-constrained transport environment.

Advance communication with the receiving facility, including trajectory updates, is a direct clinical intervention improving care on arrival.

# CHAPTER 18: METABOLIC AND ENDOCRINE EMERGENCIES IN TRANSIT

**Learning Objectives**

1. Apply disease-specific assessment, monitoring, and management principles for diabetic ketoacidosis, hyperosmolar hyperglycemic state, adrenal crisis, and thyroid storm management adapted to the transport environment.
2. Recognize transport-specific deterioration patterns and distinguish them from primary disease progression.
3. Coordinate advance communication with receiving facilities to optimize preparedness for the patient's arrival.
4. Manage pharmacologic interventions within the monitoring and resource constraints of critical care transport.

**Chapter Outline**

This chapter addresses diabetic ketoacidosis, hyperosmolar hyperglycemic state, adrenal crisis, and thyroid storm management as encountered in critical care transport, extending the foundational assessment, monitoring, pharmacologic, and equipment frameworks from earlier chapters to the specific challenges of managing these conditions during interfacility transport.

## Pathophysiology and Transport-Specific Considerations

## Diabetic Ketoacidosis and Hyperosmolar Hyperglycemic State

### DKA Pathophysiology and Transport-Specific Fluid Management

Diabetic ketoacidosis results from absolute or relative insulin deficiency producing unrestrained lipolysis, ketogenesis, and a progressive metabolic acidosis that drives the characteristic presentation of altered mentation, Kussmaul respirations, abdominal pain, and volume depletion. The transport clinician inheriting a DKA patient from a sending facility should confirm the current insulin infusion rate, the most recent glucose and anion gap values and their trends, the potassium level and its replacement status, and the volume of crystalloid already administered, since each of these parameters changes dynamically over hours and the transport crew's management must be a seamless continuation of the resuscitation trajectory rather than a restart from a new baseline.

### Insulin Infusion Continuity as the Primary Transport Priority

The continuous insulin infusion is the definitive treatment for DKA, and its uninterrupted delivery during transport is as clinically critical as vasopressor continuity in septic shock. The infusion transition considerations from Chapter 4 apply with particular force: the transport team's insulin concentration must be verified against the sending facility's concentration before a rate-equivalent transition, since a concentration mismatch will produce either underdosing (with rebound ketoacidosis) or overdosing (with hypoglycemia) that is invisible on the pump display. Point-of-care glucose monitoring should be performed at thirty-to-sixty-minute intervals during transport, with a clear protocol for transitioning from insulin to dextrose-containing fluids once the glucose falls below a defined threshold, since continuing a fixed insulin rate without glucose monitoring risks iatrogenic hypoglycemia that is entirely preventable.

### Potassium Replacement: The Hidden Danger of DKA Resuscitation

Potassium management in DKA is the single most dangerous pharmacologic task during transport, because the serum potassium level at presentation is a poor reflection of total body potassium stores: insulin therapy drives potassium intracellularly, acidosis correction shifts potassium into cells, and volume resuscitation dilutes the remaining extracellular potassium, all of which can produce a precipitous hypokalemia that triggers fatal cardiac arrhythmias. The transport clinician should obtain a potassium level before departure, should not initiate insulin therapy if the potassium is below a specific threshold (typically 3.3 mEq/L) until potassium replacement has been given, and should continue potassium replacement throughout the transport with monitoring at each reassessment interval. Continuous cardiac monitoring is mandatory for any patient receiving intravenous potassium replacement, since the ECG changes of hypokalemia (U waves, QT prolongation, ST depression) may appear before the next laboratory measurement is available.

**CAUTION:** Never initiate or continue an insulin infusion in DKA if the serum potassium is critically low; insulin-driven intracellular potassium shift superimposed on an already depleted total body potassium can produce fatal hypokalemic cardiac arrest.

## Adrenal Crisis and Thyroid Storm Management

### Adrenal Crisis: Recognition and Emergent Steroid Replacement

Acute adrenal crisis presents with refractory hypotension, hypoglycemia, hyponatremia, and altered mentation in a patient with known adrenal insufficiency or chronic steroid use who has encountered a physiologic stressor--surgery, infection, trauma, or the transport itself--that exceeds the adrenal gland's capacity to mount an appropriate cortisol response. The transport clinician should suspect adrenal crisis in any patient with unexplained hemodynamic instability who has a history of chronic steroid use, autoimmune disease, or pituitary/adrenal surgery, and should administer intravenous hydrocortisone empirically when the clinical picture is consistent, since the consequences of missing the diagnosis are severe and the consequences of empiric steroid administration in a patient who does not have adrenal crisis are minimal.

### Thyroid Storm: A Hypermetabolic Emergency

Thyroid storm represents the extreme end of thyrotoxicosis and presents with high fever, tachycardia disproportionate to the clinical picture, altered mentation, and cardiovascular compromise from the hypermetabolic and hyperdynamic state. The management is multi-targeted: beta-blockade (typically propranolol) for heart rate and symptom control, thionamide therapy (propylthiouracil or methimazole) to block new thyroid hormone synthesis, iodine solution to block hormone release (given at least one hour after thionamide to avoid substrate loading), hydrocortisone for the concurrent relative adrenal insufficiency that frequently accompanies thyroid storm, and aggressive fever management with acetaminophen and active cooling. The transport clinician managing a thyroid storm patient should anticipate the need for all of these interventions and should confirm which have been initiated at the sending facility, since the multi-drug regimen has a specific sequencing requirement (thionamide before iodine) that must be respected even under the time pressure of transport.

| Endocrine Emergency | Defining Feature | Immediate Transport Action |
|---|---|---|
| DKA | Metabolic acidosis with anion gap elevation and ketonemia | Verify insulin infusion continuity; monitor glucose q30-60min; replace potassium |
| HHS | Severe hyperglycemia (>600) with hyperosmolality but minimal ketosis | Aggressive volume resuscitation; insulin at lower rate than DKA; monitor sodium |
| Adrenal crisis | Refractory hypotension with hyponatremia in steroid-dependent patient | Empiric IV hydrocortisone; aggressive volume resuscitation; vasopressor support |
| Thyroid storm | Fever, extreme tachycardia, altered mentation in known hyperthyroidism | Beta-blockade, thionamide, iodine (sequence matters), hydrocortisone, cooling |

Figure 18.1: DKA Resuscitation Monitoring Framework During Transport

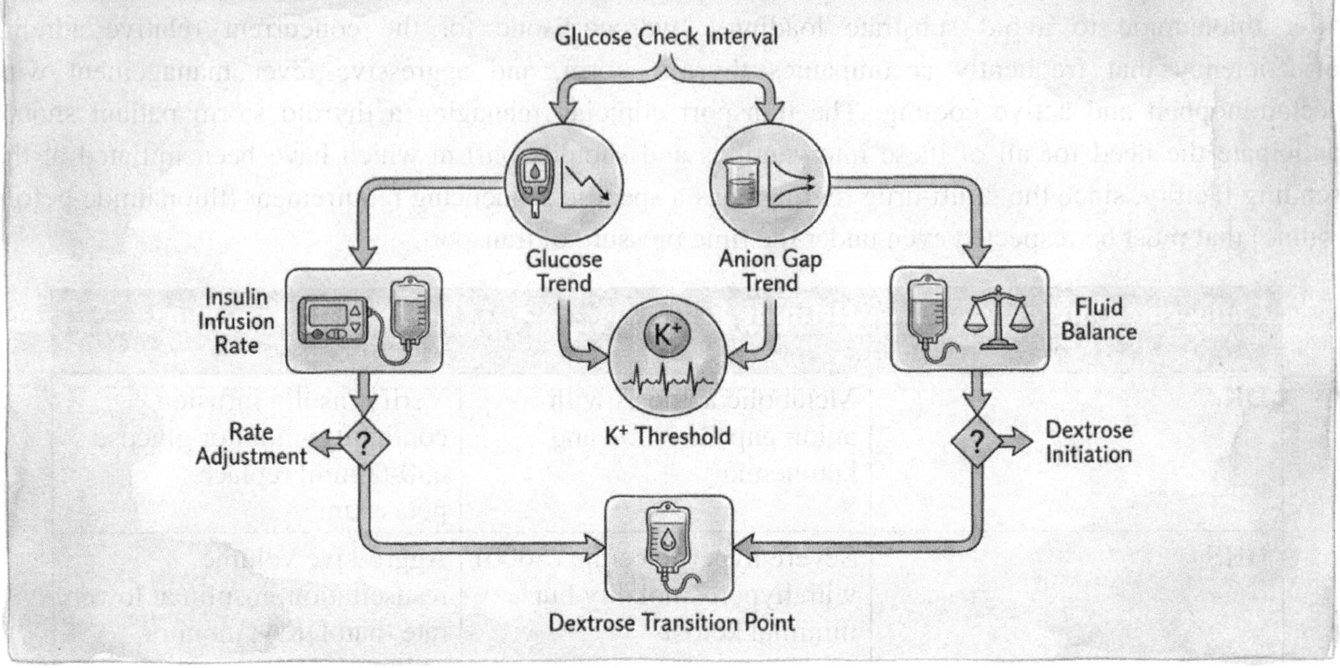


## Disease Mechanisms Relevant to the Transport Environment

The pathophysiology of the conditions addressed in this chapter interacts with the transport environment in specific, predictable ways. Altitude-related pressure and oxygenation changes, hemodynamic and monitoring constraints, pharmacologic and infusion logistics, and equipment considerations all modify the management of diabetic ketoacidosis, hyperosmolar hyperglycemic state, adrenal crisis, and thyroid storm management in ways that a purely bedside-focused clinical education does not address. The transport clinician must anticipate these interactions proactively rather than discovering them reactively when a deterioration pattern that is characteristic of the transport environment, not merely the disease itself, has already declared itself.

## Clinical Presentation and Assessment Priorities

The assessment follows the problem-based physiologic framework from Chapter 2: rapid identification of the primary derangement, establishment of a patient-specific baseline, and trend-based monitoring at fixed intervals to detect deviation before it becomes clinically obvious. The transport clinician should be particularly vigilant for the specific deterioration pattern described in the Signature introduced in this chapter, since this pattern is transport-specific and would not be encountered in the same form at the bedside.

## Management and Treatment During Transport

### Pharmacologic Management Adapted to Transport Constraints

The pharmacologic management of diabetic ketoacidosis, hyperosmolar hyperglycemic state, adrenal crisis, and thyroid storm management during transport follows the agent selection, dosing, and infusion logistics principles from Chapter 4, with disease-specific modifications. Medications with narrow therapeutic indices require closer monitoring because the environmental stressors of altitude, vibration, and temperature can alter drug metabolism, delivery, and effect. The transport clinician should confirm all active medication infusion rates, concentrations, and remaining volumes against the planned transport duration before departure.

### Procedural Interventions and Their Transport Feasibility

Any procedure anticipated as likely necessary during transport should be performed before departure whenever possible, since the benefit of early completion in a controlled environment outweighs the time cost. Procedures performed during transit should be reserved for genuinely emergent indications that cannot wait until arrival.

| Clinical Priority | Transport Action | Monitoring Focus |
|---|---|---|
| Hemodynamic stabilization | Vasoactive titration per Chapter 4 framework | Continuous arterial pressure; trend-based reassessment |
| Respiratory support | Ventilator management per Chapter 3 and 13 | SpO2, ETCO2, ventilator waveforms |
| Metabolic correction | Disease-specific therapy; infusion continuity | Point-of-care labs where available; clinical trajectory |
| Temperature management | Active warming or cooling per clinical indication | Continuous core temperature monitoring |
| Communication | Advance notification of receiving facility | Trajectory update at midpoint and pre-arrival |

Figure 18.2: Clinical Assessment Framework for Metabolic and Endocrine Emergencies in Transit

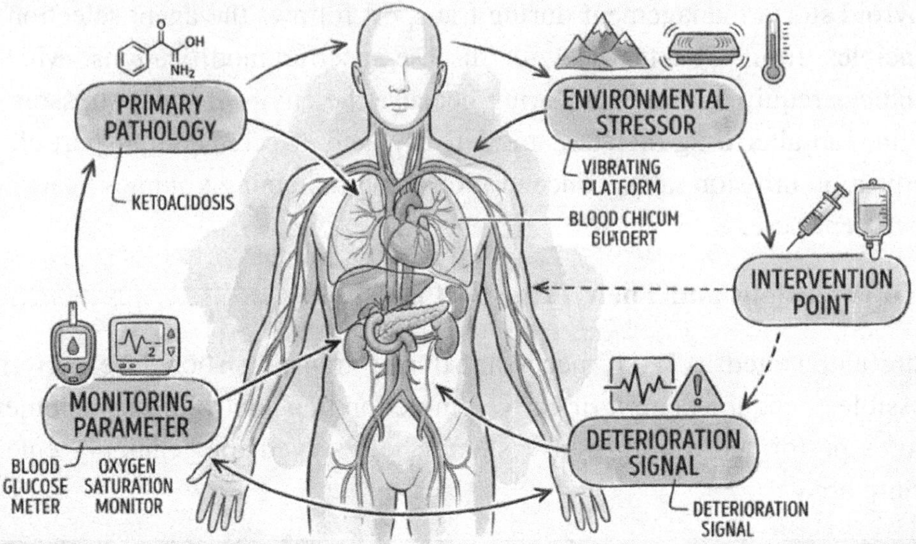


**THE IN-TRANSIT DETERIORATION SIGNATURE SYSTEM — Insulin-Infusion-Interrupted Metabolic Rebound**

**The Signature:** Progressive metabolic decompensation from an interrupted or subtherapeutic insulin infusion during transport, producing a rising anion gap and worsening acidosis that is initially attributed to disease progression rather than recognized as an iatrogenic infusion failure.

**Movement Trigger:** The transport environment introduces specific stressors that interact with the underlying disease process to produce a deterioration pattern that would not occur in the same form at the bedside.

**Early Tell:** A subtle, often indirect indicator detectable through the trend-based monitoring framework from Chapter 2, typically appearing as a discordance between improving surface-level parameters and worsening deeper physiologic indicators.

**Trap Logic:** This pattern is commonly attributed to expected disease progression or transport-related artifact rather than recognized as a specific, transport-triggered event. The discriminating feature is the temporal relationship to a transport-specific stressor and the discordance between surface and deep indicators.

**Signature Anchor:** When this pattern is suspected, address the transport-specific trigger in addition to managing the disease-specific consequences, and communicate the pattern to the receiving team.

## Special Populations and Complications

### Anticipated Complications and Contingency Planning

Each condition carries predictable complications that may develop during the transport window. The transport clinician should identify the most likely complication for the specific patient and prepare a contingency response before departure. This anticipatory approach is the practical application of the Deterioration Signature System's organizing principle: name the pattern, anticipate the trigger, and prepare the response in advance.

The conditions covered in this chapter share a common clinical theme when encountered in transport: the disease process determines the patient's baseline vulnerability, but the transport environment determines whether that vulnerability is safely managed or tipped into decompensation by altitude, movement, and resource limitation. The Signature introduced here names the most characteristic way the transport environment interacts with diabetic ketoacidosis, and the transport clinician's recognition of that interaction before it fully declares itself is the anticipatory skill this text is built to develop.

### Hyperosmolar Hyperglycemic State: Distinct From DKA Management

Hyperosmolar hyperglycemic state differs from diabetic ketoacidosis in several transport-critical respects: glucose levels are typically much higher (often exceeding six hundred milligrams per deciliter), serum osmolality is severely elevated, ketosis is minimal or absent, and the volume deficit is proportionally greater than in DKA, often exceeding nine liters. The resuscitation priority in HHS is aggressive volume replacement with isotonic crystalloid, which alone can reduce glucose substantially through hemodilution and improved renal glucose clearance, followed by insulin at a lower rate than used for DKA. The transport clinician should monitor sodium closely during HHS resuscitation, since the corrected sodium (adjusted for the glucose-induced osmotic water shift) may be substantially higher than the measured sodium and rises further as glucose is corrected, potentially reaching levels that carry a risk of osmotic demyelination if the correction is too rapid.

### Adrenal Crisis in the Steroid-Dependent Patient: A Transport Emergency

The steroid-dependent patient is a common transport population that includes patients on chronic glucocorticoid therapy for autoimmune diseases, transplant recipients on immunosuppressive protocols, and patients with known primary adrenal insufficiency. The stress of critical illness, surgery, or the transport itself can precipitate an adrenal crisis if the patient's existing steroid regimen is inadequate for the physiologic stress level, and the presentation--refractory hypotension, altered mentation, and hyponatremia--can be easily mistaken for septic shock or another cause of distributive shock. The transport clinician should specifically screen for steroid dependence in any patient with unexplained hemodynamic instability, and should administer stress-dose hydrocortisone empirically when adrenal crisis is clinically suspected, since the treatment is safe and the consequence of missing the diagnosis is a preventable death from cardiovascular collapse.

### Myxedema Coma: Recognition and Emergency Management

Myxedema coma, the extreme decompensation of hypothyroidism, presents with altered mentation, hypothermia, bradycardia, hyponatremia, and respiratory failure, and carries a mortality rate exceeding thirty percent even with treatment. The transport clinician encountering a patient with this constellation of findings should consider myxedema coma in the differential diagnosis, particularly in an older patient with a history of thyroid disease or thyroidectomy who presents with unexplained hypothermia and altered consciousness. Emergency management includes intravenous thyroid hormone replacement (levothyroxine and sometimes liothyronine), stress-dose glucocorticoids (because concurrent adrenal insufficiency is common), passive and active rewarming, and ventilatory support for the respiratory depression that typically accompanies severe myxedema. The transport clinician's role is primarily to suspect the diagnosis, initiate supportive care, and communicate the clinical suspicion to the receiving team so that thyroid function testing and hormone replacement can be initiated promptly on arrival.

### Pheochromocytoma Crisis During Transport

Pheochromocytoma crisis--paroxysmal or sustained catecholamine excess from a catecholamine-secreting tumor--presents with severe hypertension, tachycardia, diaphoresis, and headache, and can be triggered by physical stress, medication administration, or the abdominal compression that may occur during stretcher loading. The management during transport is alpha-blockade with phentolamine, followed by beta-blockade only after adequate alpha-blockade is established (beta-blockade before alpha-blockade can produce unopposed alpha-mediated vasoconstriction and paradoxical worsening of hypertension). This is one of the few clinical scenarios where the standard beta-blocker-first approach to hypertensive emergency management is specifically contraindicated, and the transport clinician should be aware of this exception.

### Additional Clinical Considerations for Transport Management

The management of patients in Chapter 18 requires attention to several additional transport-specific clinical factors that extend the principles established in the main body of the chapter. The transport clinician should be aware that the disease processes covered here interact with the transport environment in ways that are specific to the combination of the underlying pathophysiology and the particular environmental stressor encountered during a given mission, and that a management approach that is adequate for a short ground transport may be insufficient for a longer air transport at altitude, or vice versa. The serial reassessment protocol established in Chapter 2 provides the framework for detecting these interactions as they develop, and the Deterioration Signature introduced in this chapter names the most characteristic pattern by which they declare themselves.

Each patient transport is a unique combination of a specific patient's physiology, a specific set of ongoing therapies, a specific transport platform with its own environmental characteristics, and a specific mission profile with its own altitude, duration, and route constraints. The anticipatory approach to transport medicine that this text teaches is not a set of memorized responses to predetermined scenarios but a cognitive framework for analyzing the specific combination of variables present in any given transport and identifying, before departure, the most likely points of vulnerability where the transport environment will test the patient's physiologic reserve. This chapter's clinical content provides the disease-specific knowledge needed to apply that framework to the conditions covered here, while the Deterioration Signature provides the named pattern that makes the most characteristic transport-specific vulnerability explicit, recognizable, and actionable.

The receiving team's ability to continue the patient's care seamlessly after the transport crew departs depends entirely on the quality and completeness of the clinical information the transport crew provides, and for the conditions covered in this chapter, the specific information that matters most includes: the trajectory of the patient's primary condition during transport (improving, stable, or worsening, with specific details), any interventions performed during transport and their response, any new clinical findings identified by the transport crew that were not present at the sending facility, and any anticipated needs that the receiving team should prepare for based on the transport crew's clinical assessment. This information, communicated through the structured handoff format established in Chapter 2 and supplemented by the trajectory communication emphasis that is a recurring theme throughout this text, is the final clinical act of the transport and the one that determines whether the transport adds value to the patient's care continuum or merely moves the patient from one location to another without preserving the clinical narrative that only the transport crew was positioned to observe.

The transport clinician managing the conditions addressed in this chapter should develop a systematic pre-departure assessment that specifically identifies the highest-risk transport-environment interaction for each patient's specific disease process, the monitoring parameters that will detect that interaction earliest, and the intervention that will address it most effectively. This pre-departure risk analysis, adapted from the general pre-mission physiologic risk profile introduced in Chapter 1, should be specific enough to generate a concrete prediction: what is the single most likely way this specific patient's condition will interact with the specific transport environment of this specific mission? Answering that question before departure, rather than discovering the answer during transit, is the practical application of the anticipatory transport medicine framework that this entire text is designed to develop.

Clinical case presentations embedded throughout this chapter illustrate the principle that transport-specific deterioration patterns are predictable rather than random, recognizable rather than mysterious, and preventable rather than inevitable, provided the clinician applies the systematic assessment, continuous monitoring, and named-pattern recognition framework that the Deterioration Signature System codifies. Each case demonstrates the same three-part sequence: a patient with a specific disease process encounters a specific transport-environment stressor, produces a specific clinical change that could be attributed to either the disease or the environment, and is correctly managed because the transport clinician recognized the specific named Signature and applied the correct transport-specific intervention rather than the generic disease-specific response that would have been appropriate at the bedside but is insufficient or incorrect in the transport context.

The evidence base for transport-specific management of the conditions in this chapter continues to evolve, with ongoing research into optimal monitoring strategies, transport-adapted treatment protocols, and outcome data that will refine the recommendations presented here. The transport clinician should maintain awareness of emerging evidence through continuing education, program-sponsored journal clubs, and the quality improvement processes described in Chapter 24, since the standard of care for transport medicine is not static and the recommendations in any textbook represent a snapshot of evidence at the time of writing rather than a permanent standard. The principles, however, are durable: anticipate rather than react, monitor trends rather than thresholds, communicate trajectories rather than snapshots, and recognize that the transport environment is a clinical variable that acts on every patient's physiology, not a neutral conduit between two points of care.

Finally, the transport clinician should recognize that the clinical expertise required to manage these conditions during transport represents a distinct competency that builds on but extends beyond the bedside critical care training that most transport clinicians bring to their role. A clinician who is expert in managing these conditions in the intensive care unit is not automatically expert in managing them during transport, because the environmental, equipment, monitoring, and resource constraints of transport introduce variables that bedside practice never encounters. Conversely, a transport clinician who has mastered the anticipatory, environment-aware management approach described in this text brings a perspective to patient care that the bedside clinician lacks: the ability to see the patient's physiology not as a fixed state being managed in a controlled environment, but as a dynamic process interacting continuously with an environment that is itself changing throughout the transport. This dual awareness--of the disease and of the environment acting on it--is the defining competency of transport critical care medicine, and it is what this text, from its first chapter through its last, is designed to develop.

## THE IN-TRANSIT DETERIORATION SIGNATURE SYSTEM — Insulin-Infusion-Interrupted Metabolic Rebound Patterns

**Signature Introduced This Chapter:** Insulin-Infusion-Interrupted Metabolic Rebound -- a transport-specific deterioration pattern unique to diabetic ketoacidosis.

**Pattern Logic:** This Signature extends the foundational transport-physiology principles from Chapter 1 and the assessment framework from Chapter 2 into this disease domain.

**Cross-Reference Forward:** This Signature is indexed in the Anchor Section's Master Signature Atlas by organ system and clinical category.

## Summary and Key Concepts

The transport environment modifies the management of diabetic ketoacidosis, hyperosmolar hyperglycemic state, adrenal crisis, and thyroid storm management in specific, predictable ways beyond what bedside training addresses.

Trend-based monitoring at fixed intervals is the primary tool for detecting the disease-specific deterioration patterns described in this chapter's Signature.

Pharmacologic management follows the Chapter 4 framework with disease-specific modifications; infusion continuity requires particular attention.

Anticipatory contingency planning for the most likely complications is more effective than reactive management in the resource-constrained transport environment.

Advance communication with the receiving facility, including trajectory updates, is a direct clinical intervention improving care on arrival.

# CHAPTER 19: ELECTROLYTE DERANGEMENTS AND ACID-BASE DISORDERS IN TRANSIT

**Learning Objectives**

1. Apply disease-specific assessment, monitoring, and management principles for severe electrolyte abnormalities, acid-base interpretation, and renal failure management adapted to the transport environment.
2. Recognize transport-specific deterioration patterns and distinguish them from primary disease progression.
3. Coordinate advance communication with receiving facilities to optimize preparedness for the patient's arrival.
4. Manage pharmacologic interventions within the monitoring and resource constraints of critical care transport.

**Chapter Outline**

This chapter addresses severe electrolyte abnormalities, acid-base interpretation, and renal failure management as encountered in critical care transport, extending the foundational assessment, monitoring, pharmacologic, and equipment frameworks from earlier chapters to the specific challenges of managing these conditions during interfacility transport.

## Pathophysiology and Transport-Specific Considerations

## Severe Hyperkalemia Management During Transport

### ECG Recognition and Emergency Treatment Sequence

Severe hyperkalemia is the most immediately life-threatening electrolyte emergency encountered in transport, producing a predictable ECG progression from peaked T-waves through PR prolongation and QRS widening to a sine-wave pattern and ultimately ventricular fibrillation or asystole. The treatment sequence is time-critical and follows a fixed priority: intravenous calcium for immediate cardiac membrane stabilization (effect within one to three minutes), followed by insulin with dextrose to drive potassium intracellularly (effect within fifteen to thirty minutes), sodium bicarbonate if acidosis is present (effect within fifteen to thirty minutes), and nebulized albuterol as an adjunctive intracellular shift agent. The transport clinician should have calcium chloride or calcium gluconate drawn up and immediately available for any patient with a known potassium elevation or ECG changes suggestive of hyperkalemia, and should not delay treatment to obtain a confirmatory laboratory value when the ECG changes are present and the clinical context supports the diagnosis.

### Renal Failure and Dialysis-Dependent Patient Transport Considerations

Patients with end-stage renal disease who have missed dialysis sessions are at particular risk for hyperkalemia, volume overload, and uremic complications during transport, and the transport clinician should assess the number of missed sessions, the most recent dialysis adequacy (if known), and the current fluid and electrolyte status before departure. Volume overload may present as pulmonary edema requiring noninvasive ventilation or intubation during transport, and the transport clinician should be prepared to manage this with nitroglycerin for afterload reduction and, if available, continuous renal replacement therapy or ultrafiltration, though these modalities are rarely available during transport and the management is typically supportive until definitive dialysis can be provided at the receiving facility.

### Severe Hyponatremia: Risks of Overcorrection

Severe hyponatremia with neurologic symptoms--seizures, altered mentation, or signs of cerebral edema--requires emergent treatment with hypertonic saline to raise the serum sodium by a small, defined increment sufficient to reverse the life-threatening neurologic symptoms without overcorrecting. The danger of overcorrection is osmotic demyelination syndrome, a catastrophic and largely irreversible neurologic injury, and the transport clinician must monitor the rate of sodium correction closely if hypertonic saline is being administered during transport. The target is a rise of no more than ten to twelve milliequivalents per liter in the first twenty-four hours, and in practice the transport clinician's role is typically to administer a single bolus to arrest acute neurologic deterioration and then defer further correction to the receiving facility's controlled monitoring environment.

## Acid-Base Disturbance Interpretation in Transit

### Systematic Approach to Arterial Blood Gas Interpretation

A systematic approach to arterial blood gas interpretation during transport follows a fixed sequence: identify the primary process (metabolic acidosis, metabolic alkalosis, respiratory acidosis, or respiratory alkalosis), assess the degree of compensation (using the expected compensation formulas), and calculate the anion gap to classify metabolic acidosis as gap or non-gap, since each classification points to a different underlying etiology and management strategy. The transport clinician should be able to perform this interpretation rapidly from a point-of-care blood gas result and translate it into a management decision: a rising anion gap in a DKA patient suggests inadequate insulin delivery (connecting to Chapter 18's Insulin-Infusion-Interrupted Signature), while a new respiratory acidosis in a ventilated patient suggests hypoventilation or increasing dead space requiring ventilator adjustment.

### Mixed Acid-Base Disorders in the Transport Population

Transport patients frequently present with mixed acid-base disorders--the septic patient with both a metabolic acidosis from lactic acid production and a respiratory alkalosis from compensatory hyperventilation, or the COPD patient with a chronic respiratory acidosis complicated by a new metabolic acidosis from acute kidney injury. Recognizing these mixed disorders during transport is important because the appropriate intervention depends on which component is primary and which is compensatory:

treating the compensatory hyperventilation of a metabolic acidosis by sedating the patient and reducing the respiratory rate, for example, would worsen the acidosis by removing the body's compensatory mechanism, while treating the metabolic acidosis with volume resuscitation and source control allows the respiratory compensation to resolve on its own.

| Electrolyte Emergency | ECG Finding | Immediate Treatment | Transport Monitoring |
|---|---|---|---|
| Hyperkalemia | Peaked T-waves, wide QRS, sine wave | IV calcium, insulin+dextrose, albuterol neb | Continuous ECG; repeat POC K+ if available |
| Hypokalemia | U waves, ST depression, QT prolongation | IV potassium replacement | Continuous ECG; infusion rate monitoring |
| Hypocalcemia | Prolonged QT interval | IV calcium gluconate | QT interval monitoring |
| Severe hyponatremia | Not specific; seizures are clinical | Hypertonic saline (controlled bolus) | Sodium level tracking; rate of correction |
| Hypermagnesemia | Prolonged PR, wide QRS, bradycardia | IV calcium; hold magnesium-containing meds | ECG and deep tendon reflexes |

**Figure 19.1: Systematic Arterial Blood Gas Interpretation Algorithm**

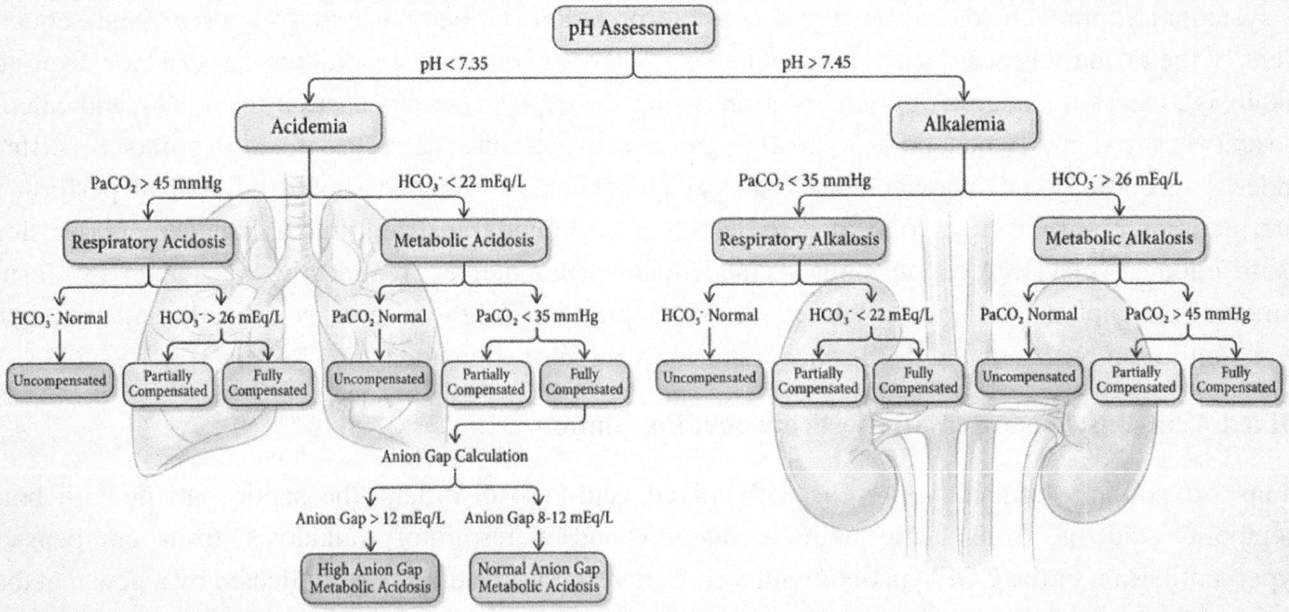

### Disease Mechanisms Relevant to the Transport Environment

The pathophysiology of the conditions addressed in this chapter interacts with the transport environment in specific, predictable ways. Altitude-related pressure and oxygenation changes, hemodynamic and monitoring constraints, pharmacologic and infusion logistics, and equipment considerations all modify the management of severe electrolyte abnormalities, acid-base interpretation, and renal failure management in ways that a purely bedside-focused clinical education does not address. The transport clinician must anticipate these interactions proactively rather than discovering them reactively when a deterioration pattern that is characteristic of the transport environment, not merely the disease itself, has already declared itself.

### Clinical Presentation and Assessment Priorities

The assessment follows the problem-based physiologic framework from Chapter 2: rapid identification of the primary derangement, establishment of a patient-specific baseline, and trend-based monitoring at fixed intervals to detect deviation before it becomes clinically obvious. The transport clinician should be particularly vigilant for the specific deterioration pattern described in the Signature introduced in this chapter, since this pattern is transport-specific and would not be encountered in the same form at the bedside.

## Management and Treatment During Transport

### Pharmacologic Management Adapted to Transport Constraints

The pharmacologic management of severe electrolyte abnormalities, acid-base interpretation, and renal failure management during transport follows the agent selection, dosing, and infusion logistics principles from Chapter 4, with disease-specific modifications. Medications with narrow therapeutic indices require closer monitoring because the environmental stressors of altitude, vibration, and temperature can alter drug metabolism, delivery, and effect. The transport clinician should confirm all active medication infusion rates, concentrations, and remaining volumes against the planned transport duration before departure.

### Procedural Interventions and Their Transport Feasibility

Any procedure anticipated as likely necessary during transport should be performed before departure whenever possible, since the benefit of early completion in a controlled environment outweighs the time cost. Procedures performed during transit should be reserved for genuinely emergent indications that cannot wait until arrival.

| Clinical Priority | Transport Action | Monitoring Focus |
|---|---|---|
| Hemodynamic stabilization | Vasoactive titration per Chapter 4 framework | Continuous arterial pressure; trend-based reassessment |
| Respiratory support | Ventilator management per Chapter 3 and 13 | SpO2, ETCO2, ventilator waveforms |

| | | |
|---|---|---|
| Metabolic correction | Disease-specific therapy; infusion continuity | Point-of-care labs where available; clinical trajectory |
| Temperature management | Active warming or cooling per clinical indication | Continuous core temperature monitoring |
| Communication | Advance notification of receiving facility | Trajectory update at midpoint and pre-arrival |

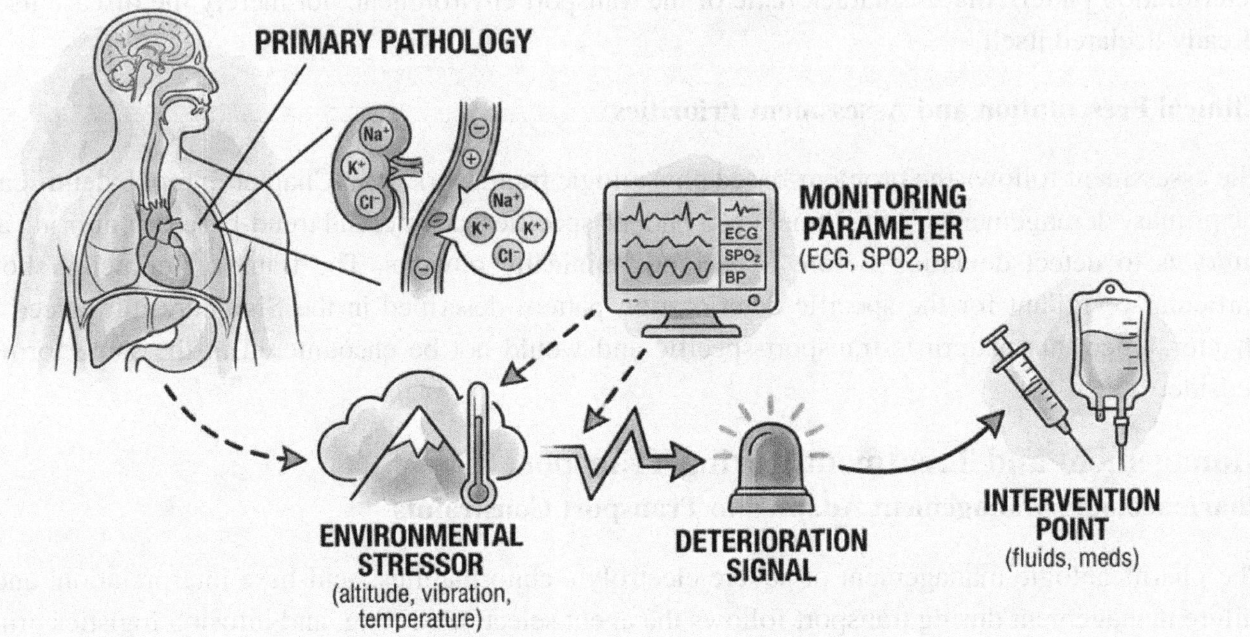


Figure 19.2: Clinical Assessment Framework for Electrolyte Derangements and Acid-Base Disorders in Transit

**THE IN-TRANSIT DETERIORATION SIGNATURE SYSTEM — Temperature-Shifted Electrolyte Toxicity**

**The Signature:** An electrolyte-driven cardiac or neuromuscular event that develops during transport as hypothermia or rewarming alters the distribution of potassium, calcium, or magnesium across cell membranes, producing a functional electrolyte toxicity at a serum level that was previously tolerated at a different body temperature.

**Movement Trigger:** The transport environment introduces specific stressors that interact with the underlying disease process to produce a deterioration pattern that would not occur in the same form at the bedside.

**Early Tell:** A subtle, often indirect indicator detectable through the trend-based monitoring framework from Chapter 2, typically appearing as a discordance between improving surface-level parameters and worsening deeper physiologic indicators.

**Trap Logic:** This pattern is commonly attributed to expected disease progression or transport-related artifact rather than recognized as a specific, transport-triggered event. The discriminating feature is the temporal relationship to a transport-specific stressor and the discordance between surface and deep indicators.

**Signature Anchor:** When this pattern is suspected, address the transport-specific trigger in addition to managing the disease-specific consequences, and communicate the pattern to the receiving team.

## Special Populations and Complications

### Anticipated Complications and Contingency Planning

Each condition carries predictable complications that may develop during the transport window. The transport clinician should identify the most likely complication for the specific patient and prepare a contingency response before departure. This anticipatory approach is the practical application of the Deterioration Signature System's organizing principle: name the pattern, anticipate the trigger, and prepare the response in advance.

The conditions covered in this chapter share a common clinical theme when encountered in transport: the disease process determines the patient's baseline vulnerability, but the transport environment determines whether that vulnerability is safely managed or tipped into decompensation by altitude, movement, and resource limitation. The Signature introduced here names the most characteristic way the transport environment interacts with severe electrolyte abnormalities, and the transport clinician's recognition of that interaction before it fully declares itself is the anticipatory skill this text is built to develop.

### Calcium Disorders: Hypercalcemia and Hypocalcemia

Severe hypercalcemia produces altered mentation, shortened QT interval, and renal dysfunction, and the emergency management during transport is aggressive volume resuscitation with isotonic saline to promote renal calcium excretion, followed by loop diuretics only after adequate volume repletion is achieved (loop diuretics administered to a dehydrated patient worsen the volume deficit without effectively lowering calcium). Calcitonin provides a modest and temporary calcium-lowering effect that begins within hours and can be administered during transport as an adjunct. Severe hypocalcemia, conversely, produces circumoral and extremity paresthesias, muscle spasms (carpopedal spasm, Trousseau sign, Chvostek sign), prolonged QT interval, and at its extreme, seizures and cardiac arrest. Intravenous calcium replacement must be administered slowly and with continuous cardiac monitoring, since rapid calcium infusion can produce bradycardia and cardiac arrest, and the specific formulation (calcium gluconate for peripheral administration, calcium chloride for central access) must match the available vascular access.

### Magnesium Disorders and Their Cardiac Implications

Hypomagnesemia frequently accompanies hypokalemia and hypocalcemia, and refractory hypokalemia that does not respond to potassium replacement alone should prompt the transport clinician to consider and treat concurrent magnesium depletion, since the renal potassium-wasting mechanism of hypomagnesemia prevents effective potassium repletion until the magnesium deficit is corrected. Hypermagnesemia, most commonly seen in the setting of magnesium sulfate therapy for preeclampsia or renal failure with magnesium-containing medication use, produces a predictable clinical progression: loss of deep tendon reflexes at mild elevation, respiratory depression at moderate elevation, and cardiac arrest at severe elevation. The antidote is intravenous calcium, which opposes magnesium's neuromuscular and cardiac effects, and should be immediately available whenever magnesium sulfate is being infused.

### Phosphate Disorders in the Transport Population

Severe hypophosphatemia, most commonly seen during refeeding syndrome in the malnourished patient and during DKA treatment as insulin drives phosphate intracellularly, can produce respiratory muscle weakness, cardiac dysfunction, and hemolytic anemia, and should be considered in any patient with unexplained respiratory or cardiac deterioration during treatment of malnutrition or DKA. Intravenous phosphate replacement must be administered slowly to avoid hypocalcemia from calcium-phosphate precipitation, and the rate should be adjusted based on renal function since the kidneys are the primary route of phosphate clearance. Hyperphosphatemia, most commonly seen in renal failure, contributes to hypocalcemia through calcium-phosphate binding and is managed primarily through dialysis at the receiving facility.

### Sodium Disorders: The Correction Rate as the Critical Variable

In both severe hyponatremia and severe hypernatremia, the rate of sodium correction is as clinically important as the direction of correction, because overly rapid correction of either abnormality produces a specific, devastating neurologic injury. Rapid correction of hyponatremia (more than ten to twelve milliequivalents per liter in twenty-four hours) produces osmotic demyelination syndrome, while rapid correction of hypernatremia produces cerebral edema. The transport clinician managing either condition should know the current sodium level, the rate of change over the preceding hours, and the specific correction target and rate prescribed by the sending or receiving team, and should monitor sodium at intervals sufficient to detect an overly rapid correction before it produces irreversible injury. For hyponatremia specifically, the transport clinician should be aware that certain interventions commonly performed during transport--volume resuscitation with isotonic saline, desmopressin administration for diabetes insipidus--can produce a rapid sodium change that overshoots the intended correction rate if not monitored carefully.

### Additional Clinical Considerations for Transport Management

The management of patients in Chapter 19 requires attention to several additional transport-specific clinical factors that extend the principles established in the main body of the chapter. The transport clinician should be aware that the disease processes covered here interact with the transport environment in ways that are specific to the combination of the underlying pathophysiology and the particular environmental stressor encountered during a given mission, and that a management approach that is adequate for a short ground transport may be insufficient for a longer air transport at altitude, or vice versa.

The serial reassessment protocol established in Chapter 2 provides the framework for detecting these interactions as they develop, and the Deterioration Signature introduced in this chapter names the most characteristic pattern by which they declare themselves.

Each patient transport is a unique combination of a specific patient's physiology, a specific set of ongoing therapies, a specific transport platform with its own environmental characteristics, and a specific mission profile with its own altitude, duration, and route constraints. The anticipatory approach to transport medicine that this text teaches is not a set of memorized responses to predetermined scenarios but a cognitive framework for analyzing the specific combination of variables present in any given transport and identifying, before departure, the most likely points of vulnerability where the transport environment will test the patient's physiologic reserve. This chapter's clinical content provides the disease-specific knowledge needed to apply that framework to the conditions covered here, while the Deterioration Signature provides the named pattern that makes the most characteristic transport-specific vulnerability explicit, recognizable, and actionable.

The receiving team's ability to continue the patient's care seamlessly after the transport crew departs depends entirely on the quality and completeness of the clinical information the transport crew provides, and for the conditions covered in this chapter, the specific information that matters most includes: the trajectory of the patient's primary condition during transport (improving, stable, or worsening, with specific details), any interventions performed during transport and their response, any new clinical findings identified by the transport crew that were not present at the sending facility, and any anticipated needs that the receiving team should prepare for based on the transport crew's clinical assessment. This information, communicated through the structured handoff format established in Chapter 2 and supplemented by the trajectory communication emphasis that is a recurring theme throughout this text, is the final clinical act of the transport and the one that determines whether the transport adds value to the patient's care continuum or merely moves the patient from one location to another without preserving the clinical narrative that only the transport crew was positioned to observe.

The transport clinician managing the conditions addressed in this chapter should develop a systematic pre-departure assessment that specifically identifies the highest-risk transport-environment interaction for each patient's specific disease process, the monitoring parameters that will detect that interaction earliest, and the intervention that will address it most effectively. This pre-departure risk analysis, adapted from the general pre-mission physiologic risk profile introduced in Chapter 1, should be specific enough to generate a concrete prediction: what is the single most likely way this specific patient's condition will interact with the specific transport environment of this specific mission? Answering that question before departure, rather than discovering the answer during transit, is the practical application of the anticipatory transport medicine framework that this entire text is designed to develop.

Clinical case presentations embedded throughout this chapter illustrate the principle that transport-specific deterioration patterns are predictable rather than random, recognizable rather than mysterious, and preventable rather than inevitable, provided the clinician applies the systematic assessment, continuous monitoring, and named-pattern recognition framework that the Deterioration Signature System codifies.

Each case demonstrates the same three-part sequence: a patient with a specific disease process encounters a specific transport-environment stressor, produces a specific clinical change that could be attributed to either the disease or the environment, and is correctly managed because the transport clinician recognized the specific named Signature and applied the correct transport-specific intervention rather than the generic disease-specific response that would have been appropriate at the bedside but is insufficient or incorrect in the transport context.

The evidence base for transport-specific management of the conditions in this chapter continues to evolve, with ongoing research into optimal monitoring strategies, transport-adapted treatment protocols, and outcome data that will refine the recommendations presented here. The transport clinician should maintain awareness of emerging evidence through continuing education, program-sponsored journal clubs, and the quality improvement processes described in Chapter 24, since the standard of care for transport medicine is not static and the recommendations in any textbook represent a snapshot of evidence at the time of writing rather than a permanent standard. The principles, however, are durable: anticipate rather than react, monitor trends rather than thresholds, communicate trajectories rather than snapshots, and recognize that the transport environment is a clinical variable that acts on every patient's physiology, not a neutral conduit between two points of care.

Finally, the transport clinician should recognize that the clinical expertise required to manage these conditions during transport represents a distinct competency that builds on but extends beyond the bedside critical care training that most transport clinicians bring to their role. A clinician who is expert in managing these conditions in the intensive care unit is not automatically expert in managing them during transport, because the environmental, equipment, monitoring, and resource constraints of transport introduce variables that bedside practice never encounters. Conversely, a transport clinician who has mastered the anticipatory, environment-aware management approach described in this text brings a perspective to patient care that the bedside clinician lacks: the ability to see the patient's physiology not as a fixed state being managed in a controlled environment, but as a dynamic process interacting continuously with an environment that is itself changing throughout the transport. This dual awareness--of the disease and of the environment acting on it--is the defining competency of transport critical care medicine, and it is what this text, from its first chapter through its last, is designed to develop.

**THE IN-TRANSIT DETERIORATION SIGNATURE SYSTEM — Temperature-Shifted Electrolyte Toxicity Patterns**

---

**Signature Introduced This Chapter:** Temperature-Shifted Electrolyte Toxicity -- a transport-specific deterioration pattern unique to severe electrolyte abnormalities.

**Pattern Logic:** This Signature extends the foundational transport-physiology principles from Chapter 1 and the assessment framework from Chapter 2 into this disease domain.

**Cross-Reference Forward:** This Signature is indexed in the Anchor Section's Master Signature Atlas by organ system and clinical category.

## Summary and Key Concepts

The transport environment modifies the management of severe electrolyte abnormalities, acid-base interpretation, and renal failure management in specific, predictable ways beyond what bedside training addresses.

Trend-based monitoring at fixed intervals is the primary tool for detecting the disease-specific deterioration patterns described in this chapter's Signature.

Pharmacologic management follows the Chapter 4 framework with disease-specific modifications; infusion continuity requires particular attention.

Anticipatory contingency planning for the most likely complications is more effective than reactive management in the resource-constrained transport environment.

Advance communication with the receiving facility, including trajectory updates, is a direct clinical intervention improving care on arrival.

# CHAPTER 20: TOXICOLOGIC EMERGENCIES IN TRANSIT

**Learning Objectives**

1. Apply disease-specific assessment, monitoring, and management principles for toxidrome recognition, antidote administration, decontamination considerations, and withdrawal syndrome management adapted to the transport environment.
2. Recognize transport-specific deterioration patterns and distinguish them from primary disease progression.
3. Coordinate advance communication with receiving facilities to optimize preparedness for the patient's arrival.
4. Manage pharmacologic interventions within the monitoring and resource constraints of critical care transport.

**Chapter Outline**

This chapter addresses toxidrome recognition, antidote administration, decontamination considerations, and withdrawal syndrome management as encountered in critical care transport, extending the foundational assessment, monitoring, pharmacologic, and equipment frameworks from earlier chapters to the specific challenges of managing these conditions during interfacility transport.

## Pathophysiology and Transport-Specific Considerations

## Common Toxidrome Recognition

### The Five Classic Toxidromes and Their Transport Relevance

Toxicologic emergencies in transport are organized by toxidrome--a constellation of signs and symptoms produced by a class of toxic agents--because the toxidrome directs the antidotal therapy and supportive management even when the specific agent is unknown. The five classic toxidromes are sympathomimetic (tachycardia, hypertension, hyperthermia, mydriasis, diaphoresis, agitation), anticholinergic (tachycardia, hyperthermia, mydriasis, dry skin, urinary retention, delirium), cholinergic (bradycardia, miosis, salivation, lacrimation, urination, defecation, diaphoresis, bronchorrhea), opioid (respiratory depression, miosis, decreased level of consciousness), and sedative-hypnotic (respiratory depression, decreased consciousness, hypotension). The transport clinician should perform a deliberate toxidrome assessment at departure and at each reassessment interval, since the clinical picture of a toxic ingestion evolves as the substance is absorbed and metabolized, and a toxidrome that was not fully declared at the sending facility may become apparent during the transport window.

### Delayed-Onset Toxicity and the Extended Transport Window

Certain ingestions have delayed toxicity profiles that make the transport window a period of particular vulnerability: acetaminophen produces minimal symptoms in the first twenty-four hours despite ongoing hepatotoxicity, sustained-release medication formulations produce delayed absorption that can shift the peak clinical effect into the transport window, and coingestants may interact to produce a clinical syndrome different from either substance alone. The transport clinician should be aware of the time of ingestion relative to the current transport window and should not assume that a patient who is clinically well at departure will remain so throughout transport, particularly for the sustained-release and delayed-toxicity agents.

## Antidote Administration and Decontamination Considerations

### Specific Antidotes Available in the Transport Setting

Transport programs should carry a limited but targeted antidote formulary that covers the most immediately life-threatening toxic exposures: naloxone for opioid toxicity, atropine for organophosphate or nerve agent cholinergic crisis, sodium bicarbonate for sodium channel blocker (tricyclic antidepressant) cardiotoxicity, intralipid emulsion for local anesthetic systemic toxicity, calcium for calcium channel blocker or hydrofluoric acid exposure, and glucagon for beta-blocker toxicity. Each antidote should be immediately accessible without searching through a general medication supply, pre-dosed or with a dosing reference immediately attached, and the crew should be trained in the indications, dose, and expected response for each agent.

### Cardiotoxic Ingestion Management During Transport

Cardiotoxic ingestions--tricyclic antidepressants, sodium channel blockers, beta-blockers, calcium channel blockers, and digoxin--represent the highest-acuity toxicologic emergencies in transport because they produce cardiac arrhythmias and hemodynamic instability that can deteriorate rapidly to cardiac arrest. The management of each is antidote-specific rather than generic: tricyclic cardiotoxicity is treated with sodium bicarbonate (to overcome the sodium channel blockade), beta-blocker toxicity with glucagon and high-dose insulin-dextrose, calcium channel blocker toxicity with calcium and high-dose insulin-dextrose, and digoxin toxicity with digoxin-specific antibody fragments. The transport clinician must recognize the specific cardiotoxic pattern on the ECG and initiate the correct antidote rather than defaulting to a generic ACLS approach that may be ineffective or harmful for the specific toxin.

| Toxidrome | Key Clinical Features | Primary Antidote | Transport Priority |
|---|---|---|---|
| Sympathomimetic | Tachycardia, hypertension, hyperthermia, agitation | Benzodiazepines for agitation; active cooling | Temperature and agitation control |

| | | | |
|---|---|---|---|
| Anticholinergic | Tachycardia, dry hot skin, mydriasis, delirium | Physostigmine (select cases only) | Seizure readiness; temperature monitoring |
| Cholinergic | SLUDGE (salivation, lacrimation, urination, defecation, GI, emesis), bradycardia, miosis | Atropine (high-dose, repeated) | Airway protection; massive atropine may be needed |
| Opioid | Respiratory depression, miosis, obtundation | Naloxone | Airway management; redosing may be needed for long-acting opioids |
| Sedative-hypnotic | Respiratory depression, obtundation, hypotension | Flumazenil (benzodiazepines only, with caution) | Airway protection; supportive care |

## Withdrawal Syndromes During Transport

### Alcohol and Benzodiazepine Withdrawal

Alcohol and benzodiazepine withdrawal can produce seizures, autonomic instability, and delirium tremens that are immediately life-threatening and that may declare themselves during the transport window if the patient's last intake was recent enough that withdrawal symptoms are still evolving. The transport clinician should assess the risk of withdrawal in any patient with a history of alcohol or benzodiazepine dependence, should continue any benzodiazepine prophylaxis initiated at the sending facility without interruption, and should have additional benzodiazepine doses immediately available for breakthrough symptoms. The pharmacologic management from Chapter 4 applies directly, with the specific consideration that benzodiazepine doses for withdrawal may be substantially higher than those used for procedural sedation, and the clinician should titrate to clinical effect rather than adhering to a fixed dose that may be inadequate for the specific patient's withdrawal severity.

### Opioid Withdrawal Considerations

Opioid withdrawal, while intensely uncomfortable, is not immediately life-threatening in the same way that alcohol and benzodiazepine withdrawal are, and the transport management is primarily symptomatic: antiemetics for nausea and vomiting, antidiarrheals, and comfort measures. However, opioid withdrawal in a critically ill patient can produce significant hemodynamic instability through catecholamine surge, tachycardia, and hypertension that complicate the management of concurrent conditions, and the transport clinician should consider whether the patient's current hemodynamic or symptom trajectory is being driven by withdrawal rather than by the primary condition for which they are being transported.

Figure 20.1: Toxidrome Recognition Assessment Framework

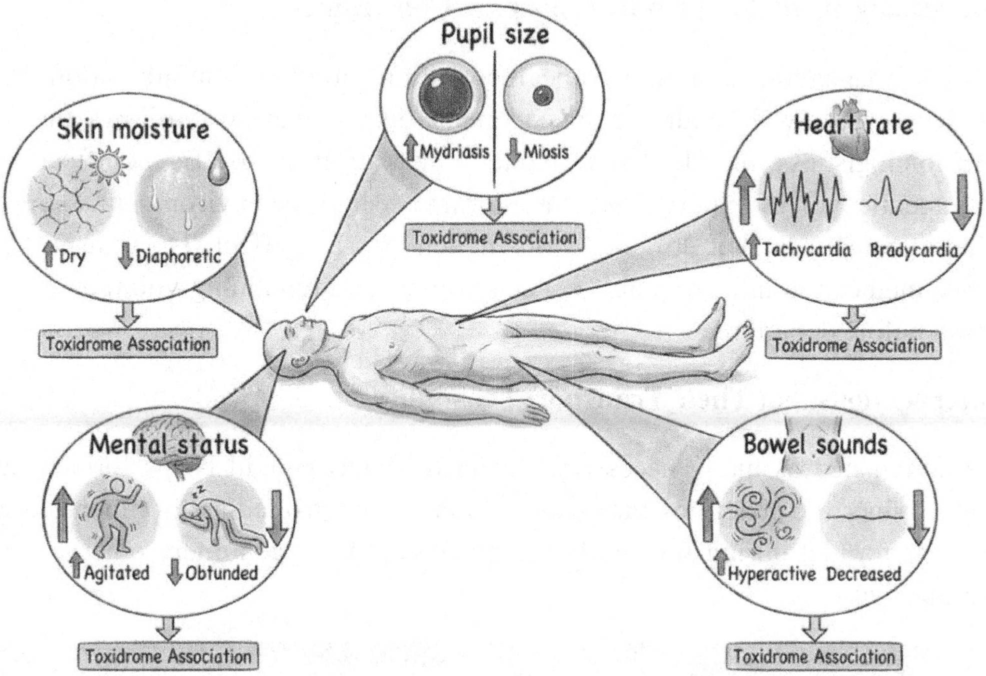


**Disease Mechanisms Relevant to the Transport Environment**

The pathophysiology of the conditions addressed in this chapter interacts with the transport environment in specific, predictable ways. Altitude-related pressure and oxygenation changes, hemodynamic and monitoring constraints, pharmacologic and infusion logistics, and equipment considerations all modify the management of toxidrome recognition, antidote administration, decontamination considerations, and withdrawal syndrome management in ways that a purely bedside-focused clinical education does not address. The transport clinician must anticipate these interactions proactively rather than discovering them reactively when a deterioration pattern that is characteristic of the transport environment, not merely the disease itself, has already declared itself.

**Clinical Presentation and Assessment Priorities**

The assessment follows the problem-based physiologic framework from Chapter 2: rapid identification of the primary derangement, establishment of a patient-specific baseline, and trend-based monitoring at fixed intervals to detect deviation before it becomes clinically obvious. The transport clinician should be particularly vigilant for the specific deterioration pattern described in the Signature introduced in this chapter, since this pattern is transport-specific and would not be encountered in the same form at the bedside.

## Management and Treatment During Transport

### Pharmacologic Management Adapted to Transport Constraints

The pharmacologic management of toxidrome recognition, antidote administration, decontamination considerations, and withdrawal syndrome management during transport follows the agent selection, dosing, and infusion logistics principles from Chapter 4, with disease-specific modifications. Medications with narrow therapeutic indices require closer monitoring because the environmental stressors of altitude, vibration, and temperature can alter drug metabolism, delivery, and effect. The transport clinician should confirm all active medication infusion rates, concentrations, and remaining volumes against the planned transport duration before departure.

### Procedural Interventions and Their Transport Feasibility

Any procedure anticipated as likely necessary during transport should be performed before departure whenever possible, since the benefit of early completion in a controlled environment outweighs the time cost. Procedures performed during transit should be reserved for genuinely emergent indications that cannot wait until arrival.

| Clinical Priority | Transport Action | Monitoring Focus |
|---|---|---|
| Hemodynamic stabilization | Vasoactive titration per Chapter 4 framework | Continuous arterial pressure; trend-based reassessment |
| Respiratory support | Ventilator management per Chapter 3 and 13 | SpO2, ETCO2, ventilator waveforms |
| Metabolic correction | Disease-specific therapy; infusion continuity | Point-of-care labs where available; clinical trajectory |
| Temperature management | Active warming or cooling per clinical indication | Continuous core temperature monitoring |
| Communication | Advance notification of receiving facility | Trajectory update at midpoint and pre-arrival |

Figure 20.2: Clinical Assessment Framework for Toxicologic Emergencies in Transit

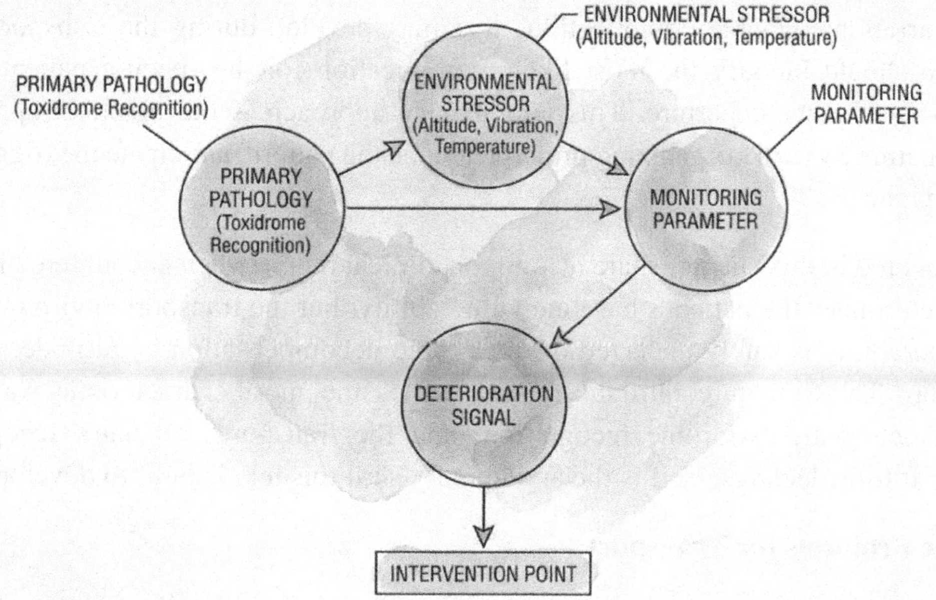


**THE IN-TRANSIT DETERIORATION SIGNATURE SYSTEM — Delayed Toxidrome Declaration During Extended Transport**

**The Signature:** A toxic ingestion whose clinical syndrome does not fully declare itself until the transport is already underway, because the time-to-peak-effect of the ingested substance extends beyond the pre-departure assessment window.

**Movement Trigger:** The transport environment introduces specific stressors that interact with the underlying disease process to produce a deterioration pattern that would not occur in the same form at the bedside.

**Early Tell:** A subtle, often indirect indicator detectable through the trend-based monitoring framework from Chapter 2, typically appearing as a discordance between improving surface-level parameters and worsening deeper physiologic indicators.

**Trap Logic:** This pattern is commonly attributed to expected disease progression or transport-related artifact rather than recognized as a specific, transport-triggered event. The discriminating feature is the temporal relationship to a transport-specific stressor and the discordance between surface and deep indicators.

**Signature Anchor:** When this pattern is suspected, address the transport-specific trigger in addition to managing the disease-specific consequences, and communicate the pattern to the receiving team.

## Special Populations and Complications

### Anticipated Complications and Contingency Planning

Each condition carries predictable complications that may develop during the transport window. The transport clinician should identify the most likely complication for the specific patient and prepare a contingency response before departure. This anticipatory approach is the practical application of the Deterioration Signature System's organizing principle: name the pattern, anticipate the trigger, and prepare the response in advance.

The conditions covered in this chapter share a common clinical theme when encountered in transport: the disease process determines the patient's baseline vulnerability, but the transport environment determines whether that vulnerability is safely managed or tipped into decompensation by altitude, movement, and resource limitation. The Signature introduced here names the most characteristic way the transport environment interacts with toxidrome recognition, and the transport clinician's recognition of that interaction before it fully declares itself is the anticipatory skill this text is built to develop.

### Specific Antidote Protocols for Transport

The transport formulary should include specific antidotes for the most commonly encountered and most immediately life-threatening toxic exposures, with pre-calculated dosing references attached to each antidote to enable rapid, accurate administration under stress. Naloxone for opioid reversal should be titrated to restore adequate respiratory drive without precipitating full reversal, since abrupt full reversal in an opioid-dependent patient can produce acute withdrawal, catecholamine surge, and pulmonary edema that is as dangerous as the opioid toxicity itself. The starting dose should be small (0.04 to 0.1 milligrams intravenously) and titrated upward until respiratory rate and tidal volume improve, rather than administering the full 2-milligram dose that was historically taught.

### Organophosphate and Nerve Agent Poisoning

Organophosphate poisoning from agricultural pesticide exposure or, in mass-casualty scenarios, nerve agent exposure, produces a cholinergic crisis characterized by the SLUDGE mnemonic (salivation, lacrimation, urination, defecation, gastrointestinal distress, emesis) plus bronchorrhea, bronchospasm, bradycardia, and muscular fasciculations progressing to paralysis. The management requires large and sometimes enormous doses of atropine--far exceeding the standard cardiac doses--titrated to the drying of airway secretions rather than to heart rate, followed by pralidoxime to reactivate acetylcholinesterase if administered before the enzyme-inhibitor bond has aged beyond reactivation. The transport clinician should carry atropine in quantities sufficient for the high-dose administration this toxidrome requires (total doses of ten to twenty milligrams or more are not uncommon in severe organophosphate poisoning) and should not be deterred by doses that would be considered massive in any other clinical context.

## Cyanide Poisoning: A Time-Critical Antidote Decision

Cyanide poisoning, encountered in fire victims from the combustion of synthetic materials and in industrial exposures, produces a rapidly lethal cellular asphyxia that presents with altered mentation, lactic acidosis, and characteristic cherry-red skin coloration (though this sign is unreliable and often absent). Hydroxocobalamin (Cyanokit) is the preferred antidote for transport administration because it is safe, effective, has minimal hemodynamic side effects compared to the older sodium nitrite-sodium thiosulfate combination, and can be administered empirically in a fire victim with unexplained altered mentation and lactic acidosis without waiting for confirmatory cyanide levels (which are not available in the transport setting). The transport clinician should administer hydroxocobalamin early in any fire victim with suspected cyanide exposure, since the cellular injury from cyanide poisoning is time-dependent and the antidote's safety profile makes empiric administration a reasonable clinical choice.

## Carbon Monoxide Poisoning and Hyperbaric Oxygen Considerations

Carbon monoxide poisoning produces tissue hypoxia by displacing oxygen from hemoglobin (forming carboxyhemoglobin) and by binding to cytochrome oxidase in the mitochondrial electron transport chain, and the treatment is high-concentration oxygen to accelerate carbon monoxide dissociation. The half-life of carboxyhemoglobin is approximately four to six hours at room air, approximately sixty to ninety minutes at one hundred percent oxygen at sea level, and approximately twenty to thirty minutes under hyperbaric oxygen conditions, which is the basis for transferring severe carbon monoxide poisoning patients to facilities with hyperbaric capability. The transport clinician should administer one hundred percent oxygen by non-rebreather mask or mechanical ventilation throughout the transport and should be aware that pulse oximetry is unreliable in carbon monoxide poisoning because standard pulse oximeters cannot distinguish carboxyhemoglobin from oxyhemoglobin, producing a falsely normal or near-normal saturation reading despite severely impaired oxygen delivery.

**CAUTION:** Standard pulse oximetry cannot detect carboxyhemoglobin and will display a falsely normal or near-normal $SpO_2$ in carbon monoxide poisoning; co-oximetry or a carboxyhemoglobin-specific measurement is required for accurate assessment.

## Additional Clinical Considerations for Transport Management

The management of patients in Chapter 20 requires attention to several additional transport-specific clinical factors that extend the principles established in the main body of the chapter. The transport clinician should be aware that the disease processes covered here interact with the transport environment in ways that are specific to the combination of the underlying pathophysiology and the particular environmental stressor encountered during a given mission, and that a management approach that is adequate for a short ground transport may be insufficient for a longer air transport at altitude, or vice versa. The serial reassessment protocol established in Chapter 2 provides the framework for detecting these interactions as they develop, and the Deterioration Signature introduced in this chapter names the most characteristic pattern by which they declare themselves.

Each patient transport is a unique combination of a specific patient's physiology, a specific set of ongoing therapies, a specific transport platform with its own environmental characteristics, and a specific mission profile with its own altitude, duration, and route constraints. The anticipatory approach to transport medicine that this text teaches is not a set of memorized responses to predetermined scenarios but a cognitive framework for analyzing the specific combination of variables present in any given transport and identifying, before departure, the most likely points of vulnerability where the transport environment will test the patient's physiologic reserve. This chapter's clinical content provides the disease-specific knowledge needed to apply that framework to the conditions covered here, while the Deterioration Signature provides the named pattern that makes the most characteristic transport-specific vulnerability explicit, recognizable, and actionable.

The receiving team's ability to continue the patient's care seamlessly after the transport crew departs depends entirely on the quality and completeness of the clinical information the transport crew provides, and for the conditions covered in this chapter, the specific information that matters most includes: the trajectory of the patient's primary condition during transport (improving, stable, or worsening, with specific details), any interventions performed during transport and their response, any new clinical findings identified by the transport crew that were not present at the sending facility, and any anticipated needs that the receiving team should prepare for based on the transport crew's clinical assessment. This information, communicated through the structured handoff format established in Chapter 2 and supplemented by the trajectory communication emphasis that is a recurring theme throughout this text, is the final clinical act of the transport and the one that determines whether the transport adds value to the patient's care continuum or merely moves the patient from one location to another without preserving the clinical narrative that only the transport crew was positioned to observe.

The transport clinician managing the conditions addressed in this chapter should develop a systematic pre-departure assessment that specifically identifies the highest-risk transport-environment interaction for each patient's specific disease process, the monitoring parameters that will detect that interaction earliest, and the intervention that will address it most effectively. This pre-departure risk analysis, adapted from the general pre-mission physiologic risk profile introduced in Chapter 1, should be specific enough to generate a concrete prediction: what is the single most likely way this specific patient's condition will interact with the specific transport environment of this specific mission? Answering that question before departure, rather than discovering the answer during transit, is the practical application of the anticipatory transport medicine framework that this entire text is designed to develop.

Clinical case presentations embedded throughout this chapter illustrate the principle that transport-specific deterioration patterns are predictable rather than random, recognizable rather than mysterious, and preventable rather than inevitable, provided the clinician applies the systematic assessment, continuous monitoring, and named-pattern recognition framework that the Deterioration Signature System codifies. Each case demonstrates the same three-part sequence: a patient with a specific disease process encounters a specific transport-environment stressor, produces a specific clinical change that could be attributed to either the disease or the environment, and is correctly managed because the transport clinician recognized the specific named Signature and applied the correct transport-specific intervention rather than the generic

disease-specific response that would have been appropriate at the bedside but is insufficient or incorrect in the transport context.

The evidence base for transport-specific management of the conditions in this chapter continues to evolve, with ongoing research into optimal monitoring strategies, transport-adapted treatment protocols, and outcome data that will refine the recommendations presented here. The transport clinician should maintain awareness of emerging evidence through continuing education, program-sponsored journal clubs, and the quality improvement processes described in Chapter 24, since the standard of care for transport medicine is not static and the recommendations in any textbook represent a snapshot of evidence at the time of writing rather than a permanent standard. The principles, however, are durable: anticipate rather than react, monitor trends rather than thresholds, communicate trajectories rather than snapshots, and recognize that the transport environment is a clinical variable that acts on every patient's physiology, not a neutral conduit between two points of care.

Finally, the transport clinician should recognize that the clinical expertise required to manage these conditions during transport represents a distinct competency that builds on but extends beyond the bedside critical care training that most transport clinicians bring to their role. A clinician who is expert in managing these conditions in the intensive care unit is not automatically expert in managing them during transport, because the environmental, equipment, monitoring, and resource constraints of transport introduce variables that bedside practice never encounters. Conversely, a transport clinician who has mastered the anticipatory, environment-aware management approach described in this text brings a perspective to patient care that the bedside clinician lacks: the ability to see the patient's physiology not as a fixed state being managed in a controlled environment, but as a dynamic process interacting continuously with an environment that is itself changing throughout the transport. This dual awareness--of the disease and of the environment acting on it--is the defining competency of transport critical care medicine, and it is what this text, from its first chapter through its last, is designed to develop.

### THE IN-TRANSIT DETERIORATION SIGNATURE SYSTEM — Delayed Toxidrome Declaration During Extended Transport Patterns

**Signature Introduced This Chapter:** Delayed Toxidrome Declaration During Extended Transport -- a transport-specific deterioration pattern unique to toxidrome recognition.

**Pattern Logic:** This Signature extends the foundational transport-physiology principles from Chapter 1 and the assessment framework from Chapter 2 into this disease domain.

**Cross-Reference Forward:** This Signature is indexed in the Anchor Section's Master Signature Atlas by organ system and clinical category.

## Summary and Key Concepts

The transport environment modifies the management of toxidrome recognition, antidote administration, decontamination considerations, and withdrawal syndrome management in specific, predictable ways beyond what bedside training addresses.

Trend-based monitoring at fixed intervals is the primary tool for detecting the disease-specific deterioration patterns described in this chapter's Signature.

Pharmacologic management follows the Chapter 4 framework with disease-specific modifications; infusion continuity requires particular attention.

Anticipatory contingency planning for the most likely complications is more effective than reactive management in the resource-constrained transport environment.

Advance communication with the receiving facility, including trajectory updates, is a direct clinical intervention improving care on arrival.

# CHAPTER 21: OBSTETRIC AND HIGH-RISK PREGNANCY EMERGENCIES IN TRANSIT

**Learning Objectives**

1. Apply the principles of hypertensive disorders of pregnancy, obstetric hemorrhage, preterm labor, and maternal cardiac arrest in the critical care transport environment.
2. Recognize transport-specific deterioration patterns and apply the Deterioration Signature System to anticipate and prevent them.
3. Coordinate advance communication with receiving facilities for optimal patient management on arrival.
4. Integrate the foundational transport-physiology, monitoring, and pharmacologic frameworks from earlier chapters into the management of these conditions.

**Chapter Outline**

This chapter addresses hypertensive disorders of pregnancy, obstetric hemorrhage, preterm labor, and maternal cardiac arrest as encountered in critical care transport, applying the altitude physiology from Chapter 1, the assessment and trending framework from Chapter 2, the airway and ventilator management from Chapter 3, the pharmacologic principles from Chapter 4, and the equipment and safety considerations from Chapter 5 to the specific populations and clinical scenarios covered here.

## Pathophysiology and Transport-Specific Considerations

## Hypertensive Disorders of Pregnancy and Eclampsia Management

### Preeclampsia Severity Stratification for Transport

Preeclampsia ranges from mild hypertension with proteinuria to severe disease with end-organ damage, HELLP syndrome (hemolysis, elevated liver enzymes, low platelets), and eclampsia (seizures), and the transport clinician must stratify severity at the sending bedside because the management intensity and monitoring requirements differ substantially across the spectrum. Severe preeclampsia with features--systolic pressure persistently above one hundred sixty, severe headache, visual disturbances, right upper quadrant pain, thrombocytopenia, or elevated transaminases--requires magnesium sulfate for seizure prophylaxis, antihypertensive therapy, and a high level of vigilance for progression to eclampsia during transport, while mild preeclampsia without severe features may require only blood pressure monitoring and delivery planning at the receiving facility.

### Magnesium Sulfate Infusion Management During Transport

Magnesium sulfate is the standard seizure prophylaxis and treatment agent for eclampsia, administered as a loading dose followed by a continuous infusion, and the transport clinician must maintain the infusion without interruption during transit while monitoring for magnesium toxicity. The earliest sign of magnesium toxicity is loss of deep tendon reflexes, followed by respiratory depression and ultimately cardiac arrest at markedly elevated levels, and the transport clinician should check deep tendon reflexes at each reassessment interval and should have calcium gluconate immediately available as the specific antidote for magnesium-induced cardiac or respiratory compromise.

### Blood Pressure Management: Targets and Agent Selection

Acute severe hypertension in preeclampsia (systolic above one hundred sixty or diastolic above one hundred ten) requires treatment within thirty to sixty minutes to prevent cerebrovascular complications, and the preferred transport agents are intravenous labetalol and intravenous hydralazine, both of which have extensive safety data in pregnancy. Nicardipine infusion provides a more titratable alternative and is increasingly used in the transport setting. The blood pressure target for severe preeclampsia is a reduction to the one hundred forty to one hundred fifty systolic range rather than normalization, since excessive blood pressure lowering can compromise uteroplacental blood flow and produce fetal distress.

## Obstetric Hemorrhage Recognition and Control

### Postpartum Hemorrhage: The Most Common Obstetric Emergency in Transport

Postpartum hemorrhage, defined as blood loss exceeding one thousand milliliters or any amount producing hemodynamic instability, is the most common obstetric emergency encountered during interfacility transport and follows a predictable hierarchy of causes: uterine atony (most common, responsible for approximately seventy to eighty percent of cases), retained placental tissue, genital tract lacerations, and coagulopathy. The transport clinician should confirm that the sending facility has administered uterotonic agents (oxytocin, methylergonovine, carboprost, or misoprostol) for suspected atony, should perform or confirm bimanual uterine massage, and should initiate blood product resuscitation for ongoing hemorrhage using the damage control resuscitation principles from Chapter 15.

### Placental Abruption and Placenta Previa Considerations

Antepartum hemorrhage from placental abruption or placenta previa presents a dual-patient emergency in which the transport clinician must manage maternal hemodynamic stabilization while monitoring fetal status, recognizing that maternal stabilization is always the first priority because a dead or hemodynamically unstable mother cannot sustain the fetus. Continuous fetal heart rate monitoring during transport, where equipment and training allow, provides real-time assessment of fetal tolerance of the maternal hemodynamic situation, though the transport clinician should be aware that fetal monitoring interpretation during the vibration and movement of transport is more difficult than at the bedside.

## Maternal Cardiac Arrest Modifications

### Left Lateral Uterine Displacement and Resuscitation Differences

Maternal cardiac arrest requires modified resuscitation that accounts for the pregnant anatomy: the gravid uterus compresses the inferior vena cava in the supine position, severely reducing venous return and rendering standard CPR less effective unless the uterus is displaced. Manual left lateral uterine displacement--pulling or pushing the uterus to the patient's left side--should be maintained continuously during chest compressions, and the crew member performing the displacement is a dedicated role that cannot be combined with compressions or airway management. If return of spontaneous circulation is not achieved within four minutes and the gestational age is at or above twenty weeks, perimortem cesarean delivery should be considered to relieve aortocaval compression and improve maternal resuscitation success, though this procedure is typically beyond the scope of transport crew capability and the receiving facility should be alerted for immediate surgical readiness on arrival.

| Obstetric Emergency | Primary Transport Action | Key Monitoring |
|---|---|---|
| Severe preeclampsia/eclampsia | Magnesium sulfate infusion; labetalol for BP >160 systolic | DTRs, respiratory rate, BP q5-10min |
| Postpartum hemorrhage | Uterotonic agents; bimanual massage; blood products | Fundal tone; hemodynamic trend; pad count |
| Placental abruption | Maternal hemodynamic stabilization; prepare for emergent delivery | Fetal heart tones; maternal vitals; coagulation status |
| Maternal cardiac arrest | Modified ACLS with left uterine displacement | Continuous CPR quality; perimortem cesarean readiness |

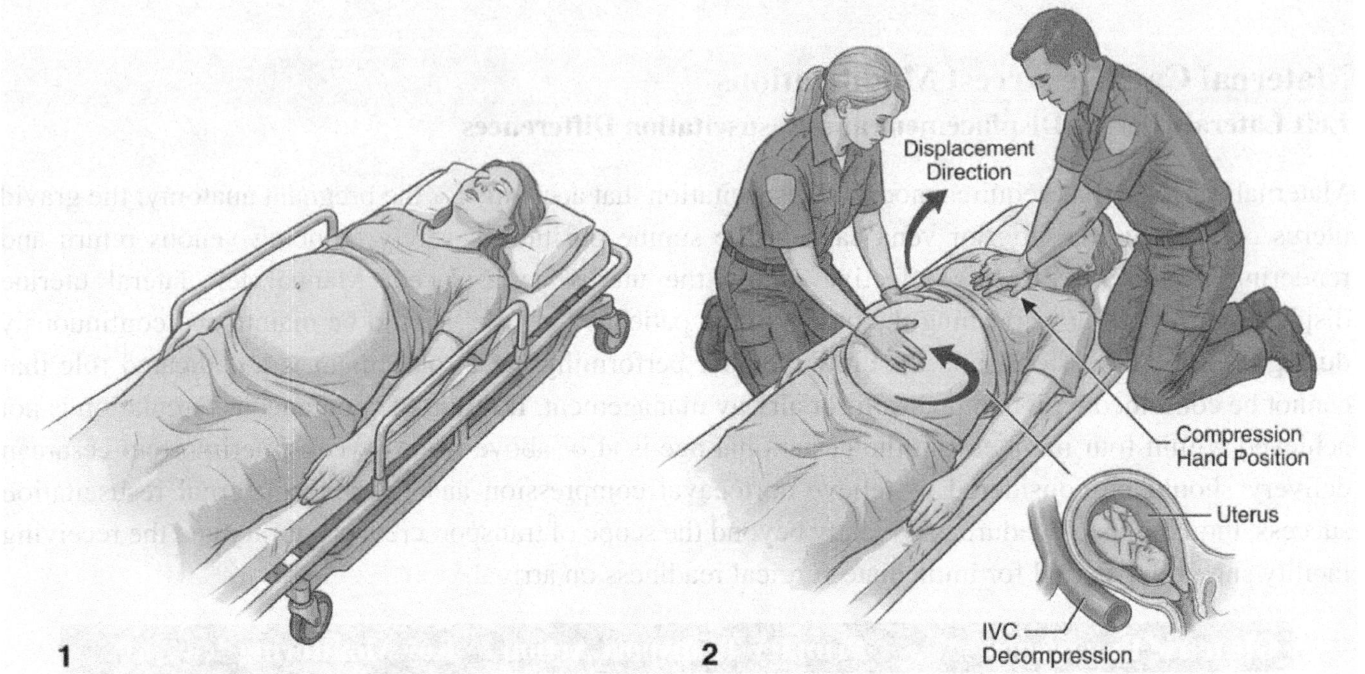


**Figure 21.1: Left Lateral Uterine Displacement Technique During Maternal Resuscitation.**

### Disease and Population-Specific Transport Vulnerabilities

The populations and conditions addressed in this chapter carry specific physiologic vulnerabilities to the transport environment that distinguish their management from adult medical transport. Hypertensive disorders of pregnancy in particular interacts with altitude, vibration, temperature, and the resource constraints of transport in ways that require anticipatory planning and disease-specific modifications to the general transport management framework.

### Clinical Presentation and Assessment Priorities

Assessment follows the problem-based physiologic framework from Chapter 2, with population-specific modifications: age-appropriate vital sign targets, weight-based medication dosing, and disease-specific monitoring parameters that may differ from the adult standards assumed elsewhere in this text. The transport clinician should establish population-appropriate baselines at departure and track trends against those baselines.

## Management and Treatment During Transport

### Pharmacologic and Procedural Management

The management of hypertensive disorders of pregnancy, obstetric hemorrhage, preterm labor, and maternal cardiac arrest during transport requires disease- and population-specific modifications to the pharmacologic and procedural frameworks from earlier chapters. Weight-based dosing, age-appropriate equipment sizing, and population-specific contraindications must be confirmed before every medication administration and every procedure, since errors in these domains carry disproportionate consequences in vulnerable populations.

**Monitoring and Communication**

Continuous monitoring follows the modality-matching principles from Chapter 2, adapted to the specific population. Advance communication with the receiving facility should include population-specific information that affects receiving-team preparation, such as gestational age, neonatal weight, or specific sub-specialty consultation needs that the receiving team should mobilize before the patient's arrival.

| Management Domain | Transport-Specific Consideration | Key Action |
|---|---|---|
| Assessment | Population-specific baselines and targets | Establish age/weight-appropriate vital sign targets at departure |
| Pharmacology | Weight-based dosing; population-specific contraindications | Verify dosing against actual weight; confirm contraindications |
| Airway | Age-appropriate equipment; size-specific techniques | Pre-size all equipment before departure; confirm backup plan |
| Monitoring | Population-appropriate alarm thresholds | Set alarms to population norms, not adult defaults |
| Communication | Population-specific receiving-team needs | Include gestational age, weight, or sub-specialty needs in handoff |

**Figure 21.2: Assessment and Management Framework for Obstetric and High-Risk Pregnancy Emergencies in Transit**

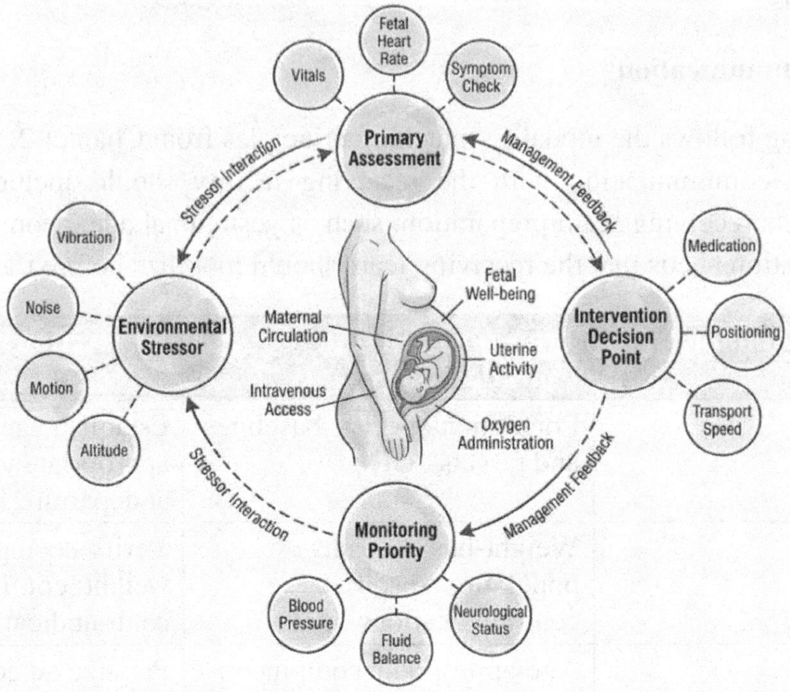


**THE IN-TRANSIT DETERIORATION SIGNATURE SYSTEM — Aortocaval Compression-Triggered Maternal Deterioration**

**The Signature:** A transport-specific deterioration pattern in which aortocaval compression triggered maternal deterioration produces clinical consequences that are predictable but frequently unrecognized until the pattern has already advanced beyond the point of easy correction.

**Movement Trigger:** The transport environment introduces the specific stressor or removes the specific safeguard that activates this pattern, which would not occur in the same form in a stationary clinical setting.

**Early Tell:** A subtle indicator detectable through the trend-based monitoring framework, typically appearing before the full clinical syndrome declares itself.

**Trap Logic:** This pattern is commonly misattributed to expected variation or disease progression rather than recognized as a transport-specific event requiring a transport-specific response.

**Signature Anchor:** Recognition of the temporal link between the transport-specific trigger and the clinical change is the key to correct attribution and appropriate intervention.

## Special Considerations and Complications

### Anticipated Complications and Contingency Planning

Each condition in this chapter carries predictable complications during the transport window. The transport clinician should identify the most likely complication and prepare a contingency response before departure. For hypertensive disorders of pregnancy, the most consequential transport-window complication is typically the one named by the Deterioration Signature above, and advance preparation for it--equipment staged, medications drawn, team roles assigned--converts a reactive emergency into an anticipated event.

The management of hypertensive disorders of pregnancy, obstetric hemorrhage, preterm labor, and maternal cardiac arrest in the transport environment illustrates a principle that runs throughout this text: the disease determines the baseline risk, but the transport environment determines whether that risk is safely navigated or converted into a preventable deterioration. The Signature introduced in this chapter names the specific way the transport environment converts baseline risk into clinical consequence for these conditions, and the clinician who recognizes the pattern before it fully declares itself is practicing the anticipatory transport medicine this text is designed to teach.

### Preterm Labor and Emergency Delivery Considerations

Preterm labor during transport presents the dual challenge of managing tocolytic therapy to inhibit contractions while preparing for the possibility that delivery will occur in the vehicle or aircraft despite tocolysis. Magnesium sulfate serves a dual role in the peripartum transport patient: as a tocolytic at higher doses and as a fetal neuroprotective agent at standard doses, and the transport clinician should confirm the specific indication and dose range with the sending obstetric team. If delivery appears imminent during transport--regular contractions with cervical change despite tocolysis, the patient reporting an urge to push, or visible fetal presenting part--the transport clinician must shift from a prevention to a delivery management posture: preparing delivery supplies, positioning the patient, and activating communication with the receiving facility for neonatal team readiness on arrival.

### Fetal Monitoring During Transport

Continuous electronic fetal monitoring during transport, where equipment and training allow, provides real-time assessment of fetal heart rate patterns that indicate fetal tolerance or distress in the face of the maternal condition. Non-reassuring fetal heart rate patterns--persistent bradycardia, absent variability, late decelerations with contractions--should prompt the transport clinician to optimize maternal oxygenation and hemodynamics, apply left lateral uterine displacement, and communicate the fetal status to the receiving team so that the obstetric and neonatal teams can be prepared for possible emergent delivery on arrival. However, the transport clinician should recognize that fetal monitoring interpretation during transport is compromised by vibration artifact, which can produce tracings that appear more abnormal than they actually are, and should avoid precipitous clinical decisions based on a single abnormal-appearing tracing without confirming the finding through a period of observation or a manual assessment.

### Amniotic Fluid Embolism: A Catastrophic Obstetric Emergency

Amniotic fluid embolism is a rare, catastrophic obstetric emergency that presents with sudden cardiovascular collapse, hypoxemia, disseminated intravascular coagulation, and seizures, typically occurring during labor, delivery, or the immediate postpartum period. There is no specific treatment;

management is entirely supportive, focusing on aggressive cardiopulmonary resuscitation, blood product replacement for the consumptive coagulopathy, and mechanical ventilation for the acute respiratory failure. The transport clinician who encounters a peripartum patient with sudden cardiovascular collapse and coagulopathy should consider amniotic fluid embolism in the differential diagnosis, initiate aggressive supportive care, and communicate the suspected diagnosis to the receiving team so that massive transfusion resources, critical care admission, and possible perimortem cesarean delivery preparation are mobilized before arrival.

**Additional Clinical Considerations for Transport Management**

The management of patients in Chapter 21 requires attention to several additional transport-specific clinical factors that extend the principles established in the main body of the chapter. The transport clinician should be aware that the disease processes covered here interact with the transport environment in ways that are specific to the combination of the underlying pathophysiology and the particular environmental stressor encountered during a given mission, and that a management approach that is adequate for a short ground transport may be insufficient for a longer air transport at altitude, or vice versa. The serial reassessment protocol established in Chapter 2 provides the framework for detecting these interactions as they develop, and the Deterioration Signature introduced in this chapter names the most characteristic pattern by which they declare themselves.

Each patient transport is a unique combination of a specific patient's physiology, a specific set of ongoing therapies, a specific transport platform with its own environmental characteristics, and a specific mission profile with its own altitude, duration, and route constraints. The anticipatory approach to transport medicine that this text teaches is not a set of memorized responses to predetermined scenarios but a cognitive framework for analyzing the specific combination of variables present in any given transport and identifying, before departure, the most likely points of vulnerability where the transport environment will test the patient's physiologic reserve. This chapter's clinical content provides the disease-specific knowledge needed to apply that framework to the conditions covered here, while the Deterioration Signature provides the named pattern that makes the most characteristic transport-specific vulnerability explicit, recognizable, and actionable.

The receiving team's ability to continue the patient's care seamlessly after the transport crew departs depends entirely on the quality and completeness of the clinical information the transport crew provides, and for the conditions covered in this chapter, the specific information that matters most includes: the trajectory of the patient's primary condition during transport (improving, stable, or worsening, with specific details), any interventions performed during transport and their response, any new clinical findings identified by the transport crew that were not present at the sending facility, and any anticipated needs that the receiving team should prepare for based on the transport crew's clinical assessment. This information, communicated through the structured handoff format established in Chapter 2 and supplemented by the trajectory communication emphasis that is a recurring theme throughout this text, is the final clinical act of the transport and the one that determines whether the transport adds value to the patient's care continuum or merely moves the patient from one location to another without preserving the clinical narrative that only the transport crew was positioned to observe.

The transport clinician managing the conditions addressed in this chapter should develop a systematic pre-departure assessment that specifically identifies the highest-risk transport-environment interaction for each patient's specific disease process, the monitoring parameters that will detect that interaction earliest, and the intervention that will address it most effectively. This pre-departure risk analysis, adapted from the general pre-mission physiologic risk profile introduced in Chapter 1, should be specific enough to generate a concrete prediction: what is the single most likely way this specific patient's condition will interact with the specific transport environment of this specific mission? Answering that question before departure, rather than discovering the answer during transit, is the practical application of the anticipatory transport medicine framework that this entire text is designed to develop.

Clinical case presentations embedded throughout this chapter illustrate the principle that transport-specific deterioration patterns are predictable rather than random, recognizable rather than mysterious, and preventable rather than inevitable, provided the clinician applies the systematic assessment, continuous monitoring, and named-pattern recognition framework that the Deterioration Signature System codifies. Each case demonstrates the same three-part sequence: a patient with a specific disease process encounters a specific transport-environment stressor, produces a specific clinical change that could be attributed to either the disease or the environment, and is correctly managed because the transport clinician recognized the specific named Signature and applied the correct transport-specific intervention rather than the generic disease-specific response that would have been appropriate at the bedside but is insufficient or incorrect in the transport context.

The evidence base for transport-specific management of the conditions in this chapter continues to evolve, with ongoing research into optimal monitoring strategies, transport-adapted treatment protocols, and outcome data that will refine the recommendations presented here. The transport clinician should maintain awareness of emerging evidence through continuing education, program-sponsored journal clubs, and the quality improvement processes described in Chapter 24, since the standard of care for transport medicine is not static and the recommendations in any textbook represent a snapshot of evidence at the time of writing rather than a permanent standard. The principles, however, are durable: anticipate rather than react, monitor trends rather than thresholds, communicate trajectories rather than snapshots, and recognize that the transport environment is a clinical variable that acts on every patient's physiology, not a neutral conduit between two points of care.

Finally, the transport clinician should recognize that the clinical expertise required to manage these conditions during transport represents a distinct competency that builds on but extends beyond the bedside critical care training that most transport clinicians bring to their role. A clinician who is expert in managing these conditions in the intensive care unit is not automatically expert in managing them during transport, because the environmental, equipment, monitoring, and resource constraints of transport introduce variables that bedside practice never encounters. Conversely, a transport clinician who has mastered the anticipatory, environment-aware management approach described in this text brings a perspective to patient care that the bedside clinician lacks: the ability to see the patient's physiology not as a fixed state being managed in a controlled environment, but as a dynamic process interacting continuously with an environment that is itself changing throughout the transport. This dual awareness--of the disease and of the environment acting on it--is the defining competency of transport critical care medicine, and it is what this text, from its first chapter through its last, is designed to develop.

**THE IN-TRANSIT DETERIORATION SIGNATURE SYSTEM — Aortocaval Compression-Triggered Maternal Deterioration Patterns**

**Signature Introduced This Chapter:** Aortocaval Compression-Triggered Maternal Deterioration.

**Pattern Logic:** This Signature applies the foundational transport-physiology and assessment principles to the specific population and disease domain covered by this chapter.

**Cross-Reference Forward:** This Signature is indexed in the Anchor Section Master Signature Atlas by clinical category and population.

## Summary and Key Concepts

The management of hypertensive disorders of pregnancy, obstetric hemorrhage, preterm labor, and maternal cardiac arrest during transport requires population- and disease-specific modifications to the general transport management frameworks.

Trend-based monitoring with population-appropriate baselines and alarm thresholds is essential for detecting deterioration patterns specific to these conditions.

Weight-based dosing, age-appropriate equipment, and population-specific contraindications must be verified before every medication and procedure.

Advance communication with the receiving facility should include population-specific information that allows the receiving team to prepare appropriately.

The Deterioration Signature introduced in this chapter names the most characteristic transport-specific vulnerability for hypertensive disorders of pregnancy and provides the anticipatory framework for preventing it.

# CHAPTER 22: NEONATAL CRITICAL CARE IN TRANSIT

**Learning Objectives**

1. Apply the principles of neonatal resuscitation, thermoregulation, congenital cardiac lesion management, and respiratory distress syndrome in the critical care transport environment.
2. Recognize transport-specific deterioration patterns and apply the Deterioration Signature System to anticipate and prevent them.
3. Coordinate advance communication with receiving facilities for optimal patient management on arrival.
4. Integrate the foundational transport-physiology, monitoring, and pharmacologic frameworks from earlier chapters into the management of these conditions.

**Chapter Outline**

This chapter addresses neonatal resuscitation, thermoregulation, congenital cardiac lesion management, and respiratory distress syndrome as encountered in critical care transport, applying the altitude physiology from Chapter 1, the assessment and trending framework from Chapter 2, the airway and ventilator management from Chapter 3, the pharmacologic principles from Chapter 4, and the equipment and safety considerations from Chapter 5 to the specific populations and clinical scenarios covered here.

## Pathophysiology and Transport-Specific Considerations

## Neonatal Resuscitation and Thermoregulation in Transit

### Temperature as the Primary Neonatal Transport Priority

Temperature management is the single most consequential and most frequently under-addressed aspect of neonatal critical care transport. Neonates, particularly preterm infants, lose heat through convection, radiation, evaporation, and conduction at rates dramatically higher than adults due to their high surface-area-to-body-mass ratio, thin skin with minimal subcutaneous fat, and immature thermoregulatory capacity. Hypothermia in a neonate produces a cascade of metabolic consequences--increased oxygen consumption, metabolic acidosis, hypoglycemia, and surfactant dysfunction--each of which worsens the underlying condition for which the infant is being transported. The transport isolette must be pre-warmed, the infant must be dried and wrapped immediately, and temperature must be continuously monitored with a skin probe throughout the transport, with a target axillary or skin temperature of 36.5 to 37.5 degrees Celsius.

### Neonatal Airway Management Differences

Neonatal airway anatomy differs fundamentally from the adult airway: the proportionally large occiput flexes the neck into an anterior position, the tongue is relatively larger, the epiglottis is omega-shaped and floppy, and the subglottic space at the cricoid ring is the narrowest point (versus the glottis in adults), making uncuffed endotracheal tubes standard for neonates and the appropriate tube size critically dependent on the infant's weight or gestational age. The transport clinician should confirm endotracheal tube size, depth at the lip, and fixation security before departure, and should have at least one size smaller and one size larger tube immediately available, since a tube that is appropriate at departure may become obstructed by secretions or dislodged during the movement of transport.

### Neonatal Vascular Access and Fluid Management

Vascular access in neonates is challenging in the best of circumstances and is substantially more difficult in a moving transport vehicle, which argues strongly for establishing secure access before departure rather than attempting it en route. Umbilical venous and arterial catheterization, where the infant still has a patent umbilicus, provides reliable central access that is unique to the neonatal population and should be considered before departure for any infant requiring vasoactive support, parenteral nutrition, or frequent laboratory monitoring. Peripheral intravenous access, while easier to obtain, is fragile in neonates and prone to infiltration, and should be supplemented by a backup access plan (intraosseous access in the proximal tibia is the neonatal rescue access site) before departure.

## Congenital Cardiac Lesion Considerations

### Ductal-Dependent Lesions and Prostaglandin Infusion Management

Neonates with ductal-dependent congenital heart lesions require continuous prostaglandin E1 infusion to maintain patency of the ductus arteriosus, and interruption of this infusion during transport can produce rapid, fatal cardiovascular collapse as the ductus closes and the infant loses the only pathway maintaining either systemic or pulmonary blood flow. The prostaglandin infusion is the single most critical medication to protect during neonatal cardiac transport, and the infusion management principles from Chapter 4--concentration verification, line security, pump battery reserve, and replacement syringe pre-preparation--apply with absolute, non-negotiable force. The transport clinician should also be aware that prostaglandin produces apnea as a predictable side effect, particularly in preterm infants, and should be prepared to provide ventilatory support throughout the transport.

### Balancing Systemic and Pulmonary Blood Flow

In neonates with mixing lesions or parallel circulations, the balance between systemic and pulmonary blood flow is determined by the relative resistance of the two circuits, and the transport clinician's oxygenation and ventilation management directly affects this balance. Excessive supplemental oxygen can reduce pulmonary vascular resistance and produce pulmonary overcirculation at the expense of systemic blood flow, a scenario that presents as improving oxygen saturation with worsening systemic perfusion--a pattern that is counterintuitive to the transport clinician accustomed to treating hypoxemia with more oxygen. The target oxygen saturation for many ductal-dependent and mixing lesions is deliberately lower than for other patient populations, typically seventy-five to eighty-five percent, and the transport clinician must confirm the cardiologist-specified saturation target before departure rather than defaulting to the ninety-four percent or higher target used for most other transport patients.

| Neonatal Transport Priority | Key Action | Risk if Omitted |
|---|---|---|
| Temperature maintenance | Pre-warm isolette; continuous skin temp monitoring | Hypothermia cascade: acidosis, hypoglycemia, surfactant dysfunction |
| Prostaglandin continuity (if ductal-dependent) | Verify infusion rate, concentration, line security, pump battery | Ductal closure with fatal cardiovascular collapse |
| Airway security | Confirm ETT size, depth, fixation; backup tubes available | Tube dislodgement in an infant whose reintubation is extremely difficult in transit |
| Glucose monitoring | Point-of-care glucose q30-60min | Neonatal hypoglycemia causing seizures and brain injury |
| Target SpO2 (cardiac lesions) | Confirm cardiologist-specified target; may be 75-85% | Excessive O2 producing pulmonary overcirculation and systemic hypoperfusion |

Figure 22.1: Neonatal Transport Isolette Configuration and Monitoring

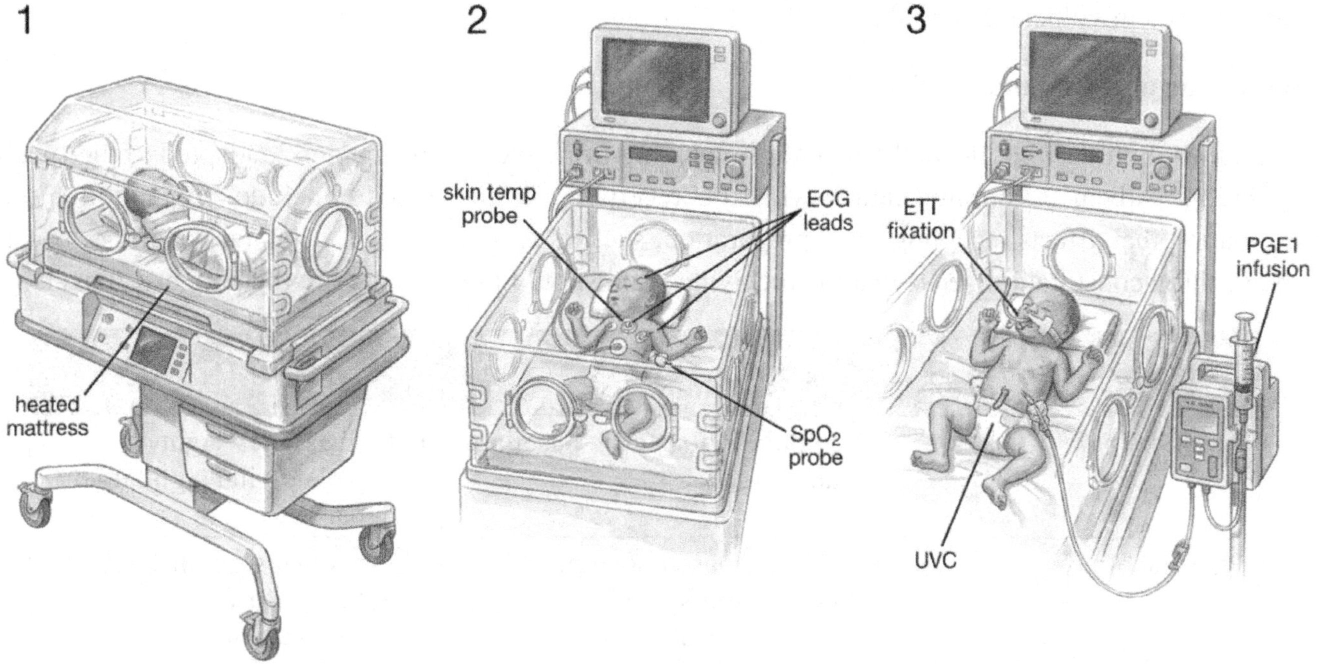

### Disease and Population-Specific Transport Vulnerabilities

The populations and conditions addressed in this chapter carry specific physiologic vulnerabilities to the transport environment that distinguish their management from adult medical transport. Neonatal resuscitation in particular interacts with altitude, vibration, temperature, and the resource constraints of transport in ways that require anticipatory planning and disease-specific modifications to the general transport management framework.

### Clinical Presentation and Assessment Priorities

Assessment follows the problem-based physiologic framework from Chapter 2, with population-specific modifications: age-appropriate vital sign targets, weight-based medication dosing, and disease-specific monitoring parameters that may differ from the adult standards assumed elsewhere in this text. The transport clinician should establish population-appropriate baselines at departure and track trends against those baselines.

## Management and Treatment During Transport

### Pharmacologic and Procedural Management

The management of neonatal resuscitation, thermoregulation, congenital cardiac lesion management, and respiratory distress syndrome during transport requires disease- and population-specific modifications to the pharmacologic and procedural frameworks from earlier chapters. Weight-based dosing, age-appropriate equipment sizing, and population-specific contraindications must be confirmed before every medication administration and every procedure, since errors in these domains carry disproportionate consequences in vulnerable populations.

### Monitoring and Communication

Continuous monitoring follows the modality-matching principles from Chapter 2, adapted to the specific population. Advance communication with the receiving facility should include population-specific information that affects receiving-team preparation, such as gestational age, neonatal weight, or specific sub-specialty consultation needs that the receiving team should mobilize before the patient's arrival.

| Management Domain | Transport-Specific Consideration | Key Action |
|---|---|---|
| Assessment | Population-specific baselines and targets | Establish age/weight-appropriate vital sign targets at departure |
| Pharmacology | Weight-based dosing; population-specific contraindications | Verify dosing against actual weight; confirm contraindications |

| | | |
|---|---|---|
| Airway | Age-appropriate equipment; size-specific techniques | Pre-size all equipment before departure; confirm backup plan |
| Monitoring | Population-appropriate alarm thresholds | Set alarms to population norms, not adult defaults |
| Communication | Population-specific receiving-team needs | Include gestational age, weight, or sub-specialty needs in handoff |

**Figure 22.2: Assessment and Management Framework for Neonatal Critical Care in Transit**

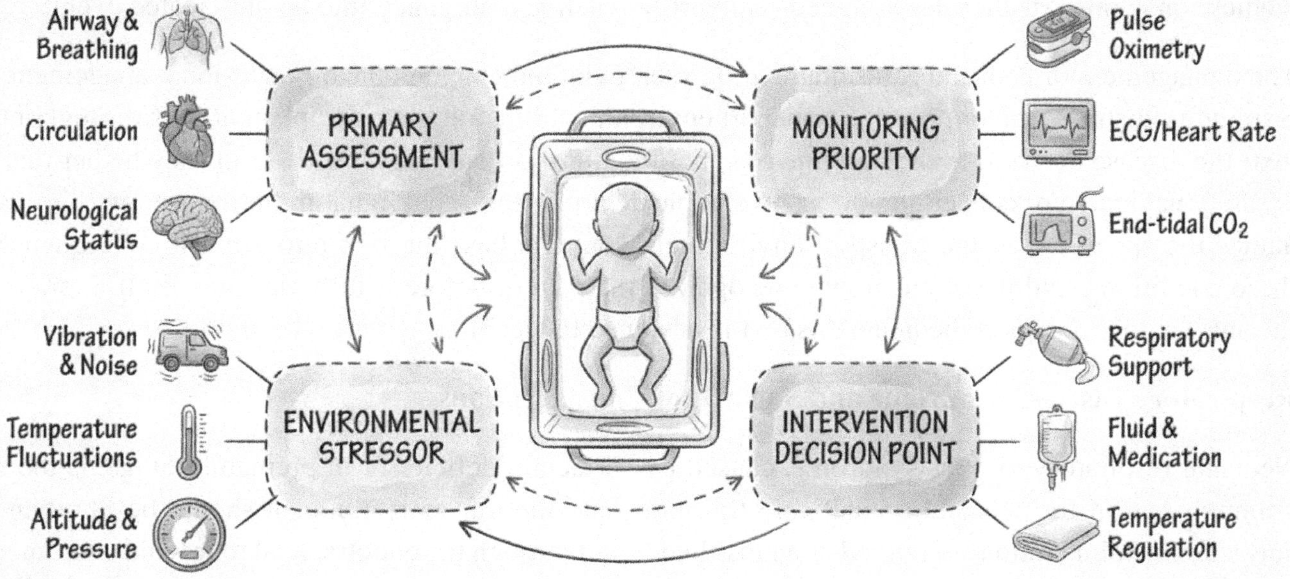


**THE IN-TRANSIT DETERIORATION SIGNATURE SYSTEM — Thermoregulatory Failure Cascade in the Transported Neonate**

**The Signature:** A transport-specific deterioration pattern in which thermoregulatory failure cascade in the transported neonate produces clinical consequences that are predictable but frequently unrecognized until the pattern has already advanced beyond the point of easy correction.

**Movement Trigger:** The transport environment introduces the specific stressor or removes the specific safeguard that activates this pattern, which would not occur in the same form in a stationary clinical setting.

**Early Tell:** A subtle indicator detectable through the trend-based monitoring framework, typically appearing before the full clinical syndrome declares itself.

**Trap Logic:** This pattern is commonly misattributed to expected variation or disease progression rather than recognized as a transport-specific event requiring a transport-specific response.

**Signature Anchor:** Recognition of the temporal link between the transport-specific trigger and the clinical change is the key to correct attribution and appropriate intervention.

## Special Considerations and Complications

### Anticipated Complications and Contingency Planning

Each condition in this chapter carries predictable complications during the transport window. The transport clinician should identify the most likely complication and prepare a contingency response before departure. For neonatal resuscitation, the most consequential transport-window complication is typically the one named by the Deterioration Signature above, and advance preparation for it--equipment staged, medications drawn, team roles assigned--converts a reactive emergency into an anticipated event.

The management of neonatal resuscitation, thermoregulation, congenital cardiac lesion management, and respiratory distress syndrome in the transport environment illustrates a principle that runs throughout this text: the disease determines the baseline risk, but the transport environment determines whether that risk is safely navigated or converted into a preventable deterioration. The Signature introduced in this chapter names the specific way the transport environment converts baseline risk into clinical consequence for these conditions, and the clinician who recognizes the pattern before it fully declares itself is practicing the anticipatory transport medicine this text is designed to teach.

### Respiratory Distress Syndrome and Surfactant Considerations

Neonatal respiratory distress syndrome, caused by surfactant deficiency in premature lungs, is the most common reason for neonatal critical care transport, and the transport clinician should be familiar with surfactant administration--delivered as an instilled liquid through the endotracheal tube--and its immediate effects on pulmonary compliance and oxygenation. After surfactant administration, the infant's lung compliance may improve rapidly, and the transport clinician must be prepared to reduce ventilator pressures promptly to avoid overventilation and air leak syndrome (pneumothorax, pulmonary interstitial emphysema) that can result from ventilating newly compliant lungs at pressures that were appropriate for the pre-surfactant stiff lung but are excessive afterward.

### Persistent Pulmonary Hypertension of the Newborn

Persistent pulmonary hypertension of the newborn results from failure of the normal postnatal decline in pulmonary vascular resistance, producing right-to-left shunting through the patent foramen ovale and ductus arteriosus with resulting severe hypoxemia that is refractory to supplemental oxygen alone. The management during transport includes high-concentration oxygen, gentle ventilation (avoiding overdistention that increases pulmonary vascular resistance), and inhaled nitric oxide where available, and the transport clinician should be aware that this condition responds to specific interventions that reduce pulmonary vascular resistance rather than to escalating FiO2 alone.

## Neonatal Seizures: Recognition and Transport-Specific Management

Neonatal seizures may be subtle and easily overlooked during transport: repetitive eye deviations, lip smacking, cycling movements of the extremities, and apneic episodes may all represent seizure activity that the transport clinician might attribute to normal neonatal behavior or to the stimulation of the transport environment. Any repetitive, stereotyped movement pattern in a neonate should be considered a possible seizure, and the management includes phenobarbital as the first-line anticonvulsant (given as a weight-based loading dose), glucose correction if hypoglycemia is present, and communication with the receiving neonatal team for possible continuous EEG monitoring on arrival.

## Necrotizing Enterocolitis: Transport of the Surgical Neonate

Necrotizing enterocolitis, the most common surgical emergency in the neonatal intensive care unit, presents with abdominal distention, feeding intolerance, bloody stools, and in advanced cases, pneumatosis intestinalis and portal venous gas on abdominal radiography. Neonates with suspected necrotizing enterocolitis being transported for surgical evaluation require gastric decompression with a nasogastric or orogastric tube on continuous suction, broad-spectrum antimicrobial therapy, aggressive volume resuscitation (since third-spacing from peritoneal inflammation can produce severe hypovolemia), and strict nothing-by-mouth status throughout transport. The transport clinician should monitor the abdomen for increasing distention, which may indicate progression, and should communicate any interval change to the receiving surgical team.

## Additional Clinical Considerations for Transport Management

The management of patients in Chapter 22 requires attention to several additional transport-specific clinical factors that extend the principles established in the main body of the chapter. The transport clinician should be aware that the disease processes covered here interact with the transport environment in ways that are specific to the combination of the underlying pathophysiology and the particular environmental stressor encountered during a given mission, and that a management approach that is adequate for a short ground transport may be insufficient for a longer air transport at altitude, or vice versa. The serial reassessment protocol established in Chapter 2 provides the framework for detecting these interactions as they develop, and the Deterioration Signature introduced in this chapter names the most characteristic pattern by which they declare themselves.

Each patient transport is a unique combination of a specific patient's physiology, a specific set of ongoing therapies, a specific transport platform with its own environmental characteristics, and a specific mission profile with its own altitude, duration, and route constraints. The anticipatory approach to transport medicine that this text teaches is not a set of memorized responses to predetermined scenarios but a cognitive framework for analyzing the specific combination of variables present in any given transport and identifying, before departure, the most likely points of vulnerability where the transport environment will test the patient's physiologic reserve. This chapter's clinical content provides the disease-specific knowledge needed to apply that framework to the conditions covered here, while the Deterioration

Signature provides the named pattern that makes the most characteristic transport-specific vulnerability explicit, recognizable, and actionable.

The receiving team's ability to continue the patient's care seamlessly after the transport crew departs depends entirely on the quality and completeness of the clinical information the transport crew provides, and for the conditions covered in this chapter, the specific information that matters most includes: the trajectory of the patient's primary condition during transport (improving, stable, or worsening, with specific details), any interventions performed during transport and their response, any new clinical findings identified by the transport crew that were not present at the sending facility, and any anticipated needs that the receiving team should prepare for based on the transport crew's clinical assessment. This information, communicated through the structured handoff format established in Chapter 2 and supplemented by the trajectory communication emphasis that is a recurring theme throughout this text, is the final clinical act of the transport and the one that determines whether the transport adds value to the patient's care continuum or merely moves the patient from one location to another without preserving the clinical narrative that only the transport crew was positioned to observe.

The transport clinician managing the conditions addressed in this chapter should develop a systematic pre-departure assessment that specifically identifies the highest-risk transport-environment interaction for each patient's specific disease process, the monitoring parameters that will detect that interaction earliest, and the intervention that will address it most effectively. This pre-departure risk analysis, adapted from the general pre-mission physiologic risk profile introduced in Chapter 1, should be specific enough to generate a concrete prediction: what is the single most likely way this specific patient's condition will interact with the specific transport environment of this specific mission? Answering that question before departure, rather than discovering the answer during transit, is the practical application of the anticipatory transport medicine framework that this entire text is designed to develop.

Clinical case presentations embedded throughout this chapter illustrate the principle that transport-specific deterioration patterns are predictable rather than random, recognizable rather than mysterious, and preventable rather than inevitable, provided the clinician applies the systematic assessment, continuous monitoring, and named-pattern recognition framework that the Deterioration Signature System codifies. Each case demonstrates the same three-part sequence: a patient with a specific disease process encounters a specific transport-environment stressor, produces a specific clinical change that could be attributed to either the disease or the environment, and is correctly managed because the transport clinician recognized the specific named Signature and applied the correct transport-specific intervention rather than the generic disease-specific response that would have been appropriate at the bedside but is insufficient or incorrect in the transport context.

The evidence base for transport-specific management of the conditions in this chapter continues to evolve, with ongoing research into optimal monitoring strategies, transport-adapted treatment protocols, and outcome data that will refine the recommendations presented here. The transport clinician should maintain awareness of emerging evidence through continuing education, program-sponsored journal clubs, and the quality improvement processes described in Chapter 24, since the standard of care for transport medicine is not static and the recommendations in any textbook represent a snapshot of evidence at the time of writing rather than a permanent standard. The principles, however, are durable: anticipate rather than react, monitor trends rather than thresholds, communicate trajectories rather than snapshots, and recognize that the transport environment is a clinical variable that acts on every patient's physiology, not a neutral conduit between two points of care.

Finally, the transport clinician should recognize that the clinical expertise required to manage these conditions during transport represents a distinct competency that builds on but extends beyond the bedside critical care training that most transport clinicians bring to their role. A clinician who is expert in managing these conditions in the intensive care unit is not automatically expert in managing them during transport, because the environmental, equipment, monitoring, and resource constraints of transport introduce variables that bedside practice never encounters. Conversely, a transport clinician who has mastered the anticipatory, environment-aware management approach described in this text brings a perspective to patient care that the bedside clinician lacks: the ability to see the patient's physiology not as a fixed state being managed in a controlled environment, but as a dynamic process interacting continuously with an environment that is itself changing throughout the transport. This dual awareness--of the disease and of the environment acting on it--is the defining competency of transport critical care medicine, and it is what this text, from its first chapter through its last, is designed to develop.

**THE IN-TRANSIT DETERIORATION SIGNATURE SYSTEM — Thermoregulatory Failure Cascade in the Transported Neonate Patterns**

**Signature Introduced This Chapter:** Thermoregulatory Failure Cascade in the Transported Neonate.

**Pattern Logic:** This Signature applies the foundational transport-physiology and assessment principles to the specific population and disease domain covered by this chapter.

**Cross-Reference Forward:** This Signature is indexed in the Anchor Section Master Signature Atlas by clinical category and population.

## Summary and Key Concepts

The management of neonatal resuscitation, thermoregulation, congenital cardiac lesion management, and respiratory distress syndrome during transport requires population- and disease-specific modifications to the general transport management frameworks.

Trend-based monitoring with population-appropriate baselines and alarm thresholds is essential for detecting deterioration patterns specific to these conditions.

Weight-based dosing, age-appropriate equipment, and population-specific contraindications must be verified before every medication and procedure.

Advance communication with the receiving facility should include population-specific information that allows the receiving team to prepare appropriately.

The Deterioration Signature introduced in this chapter names the most characteristic transport-specific vulnerability for neonatal resuscitation and provides the anticipatory framework for preventing it.

# CHAPTER 23: PEDIATRIC CRITICAL CARE IN TRANSIT

**Learning Objectives**

1. Apply the principles of pediatric airway management, shock recognition, weight-based dosing, and age-specific assessment in the critical care transport environment.
2. Recognize transport-specific deterioration patterns and apply the Deterioration Signature System to anticipate and prevent them.
3. Coordinate advance communication with receiving facilities for optimal patient management on arrival.
4. Integrate the foundational transport-physiology, monitoring, and pharmacologic frameworks from earlier chapters into the management of these conditions.

**Chapter Outline**

This chapter addresses pediatric airway management, shock recognition, weight-based dosing, and age-specific assessment as encountered in critical care transport, applying the altitude physiology from Chapter 1, the assessment and trending framework from Chapter 2, the airway and ventilator management from Chapter 3, the pharmacologic principles from Chapter 4, and the equipment and safety considerations from Chapter 5 to the specific populations and clinical scenarios covered here.

## Pathophysiology and Transport-Specific Considerations

## Pediatric Airway and Ventilator Management Differences

### Age-Specific Airway Anatomy and Equipment Sizing

Pediatric airway management during transport requires age- and weight-specific equipment selection that must be performed before departure rather than estimated during an airway emergency. The pediatric airway differs from the adult airway in proportionally larger tongue and occiput, higher and more anterior larynx, shorter trachea with a proportionally smaller margin for tube depth error, and, in younger children, a funnel-shaped subglottic space that is the narrowest point. Equipment sizing follows established formulas based on age or, more reliably, length-based estimation systems such as the Broselow tape, and the transport crew should have the correctly sized endotracheal tube, laryngoscope blade, suction catheter, and rescue airway device pre-selected and immediately accessible before departure, since searching for the correct size during an airway emergency in a moving vehicle wastes the seconds that determine outcome.

### Weight-Based Medication Dosing and Error Prevention

Every medication dose in pediatric transport is weight-based, and the most dangerous error in pediatric transport pharmacology is a weight-estimation error that produces a tenfold dosing error--administering an adult dose to a child, or calculating a dose based on an estimated weight that is significantly different from the actual weight. The transport clinician should weigh the child directly whenever a scale is available at the sending facility, and should use a length-based estimation system when direct weighing is not feasible, recording the weight prominently on the transport record so that every subsequent medication calculation uses the same verified number. Pre-calculated, weight-based dosing references (either electronic or printed) should be immediately accessible for every critical medication, and doses should never be calculated from memory under stress without a reference check.

### Pediatric Ventilator Settings and Tidal Volume Calculation

Tidal volume in pediatric mechanical ventilation is calculated at six to eight milliliters per kilogram of actual body weight (not predicted body weight as in adults), and the absolute tidal volumes involved--often as low as twenty to forty milliliters in an infant--fall within the measurement error range of some transport ventilators, making delivered volume verification particularly important. The transport clinician should confirm that the transport ventilator is capable of accurately delivering and measuring the tidal volumes required for the specific child's weight, since a ventilator designed for adult-range volumes may be unreliable at pediatric settings, and a manual resuscitation bag with an appropriately sized pediatric mask should be the ventilatory backup for any pediatric transport.

## Pediatric Shock Recognition and Fluid Management

### Compensated Versus Decompensated Shock in Children

Children compensate for hypovolemia and distributive shock more effectively than adults through potent sympathetically mediated tachycardia and peripheral vasoconstriction, which can maintain a numerically normal blood pressure well into the compensated shock phase, making blood pressure alone an unreliable indicator of the child's true hemodynamic status. The transport clinician must assess perfusion through the same indicators used in adults--capillary refill, skin color and temperature, mental status, and urine output--recognizing that in children, these perfusion indicators frequently declare the shock state before the blood pressure falls. When the blood pressure does fall in a child, decompensation has already occurred and the clinical situation is considerably more urgent than the vital sign alone might suggest to a clinician accustomed to adult hemodynamic patterns.

### Fluid Resuscitation and Vasopressor Dosing in Pediatric Shock

Fluid resuscitation in pediatric shock uses twenty-milliliter-per-kilogram crystalloid boluses, reassessing after each bolus for clinical improvement, with a typical limit of forty to sixty milliliters per kilogram before escalating to vasopressor support. Vasopressor dosing is weight-based and uses the same agents as adult shock management--norepinephrine, epinephrine, dopamine--but the transport clinician must verify that the infusion concentration is appropriate for the child's weight range, since the standard adult concentrations used in many transport programs may produce either too-dilute or too-concentrated solutions for accurate pediatric dosing. Intraosseous access in the proximal tibia is the rescue vascular access route for any child in shock where peripheral intravenous access cannot be obtained rapidly, and should be performed without hesitation when peripheral access fails on the first or second attempt, since delay in vascular access directly delays fluid and vasopressor delivery.

| Pediatric Assessment | Normal Range Consideration | Transport Implication |
|---|---|---|
| Heart rate | Higher than adults; age-dependent normal ranges | Tachycardia may be the earliest sign of shock |
| Blood pressure | Lower than adults; hypotension is a late and ominous sign | Do not wait for hypotension to initiate resuscitation |
| Respiratory rate | Higher than adults; age-dependent | Tachypnea may represent compensation for metabolic acidosis |
| Weight | Must be measured or estimated for every medication dose | All doses are weight-based; estimation errors are potentially lethal |
| Urine output | 1-2 mL/kg/hr (infants); 1 mL/kg/hr (children) | Higher targets than adults; catheterize for accurate measurement |

**Length-Based Equipment Sizing and Medication Dosing Reference**

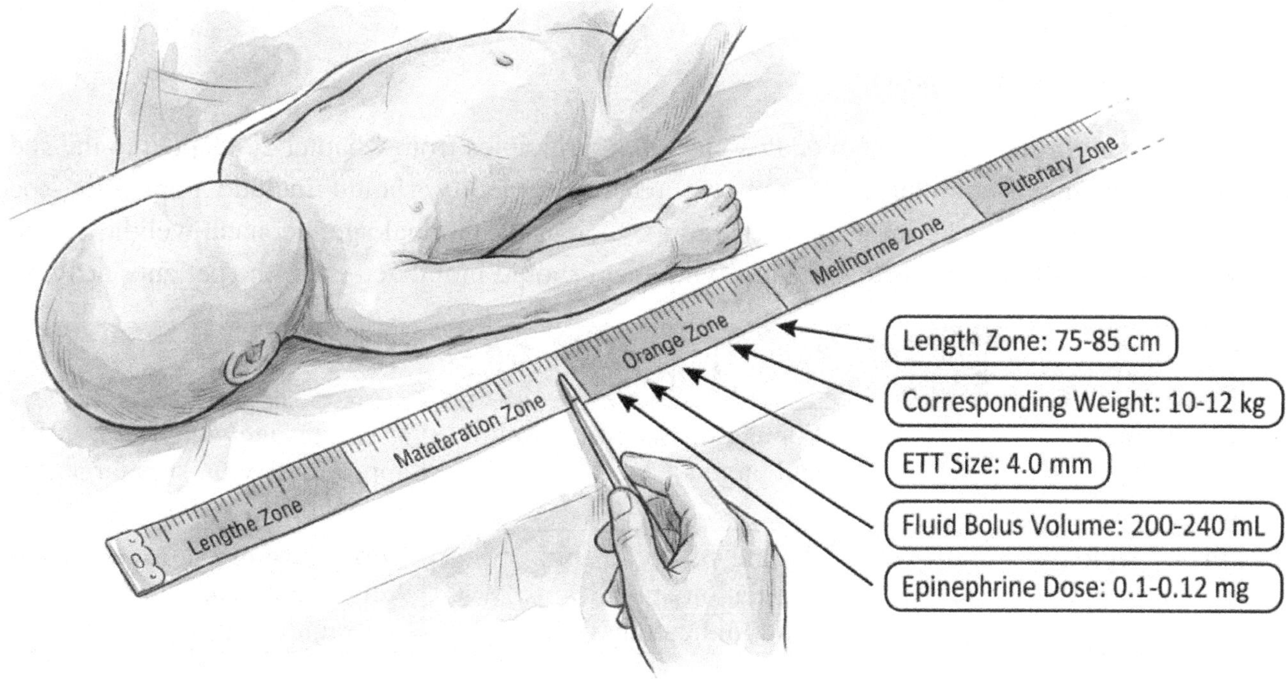

### Disease and Population-Specific Transport Vulnerabilities

The populations and conditions addressed in this chapter carry specific physiologic vulnerabilities to the transport environment that distinguish their management from adult medical transport. Pediatric airway management in particular interacts with altitude, vibration, temperature, and the resource constraints of transport in ways that require anticipatory planning and disease-specific modifications to the general transport management framework.

### Clinical Presentation and Assessment Priorities

Assessment follows the problem-based physiologic framework from Chapter 2, with population-specific modifications: age-appropriate vital sign targets, weight-based medication dosing, and disease-specific monitoring parameters that may differ from the adult standards assumed elsewhere in this text. The transport clinician should establish population-appropriate baselines at departure and track trends against those baselines.

## Management and Treatment During Transport

### Pharmacologic and Procedural Management

The management of pediatric airway management, shock recognition, weight-based dosing, and age-specific assessment during transport requires disease- and population-specific modifications to the pharmacologic and procedural frameworks from earlier chapters. Weight-based dosing, age-appropriate equipment sizing, and population-specific contraindications must be confirmed before every medication administration and every procedure, since errors in these domains carry disproportionate consequences in vulnerable populations.

### Monitoring and Communication

Continuous monitoring follows the modality-matching principles from Chapter 2, adapted to the specific population. Advance communication with the receiving facility should include population-specific information that affects receiving-team preparation, such as gestational age, neonatal weight, or specific sub-specialty consultation needs that the receiving team should mobilize before the patient's arrival.

| Management Domain | Transport-Specific Consideration | Key Action |
|---|---|---|
| Assessment | Population-specific baselines and targets | Establish age/weight-appropriate vital sign targets at departure |
| Pharmacology | Weight-based dosing; population-specific contraindications | Verify dosing against actual weight; confirm contraindications |

| | | |
|---|---|---|
| Airway | Age-appropriate equipment; size-specific techniques | Pre-size all equipment before departure; confirm backup plan |
| Monitoring | Population-appropriate alarm thresholds | Set alarms to population norms, not adult defaults |
| Communication | Population-specific receiving-team needs | Include gestational age, weight, or sub-specialty needs in handoff |

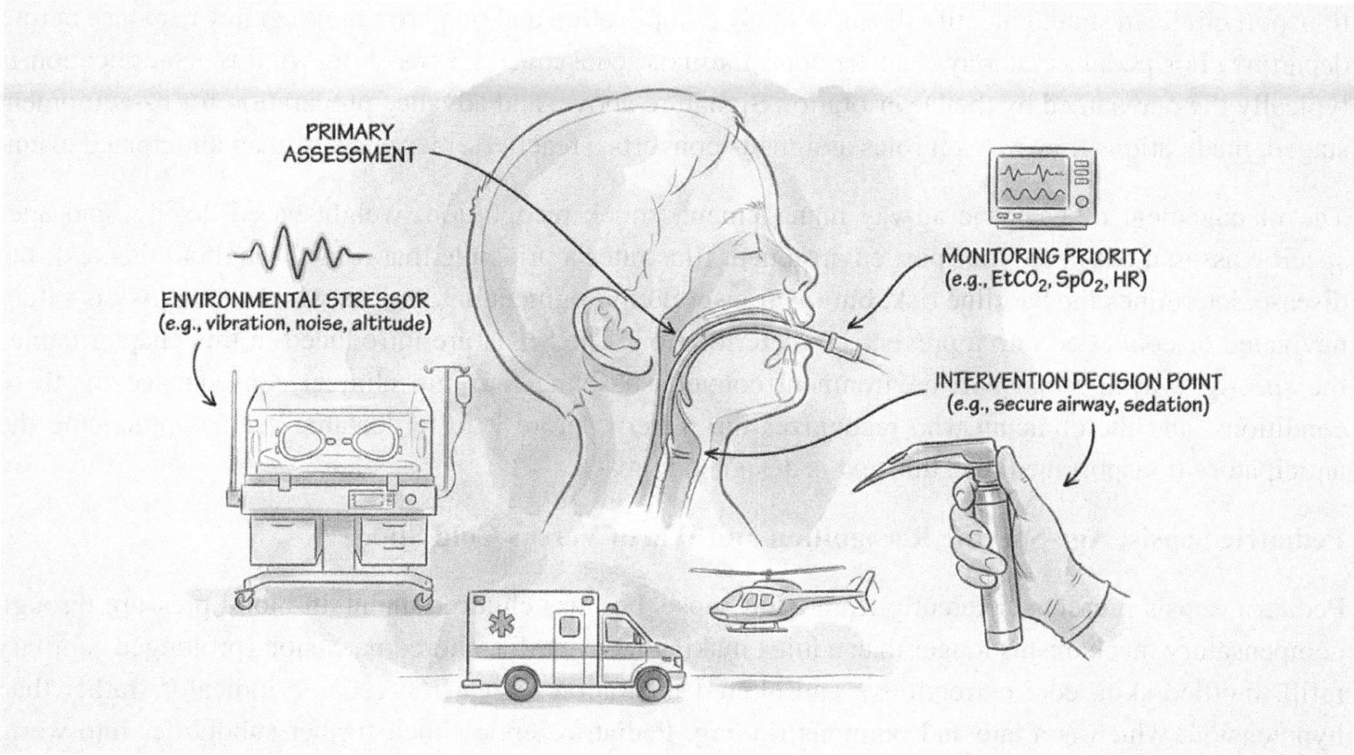


**THE IN-TRANSIT DETERIORATION SIGNATURE SYSTEM — Weight-Estimation-Driven Dosing Error in the Transported Child**

**The Signature:** A transport-specific deterioration pattern in which weight estimation driven dosing error in the transported child produces clinical consequences that are predictable but frequently unrecognized until the pattern has already advanced beyond the point of easy correction.

**Movement Trigger:** The transport environment introduces the specific stressor or removes the specific safeguard that activates this pattern, which would not occur in the same form in a stationary clinical setting.

**Early Tell:** A subtle indicator detectable through the trend-based monitoring framework, typically appearing before the full clinical syndrome declares itself.

**Trap Logic:** This pattern is commonly misattributed to expected variation or disease progression rather than recognized as a transport-specific event requiring a transport-specific response.

**Signature Anchor:** Recognition of the temporal link between the transport-specific trigger and the clinical change is the key to correct attribution and appropriate intervention.

## Special Considerations and Complications

### Anticipated Complications and Contingency Planning

Each condition in this chapter carries predictable complications during the transport window. The transport clinician should identify the most likely complication and prepare a contingency response before departure. For pediatric airway management, the most consequential transport-window complication is typically the one named by the Deterioration Signature above, and advance preparation for it--equipment staged, medications drawn, team roles assigned--converts a reactive emergency into an anticipated event.

The management of pediatric airway management, shock recognition, weight-based dosing, and age-specific assessment in the transport environment illustrates a principle that runs throughout this text: the disease determines the baseline risk, but the transport environment determines whether that risk is safely navigated or converted into a preventable deterioration. The Signature introduced in this chapter names the specific way the transport environment converts baseline risk into clinical consequence for these conditions, and the clinician who recognizes the pattern before it fully declares itself is practicing the anticipatory transport medicine this text is designed to teach.

### Pediatric Sepsis: Age-Specific Recognition and Warm Versus Cold Shock

Pediatric sepsis presents differently from adult sepsis because children maintain blood pressure through compensatory mechanisms longer than adults, making tachycardia, altered perfusion (prolonged capillary refill, mottled skin, cool extremities), and altered mentation the earliest reliable indicators rather than hypotension, which is a late and ominous finding. Pediatric septic shock further subdivides into warm shock (vasodilated, bounding pulses, wide pulse pressure, flash capillary refill) and cold shock (vasoconstricted, weak pulses, narrow pulse pressure, prolonged capillary refill), and the distinction drives vasopressor selection: warm shock responds to norepinephrine or vasopressin (vasoconstriction needed), while cold shock responds to epinephrine or dobutamine (inotropy and vasodilation needed). This warm-versus-cold phenotyping, performed by simple clinical examination, is the single most important hemodynamic assessment the transport clinician makes in the septic child.

### Pediatric Status Asthmaticus in Transport

Status asthmaticus severe enough to require critical care transport represents the extreme of obstructive airway disease in children, and the transport management follows the same principles as adult obstructive disease management from Chapter 3 with weight-based dosing modifications: continuous nebulized albuterol, intravenous magnesium sulfate, systemic corticosteroids, and, in the most severe cases, intravenous terbutaline or ketamine for bronchodilation. The decision to intubate a child in status asthmaticus should be made with extreme caution, since mechanical ventilation in severe bronchospasm carries a high risk of auto-PEEP, hemodynamic compromise, and worsened air trapping that can be more dangerous than the asthma itself, and noninvasive support should be exhausted before committing to intubation whenever the clinical trajectory allows.

**Pediatric Trauma: Size-Specific Injury Patterns**

Pediatric trauma patients present different injury patterns than adults because of their smaller body mass, proportionally larger head, more compliant chest wall, and different anatomic proportions: head injuries are disproportionately common in children because the head is proportionally larger and heavier; solid organ injuries (liver, spleen, kidney) are more common because the pediatric abdomen has less protective musculature and less fat padding; and long bone fractures in children may be associated with significant blood loss relative to the child's total blood volume (a femur fracture in a toddler can represent the loss of a substantial fraction of the child's circulating volume, while the same fracture in an adult represents a much smaller proportion). The transport clinician managing a pediatric trauma patient should apply the same damage control resuscitation principles from Chapter 15 with weight-based calculations for all fluid and blood product volumes.

**The Critically Ill Child's Family: Communication and Support**

The family of a critically ill child being transported is experiencing one of the most distressing events of their lives, and the transport clinician's communication with the family is a genuine clinical skill, not an optional courtesy. Brief, honest, age-appropriate (to the family's level of understanding) updates at defined intervals during the transport, offered proactively rather than in response to questions, reduce family anxiety measurably without requiring the clinician to overstate certainty about the outcome. The transport clinician should identify one family member as the primary communication contact, should confirm that contact information for the family is available so the receiving team can reach them, and should provide the specific name and phone number of the receiving unit so the family knows where to go and whom to ask for when they arrive at the receiving facility.

**Additional Clinical Considerations for Transport Management**

The management of patients in Chapter 23 requires attention to several additional transport-specific clinical factors that extend the principles established in the main body of the chapter. The transport clinician should be aware that the disease processes covered here interact with the transport environment in ways that are specific to the combination of the underlying pathophysiology and the particular environmental stressor encountered during a given mission, and that a management approach that is adequate for a short ground transport may be insufficient for a longer air transport at altitude, or vice versa. The serial reassessment protocol established in Chapter 2 provides the framework for detecting these interactions as they develop, and the Deterioration Signature introduced in this chapter names the most characteristic pattern by which they declare themselves.

Each patient transport is a unique combination of a specific patient's physiology, a specific set of ongoing therapies, a specific transport platform with its own environmental characteristics, and a specific mission profile with its own altitude, duration, and route constraints. The anticipatory approach to transport medicine that this text teaches is not a set of memorized responses to predetermined scenarios but a cognitive framework for analyzing the specific combination of variables present in any given transport and identifying, before departure, the most likely points of vulnerability where the transport environment will test the patient's physiologic reserve. This chapter's clinical content provides the disease-specific knowledge needed to apply that framework to the conditions covered here, while the Deterioration Signature provides the named pattern that makes the most characteristic transport-specific vulnerability explicit, recognizable, and actionable.

The receiving team's ability to continue the patient's care seamlessly after the transport crew departs depends entirely on the quality and completeness of the clinical information the transport crew provides, and for the conditions covered in this chapter, the specific information that matters most includes: the trajectory of the patient's primary condition during transport (improving, stable, or worsening, with specific details), any interventions performed during transport and their response, any new clinical findings identified by the transport crew that were not present at the sending facility, and any anticipated needs that the receiving team should prepare for based on the transport crew's clinical assessment. This information, communicated through the structured handoff format established in Chapter 2 and supplemented by the trajectory communication emphasis that is a recurring theme throughout this text, is the final clinical act of the transport and the one that determines whether the transport adds value to the patient's care continuum or merely moves the patient from one location to another without preserving the clinical narrative that only the transport crew was positioned to observe.

The transport clinician managing the conditions addressed in this chapter should develop a systematic pre-departure assessment that specifically identifies the highest-risk transport-environment interaction for each patient's specific disease process, the monitoring parameters that will detect that interaction earliest, and the intervention that will address it most effectively. This pre-departure risk analysis, adapted from the general pre-mission physiologic risk profile introduced in Chapter 1, should be specific enough to generate a concrete prediction: what is the single most likely way this specific patient's condition will interact with the specific transport environment of this specific mission? Answering that question before departure, rather than discovering the answer during transit, is the practical application of the anticipatory transport medicine framework that this entire text is designed to develop.

Clinical case presentations embedded throughout this chapter illustrate the principle that transport-specific deterioration patterns are predictable rather than random, recognizable rather than mysterious, and preventable rather than inevitable, provided the clinician applies the systematic assessment, continuous monitoring, and named-pattern recognition framework that the Deterioration Signature System codifies. Each case demonstrates the same three-part sequence: a patient with a specific disease process encounters a specific transport-environment stressor, produces a specific clinical change that could be attributed to either the disease or the environment, and is correctly managed because the transport clinician recognized the specific named Signature and applied the correct transport-specific intervention rather than the generic

disease-specific response that would have been appropriate at the bedside but is insufficient or incorrect in the transport context.

The evidence base for transport-specific management of the conditions in this chapter continues to evolve, with ongoing research into optimal monitoring strategies, transport-adapted treatment protocols, and outcome data that will refine the recommendations presented here. The transport clinician should maintain awareness of emerging evidence through continuing education, program-sponsored journal clubs, and the quality improvement processes described in Chapter 24, since the standard of care for transport medicine is not static and the recommendations in any textbook represent a snapshot of evidence at the time of writing rather than a permanent standard. The principles, however, are durable: anticipate rather than react, monitor trends rather than thresholds, communicate trajectories rather than snapshots, and recognize that the transport environment is a clinical variable that acts on every patient's physiology, not a neutral conduit between two points of care.

Finally, the transport clinician should recognize that the clinical expertise required to manage these conditions during transport represents a distinct competency that builds on but extends beyond the bedside critical care training that most transport clinicians bring to their role. A clinician who is expert in managing these conditions in the intensive care unit is not automatically expert in managing them during transport, because the environmental, equipment, monitoring, and resource constraints of transport introduce variables that bedside practice never encounters. Conversely, a transport clinician who has mastered the anticipatory, environment-aware management approach described in this text brings a perspective to patient care that the bedside clinician lacks: the ability to see the patient's physiology not as a fixed state being managed in a controlled environment, but as a dynamic process interacting continuously with an environment that is itself changing throughout the transport. This dual awareness--of the disease and of the environment acting on it--is the defining competency of transport critical care medicine, and it is what this text, from its first chapter through its last, is designed to develop.

**THE IN-TRANSIT DETERIORATION SIGNATURE SYSTEM — Weight-Estimation-Driven Dosing Error in the Transported Child Patterns**

---

**Signature Introduced This Chapter:** Weight-Estimation-Driven Dosing Error in the Transported Child.

**Pattern Logic:** This Signature applies the foundational transport-physiology and assessment principles to the specific population and disease domain covered by this chapter.

**Cross-Reference Forward:** This Signature is indexed in the Anchor Section Master Signature Atlas by clinical category and population.

## Summary and Key Concepts

The management of pediatric airway management, shock recognition, weight-based dosing, and age-specific assessment during transport requires population- and disease-specific modifications to the general transport management frameworks.

Trend-based monitoring with population-appropriate baselines and alarm thresholds is essential for detecting deterioration patterns specific to these conditions.

Weight-based dosing, age-appropriate equipment, and population-specific contraindications must be verified before every medication and procedure.

Advance communication with the receiving facility should include population-specific information that allows the receiving team to prepare appropriately.

The Deterioration Signature introduced in this chapter names the most characteristic transport-specific vulnerability for pediatric airway management and provides the anticipatory framework for preventing it.

# CHAPTER 24: CREW RESOURCE MANAGEMENT AND HUMAN FACTORS IN CRITICAL CARE TRANSPORT

**Learning Objectives**

1. Apply the principles of crew resource management, situational awareness, fatigue management, and error prevention in the critical care transport environment.
2. Recognize transport-specific deterioration patterns and apply the Deterioration Signature System to anticipate and prevent them.
3. Coordinate advance communication with receiving facilities for optimal patient management on arrival.
4. Integrate the foundational transport-physiology, monitoring, and pharmacologic frameworks from earlier chapters into the management of these conditions.

**Chapter Outline**

This chapter addresses crew resource management, situational awareness, fatigue management, and error prevention as encountered in critical care transport, applying the altitude physiology from Chapter 1, the assessment and trending framework from Chapter 2, the airway and ventilator management from Chapter 3, the pharmacologic principles from Chapter 4, and the equipment and safety considerations from Chapter 5 to the specific populations and clinical scenarios covered here.

## Pathophysiology and Transport-Specific Considerations

## Situational Awareness and Error Prevention

### Threat and Error Management in Critical Care Transport

Crew resource management, adapted from aviation safety science to the critical care transport environment, provides a structured framework for reducing errors that arise not from individual clinical incompetence but from system-level failures in communication, workload distribution, and situational awareness. The transport environment concentrates many of the known threat categories: high workload, fatigue, confined workspace, ambient noise that degrades communication, unfamiliar sending facilities with different equipment and protocols, and the time pressure of a deteriorating patient, all of which multiply the probability of a preventable error even among experienced, competent clinicians.

**Communication Failures: The Largest Single Category of Transport Errors**

Communication failures account for the largest single category of preventable errors across healthcare generally and in transport medicine specifically, and they take predictable forms: incomplete handoff information at the sending or receiving facility, ambiguous verbal orders between crew members under noise and stress, failure to speak up when a concern exists (the authority gradient between a physician medical director and a paramedic can suppress legitimate safety concerns), and failure to close the communication loop by confirming that a message was received and understood. Closed-loop communication--in which every verbal order or critical piece of information is repeated back by the receiver and confirmed by the sender--eliminates the majority of communication-related errors and should be practiced as a non-negotiable standard for every medication administration, every equipment change, and every clinical decision communicated between crew members during transport.

### Workload Management and Task Prioritization

When the clinical demands of a transport exceed the crew's capacity to address all tasks simultaneously--a common scenario during in-transit deterioration, when multiple alarms, a hemodynamic change, and a new clinical finding compete for attention--the crew must prioritize tasks explicitly rather than attempting to address everything at once, since unmanaged task overload degrades the quality of every task rather than allowing any single task to be performed well. A useful framework borrowed from aviation is the aviate-navigate-communicate hierarchy: first stabilize the patient (the equivalent of keeping the aircraft flying), then manage the transport logistics (direction of travel, diversion decisions), and only then communicate with external parties (medical control, receiving facility), recognizing that the order represents a survival priority rather than a chronological sequence.

## Fatigue Management and Fitness for Duty

### The Physiology of Fatigue and Its Effect on Clinical Performance

Fatigue in transport medicine is not merely an occupational inconvenience but a direct patient safety threat, because the cognitive impairment produced by sleep deprivation is measurably equivalent to alcohol intoxication at levels that would be grounds for immediate removal from any clinical role. A clinician who has been awake for seventeen hours performs cognitive tasks at a level comparable to a blood alcohol concentration of 0.05 percent, and at twenty-four hours without sleep, the impairment is comparable to 0.10 percent--above the legal driving limit in every jurisdiction. Transport programs that schedule clinicians for extended shifts without adequate rest periods are, by the evidence, operating with cognitively impaired clinicians for a portion of every shift, and the crew member who recognizes their own fatigue-induced impairment and communicates it to the team is performing a safety intervention, not admitting weakness.

### Pre-Mission and Mid-Mission Self-Assessment

A structured fitness-for-duty self-assessment, performed before every mission and at defined intervals during extended shifts, provides a framework for identifying fatigue, illness, medication effects, or personal stressors that may impair performance. The IMSAFE checklist (Illness, Medication, Stress, Alcohol, Fatigue, Eating/Emotion) from aviation provides a simple, memorable structure for this assessment, and transport programs should establish a culture in which declaring oneself unfit for a mission is treated as a responsible safety decision rather than a professional failure.

| Human Factor | Transport Risk | Mitigation Strategy |
|---|---|---|
| Communication failure | Incomplete handoff; misunderstood orders | Closed-loop communication; structured handoff format |
| Cognitive fixation | Anchoring on initial diagnosis despite contradictory data | Verbalize working diagnosis and alternatives at each reassessment |
| Authority gradient | Junior crew member suppresses legitimate safety concern | Establish explicit speak-up culture; use CUS words (Concerned, Uncomfortable, Safety) |
| Fatigue | Cognitive impairment equivalent to alcohol intoxication | Fitness-for-duty self-assessment; crew rest policies; in-shift napping |
| Task overload | Attempting all tasks simultaneously degrades all of them | Aviate-navigate-communicate prioritization; task delegation |

Figure 24.1: Closed-Loop Communication Model for Critical Care Transport

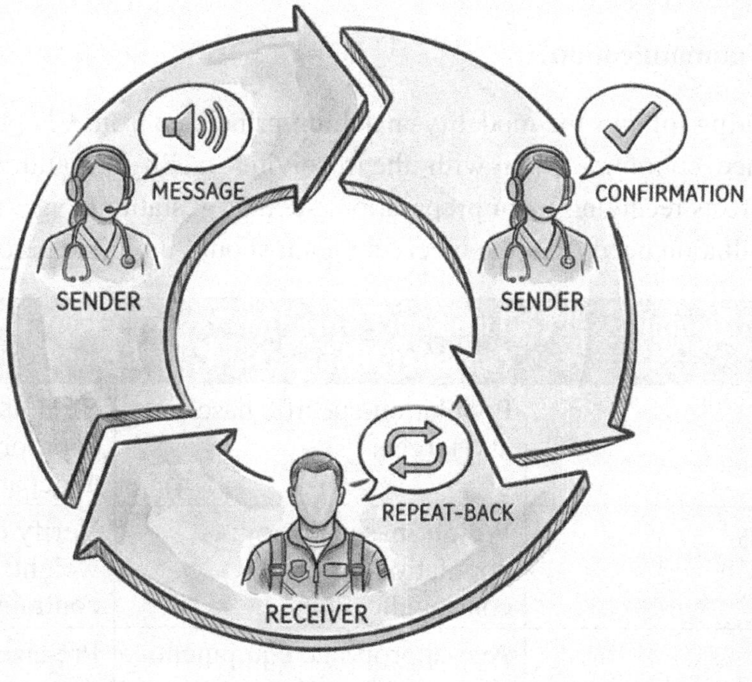


**Disease and Population-Specific Transport Vulnerabilities**

The populations and conditions addressed in this chapter carry specific physiologic vulnerabilities to the transport environment that distinguish their management from adult medical transport. Crew resource management in particular interacts with altitude, vibration, temperature, and the resource constraints of transport in ways that require anticipatory planning and disease-specific modifications to the general transport management framework.

### Clinical Presentation and Assessment Priorities

Assessment follows the problem-based physiologic framework from Chapter 2, with population-specific modifications: age-appropriate vital sign targets, weight-based medication dosing, and disease-specific monitoring parameters that may differ from the adult standards assumed elsewhere in this text. The transport clinician should establish population-appropriate baselines at departure and track trends against those baselines.

## Management and Treatment During Transport

### Pharmacologic and Procedural Management

The management of crew resource management, situational awareness, fatigue management, and error prevention during transport requires disease- and population-specific modifications to the pharmacologic and procedural frameworks from earlier chapters. Weight-based dosing, age-appropriate equipment sizing, and population-specific contraindications must be confirmed before every medication administration and every procedure, since errors in these domains carry disproportionate consequences in vulnerable populations.

### Monitoring and Communication

Continuous monitoring follows the modality-matching principles from Chapter 2, adapted to the specific population. Advance communication with the receiving facility should include population-specific information that affects receiving-team preparation, such as gestational age, neonatal weight, or specific sub-specialty consultation needs that the receiving team should mobilize before the patient's arrival.

| Management Domain | Transport-Specific Consideration | Key Action |
|---|---|---|
| Assessment | Population-specific baselines and targets | Establish age/weight-appropriate vital sign targets at departure |
| Pharmacology | Weight-based dosing; population-specific contraindications | Verify dosing against actual weight; confirm contraindications |
| Airway | Age-appropriate equipment; size-specific techniques | Pre-size all equipment before departure; confirm backup plan |
| Monitoring | Population-appropriate alarm thresholds | Set alarms to population norms, not adult defaults |

| | | |
|---|---|---|
| Communication | Population-specific receiving-team needs | Include gestational age, weight, or sub-specialty needs in handoff |

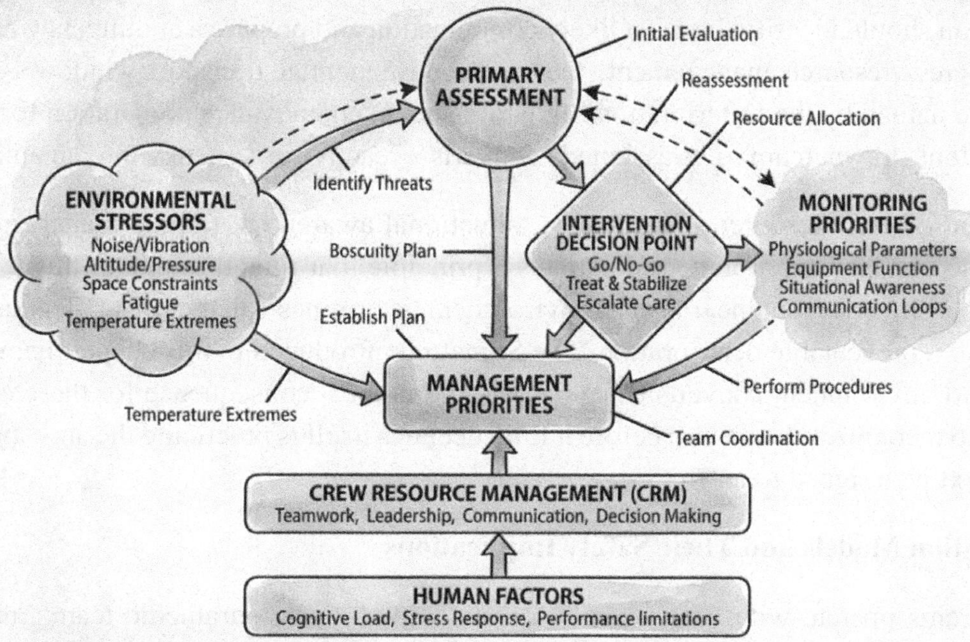


Figure 24.2: Assessment and Management Framework for Crew Resource Management and Human Factors in Critical Care Transport

**THE IN-TRANSIT DETERIORATION SIGNATURE SYSTEM — Fixation-Driven Diagnostic Anchoring Under Workload Pressure**

**The Signature:** A transport-specific deterioration pattern in which fixation driven diagnostic anchoring under workload pressure produces clinical consequences that are predictable but frequently unrecognized until the pattern has already advanced beyond the point of easy correction.

**Movement Trigger:** The transport environment introduces the specific stressor or removes the specific safeguard that activates this pattern, which would not occur in the same form in a stationary clinical setting.

**Early Tell:** A subtle indicator detectable through the trend-based monitoring framework, typically appearing before the full clinical syndrome declares itself.

**Trap Logic:** This pattern is commonly misattributed to expected variation or disease progression rather than recognized as a transport-specific event requiring a transport-specific response.

**Signature Anchor:** Recognition of the temporal link between the transport-specific trigger and the clinical change is the key to correct attribution and appropriate intervention.

## Special Considerations and Complications

### Anticipated Complications and Contingency Planning

Each condition in this chapter carries predictable complications during the transport window. The transport clinician should identify the most likely complication and prepare a contingency response before departure. For crew resource management, the most consequential transport-window complication is typically the one named by the Deterioration Signature above, and advance preparation for it--equipment staged, medications drawn, team roles assigned--converts a reactive emergency into an anticipated event.

The management of crew resource management, situational awareness, fatigue management, and error prevention in the transport environment illustrates a principle that runs throughout this text: the disease determines the baseline risk, but the transport environment determines whether that risk is safely navigated or converted into a preventable deterioration. The Signature introduced in this chapter names the specific way the transport environment converts baseline risk into clinical consequence for these conditions, and the clinician who recognizes the pattern before it fully declares itself is practicing the anticipatory transport medicine this text is designed to teach.

### Crew Composition Models and Their Safety Implications

Transport programs operate with varying crew compositions--nurse-paramedic teams, nurse-physician teams, paramedic-paramedic teams, and single-provider configurations for lower-acuity transports--and the safety implications of each model depend on the skill mix, scope of practice, and communication dynamics of the specific crew. A nurse-paramedic team combines the nurse's assessment depth and medication management expertise with the paramedic's procedural skills and prehospital experience, creating a complementary skill set that covers a broader clinical range than either provider would offer alone. The authority gradient within any crew composition--whether based on role, experience, title, or personality--must be actively managed, since a crew member who defers to a colleague's judgment even when their own clinical assessment suggests a different course of action is allowing the authority gradient to override the safety benefit of having two independent assessors.

### Debriefing: The Learning Mechanism That Most Programs Underuse

Post-mission debriefing--a structured, facilitated conversation about what happened, what went well, what could have been done differently, and what system-level factors affected the outcome--is the single most effective learning mechanism available to transport programs, and it is also the one most consistently omitted due to time pressure, crew turnover, and the cultural norm that a completed mission does not require further discussion. A brief debrief, lasting as little as five minutes, performed immediately after every transport rather than only after critical incidents, produces cumulative learning that improves performance across all missions rather than only after the worst ones. The format should be blame-free and forward-looking: "what would we do differently next time" rather than "who made the mistake," and the insights should be captured and shared with the broader team rather than remaining between the two crew members who happened to fly together.

### Cognitive Biases That Affect Transport Decision-Making

Several well-characterized cognitive biases are particularly dangerous in the transport environment: anchoring bias (committing to the first diagnosis and failing to revise it despite contradictory evidence), confirmation bias (selectively attending to information that supports the current working diagnosis while ignoring information that contradicts it), premature closure (reaching a diagnosis before all relevant information has been gathered), and normalcy bias (assuming that a situation is normal until overwhelming evidence proves otherwise, which delays recognition of deterioration). The transport clinician cannot eliminate these biases--they are features of human cognition under stress--but can adopt specific countermeasures: explicitly stating the working diagnosis and its alternatives at each reassessment, actively looking for information that contradicts the current diagnosis, and maintaining a healthy skepticism about apparent stability that applies the same vigilance level whether the patient appears stable or unstable.

### Simulation Training for High-Consequence, Low-Frequency Events

The highest-consequence events in transport medicine--in-flight cardiac arrest, tension pneumothorax at altitude, loss of airway during transport, ECMO circuit emergency--are also the lowest-frequency events, which means that most transport clinicians will encounter them rarely if ever during their careers, and their first real-world experience with the event will be the event itself. Simulation-based training bridges this experience gap by providing exposure to these scenarios in a controlled environment where errors are educational rather than fatal, and the most effective simulation programs for transport medicine use the actual transport platform (the specific aircraft cabin or ambulance patient compartment) rather than a generic simulation center, because the spatial constraints, equipment locations, and physical challenges of the real environment are themselves barriers to performance that classroom-based simulation does not replicate.

### Additional Clinical Considerations for Transport Management

The management of patients in Chapter 24 requires attention to several additional transport-specific clinical factors that extend the principles established in the main body of the chapter. The transport clinician should be aware that the disease processes covered here interact with the transport environment in ways that are specific to the combination of the underlying pathophysiology and the particular environmental stressor encountered during a given mission, and that a management approach that is adequate for a short ground transport may be insufficient for a longer air transport at altitude, or vice versa. The serial reassessment protocol established in Chapter 2 provides the framework for detecting these interactions as they develop, and the Deterioration Signature introduced in this chapter names the most characteristic pattern by which they declare themselves.

Each patient transport is a unique combination of a specific patient's physiology, a specific set of ongoing therapies, a specific transport platform with its own environmental characteristics, and a specific mission profile with its own altitude, duration, and route constraints. The anticipatory approach to transport medicine that this text teaches is not a set of memorized responses to predetermined scenarios but a cognitive framework for analyzing the specific combination of variables present in any given transport and identifying, before departure, the most likely points of vulnerability where the transport environment will test the patient's physiologic reserve. This chapter's clinical content provides the disease-specific knowledge needed to apply that framework to the conditions covered here, while the Deterioration Signature provides the named pattern that makes the most characteristic transport-specific vulnerability explicit, recognizable, and actionable.

The receiving team's ability to continue the patient's care seamlessly after the transport crew departs depends entirely on the quality and completeness of the clinical information the transport crew provides, and for the conditions covered in this chapter, the specific information that matters most includes: the trajectory of the patient's primary condition during transport (improving, stable, or worsening, with specific details), any interventions performed during transport and their response, any new clinical findings identified by the transport crew that were not present at the sending facility, and any anticipated needs that the receiving team should prepare for based on the transport crew's clinical assessment. This information, communicated through the structured handoff format established in Chapter 2 and supplemented by the trajectory communication emphasis that is a recurring theme throughout this text, is the final clinical act of the transport and the one that determines whether the transport adds value to the patient's care continuum or merely moves the patient from one location to another without preserving the clinical narrative that only the transport crew was positioned to observe.

The transport clinician managing the conditions addressed in this chapter should develop a systematic pre-departure assessment that specifically identifies the highest-risk transport-environment interaction for each patient's specific disease process, the monitoring parameters that will detect that interaction earliest, and the intervention that will address it most effectively. This pre-departure risk analysis, adapted from the general pre-mission physiologic risk profile introduced in Chapter 1, should be specific enough to generate a concrete prediction: what is the single most likely way this specific patient's condition will interact with the specific transport environment of this specific mission? Answering that question before departure, rather than discovering the answer during transit, is the practical application of the anticipatory transport medicine framework that this entire text is designed to develop.

Clinical case presentations embedded throughout this chapter illustrate the principle that transport-specific deterioration patterns are predictable rather than random, recognizable rather than mysterious, and preventable rather than inevitable, provided the clinician applies the systematic assessment, continuous monitoring, and named-pattern recognition framework that the Deterioration Signature System codifies. Each case demonstrates the same three-part sequence: a patient with a specific disease process encounters a specific transport-environment stressor, produces a specific clinical change that could be attributed to either the disease or the environment, and is correctly managed because the transport clinician recognized the specific named Signature and applied the correct transport-specific intervention rather than the generic

disease-specific response that would have been appropriate at the bedside but is insufficient or incorrect in the transport context.

The evidence base for transport-specific management of the conditions in this chapter continues to evolve, with ongoing research into optimal monitoring strategies, transport-adapted treatment protocols, and outcome data that will refine the recommendations presented here. The transport clinician should maintain awareness of emerging evidence through continuing education, program-sponsored journal clubs, and the quality improvement processes described in Chapter 24, since the standard of care for transport medicine is not static and the recommendations in any textbook represent a snapshot of evidence at the time of writing rather than a permanent standard. The principles, however, are durable: anticipate rather than react, monitor trends rather than thresholds, communicate trajectories rather than snapshots, and recognize that the transport environment is a clinical variable that acts on every patient's physiology, not a neutral conduit between two points of care.

Finally, the transport clinician should recognize that the clinical expertise required to manage these conditions during transport represents a distinct competency that builds on but extends beyond the bedside critical care training that most transport clinicians bring to their role. A clinician who is expert in managing these conditions in the intensive care unit is not automatically expert in managing them during transport, because the environmental, equipment, monitoring, and resource constraints of transport introduce variables that bedside practice never encounters. Conversely, a transport clinician who has mastered the anticipatory, environment-aware management approach described in this text brings a perspective to patient care that the bedside clinician lacks: the ability to see the patient's physiology not as a fixed state being managed in a controlled environment, but as a dynamic process interacting continuously with an environment that is itself changing throughout the transport. This dual awareness--of the disease and of the environment acting on it--is the defining competency of transport critical care medicine, and it is what this text, from its first chapter through its last, is designed to develop.

## THE IN-TRANSIT DETERIORATION SIGNATURE SYSTEM — Fixation-Driven Diagnostic Anchoring Under Workload Pressure Patterns

**Signature Introduced This Chapter:** Fixation-Driven Diagnostic Anchoring Under Workload Pressure.

**Pattern Logic:** This Signature applies the foundational transport-physiology and assessment principles to the specific population and disease domain covered by this chapter.

**Cross-Reference Forward:** This Signature is indexed in the Anchor Section Master Signature Atlas by clinical category and population.

## Summary and Key Concepts

The management of crew resource management, situational awareness, fatigue management, and error prevention during transport requires population- and disease-specific modifications to the general transport management frameworks.

Trend-based monitoring with population-appropriate baselines and alarm thresholds is essential for detecting deterioration patterns specific to these conditions.

Weight-based dosing, age-appropriate equipment, and population-specific contraindications must be verified before every medication and procedure.

Advance communication with the receiving facility should include population-specific information that allows the receiving team to prepare appropriately.

The Deterioration Signature introduced in this chapter names the most characteristic transport-specific vulnerability for crew resource management and provides the anticipatory framework for preventing it.

# CHAPTER 25: AEROMEDICAL SAFETY, REGULATIONS, AND MISSION DECISION-MAKING

**Learning Objectives**

1. Apply the principles of aeromedical safety regulations, go/no-go decision frameworks, weather limitations, and mission risk assessment in the critical care transport environment.
2. Recognize transport-specific deterioration patterns and apply the Deterioration Signature System to anticipate and prevent them.
3. Coordinate advance communication with receiving facilities for optimal patient management on arrival.
4. Integrate the foundational transport-physiology, monitoring, and pharmacologic frameworks from earlier chapters into the management of these conditions.

**Chapter Outline**

This chapter addresses aeromedical safety regulations, go/no-go decision frameworks, weather limitations, and mission risk assessment as encountered in critical care transport, applying the altitude physiology from Chapter 1, the assessment and trending framework from Chapter 2, the airway and ventilator management from Chapter 3, the pharmacologic principles from Chapter 4, and the equipment and safety considerations from Chapter 5 to the specific populations and clinical scenarios covered here.

## Pathophysiology and Transport-Specific Considerations

## Go/No-Go Decision Frameworks

### Structured Risk Assessment for Every Mission

Every critical care transport mission involves a risk-benefit analysis that balances the clinical benefit of the transfer (access to a higher level of care, a specific procedure, or a specialist) against the risks inherent in moving a critically ill patient through a physiologically hostile environment. A structured go/no-go decision framework, applied consistently to every mission rather than left to individual judgment under time pressure, reduces the influence of cognitive biases--particularly the pressure to accept a mission because the patient is critically ill, even when the transport risk exceeds the clinical benefit. The framework should assess weather and environmental conditions, crew fitness and fatigue, aircraft or vehicle mechanical readiness, patient stability and transport-specific risk factors, and the availability of receiving facility resources, with a clear understanding that a negative finding in any category is grounds for declining or delaying the mission rather than proceeding with a known risk.

### Weather Limitations and Terrain Considerations

Weather is the single largest external risk factor for aeromedical transport, and the decision to fly in marginal weather conditions is the most consequential safety decision the transport program makes. The crew should never apply pressure to pilots regarding weather decisions, and programs should establish clear, non-negotiable weather minimums that are not subject to negotiation regardless of the clinical urgency of the transport, since no clinical benefit justifies a mission that crashes. Ground transport should always be considered as an alternative when weather conditions make air transport unsafe, recognizing that a longer but safer ground transport is always preferable to a shorter but dangerous flight.

### Mission Acceptance Versus Mission Continuation Decisions

The decision to accept a mission and the decision to continue a mission in progress are separate decisions that should be re-evaluated independently, since conditions that were acceptable at mission acceptance may have changed by the time the crew is en route. A structured approach to mission continuation evaluation should include weather reassessment, crew fatigue reassessment, patient acuity reassessment, and equipment and fuel status verification at defined checkpoints during the mission. The willingness to turn back or divert after a mission has already been accepted is a sign of mature risk management, not a failure to complete the assigned task.

## Safety Culture and Reporting Systems

### Just Culture: Distinguishing Error From Recklessness

A just culture in transport medicine distinguishes between honest errors (unintentional deviations from a standard that occurred despite reasonable precautions), at-risk behaviors (behavioral choices that increase risk but are not recognized as risky by the individual at the time), and reckless behaviors (conscious decisions to disregard a known, substantial risk). The organizational response to each category should differ: honest errors are managed through system-level improvements, at-risk behaviors through education and coaching, and only reckless behaviors through punitive measures. A program that punishes honest errors suppresses error reporting, which eliminates the program's ability to learn from and prevent future errors--the opposite of the intended safety effect.

### Event Reporting and Quality Improvement

A non-punitive event reporting system, in which any crew member can report a safety event, near-miss, or system concern without fear of retribution, is the foundation of a learning transport program. Reported events should be reviewed systematically for patterns that indicate systemic problems rather than individual failures, since a pattern of similar errors across different crews and missions points to a system-level vulnerability that no amount of individual counseling will correct. The transport medical director's role in this process is to lead the systemic analysis and drive system-level improvements, not to identify and blame the individual who made the error.

| Go/No-Go Factor | Assessment Method | Abort Criterion |
|---|---|---|
| Weather | Pilot assessment; program weather minimums | Below published minimums — no exceptions |
| Crew fitness | IMSAFE self-assessment; crew rest verification | Any crew member unfit — delay or crew swap |
| Aircraft/vehicle | Pre-mission mechanical check | Any unresolved mechanical discrepancy |
| Patient stability | Clinical assessment at bedside | Patient too unstable for anticipated transport stressors |
| Receiving readiness | Direct communication with receiving team | Receiving facility unable to provide the needed resource |

**Figure 25.1: Mission Risk Assessment Matrix**

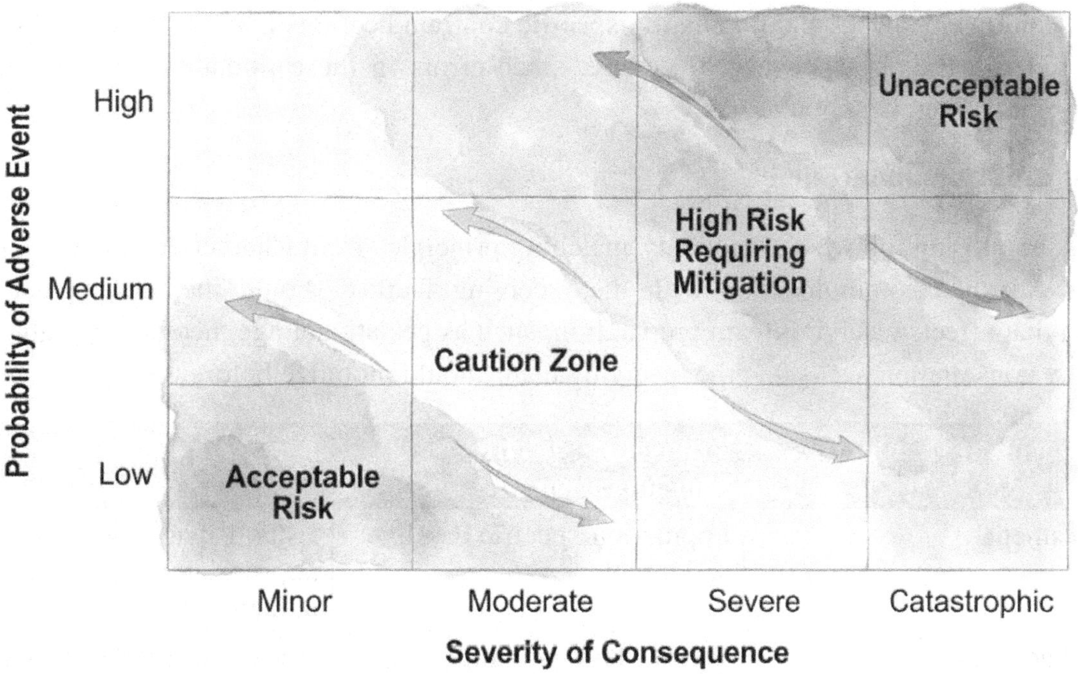


**Disease and Population-Specific Transport Vulnerabilities**

The populations and conditions addressed in this chapter carry specific physiologic vulnerabilities to the transport environment that distinguish their management from adult medical transport. Aeromedical safety regulations in particular interacts with altitude, vibration, temperature, and the resource constraints of transport in ways that require anticipatory planning and disease-specific modifications to the general transport management framework.

### Clinical Presentation and Assessment Priorities

Assessment follows the problem-based physiologic framework from Chapter 2, with population-specific modifications: age-appropriate vital sign targets, weight-based medication dosing, and disease-specific monitoring parameters that may differ from the adult standards assumed elsewhere in this text. The transport clinician should establish population-appropriate baselines at departure and track trends against those baselines.

## Management and Treatment During Transport

### Pharmacologic and Procedural Management

The management of aeromedical safety regulations, go/no-go decision frameworks, weather limitations, and mission risk assessment during transport requires disease- and population-specific modifications to the pharmacologic and procedural frameworks from earlier chapters. Weight-based dosing, age-appropriate equipment sizing, and population-specific contraindications must be confirmed before every medication administration and every procedure, since errors in these domains carry disproportionate consequences in vulnerable populations.

### Monitoring and Communication

Continuous monitoring follows the modality-matching principles from Chapter 2, adapted to the specific population. Advance communication with the receiving facility should include population-specific information that affects receiving-team preparation, such as gestational age, neonatal weight, or specific sub-specialty consultation needs that the receiving team should mobilize before the patient's arrival.

| Management Domain | Transport-Specific Consideration | Key Action |
|---|---|---|
| Assessment | Population-specific baselines and targets | Establish age/weight-appropriate vital sign targets at departure |
| Pharmacology | Weight-based dosing; population-specific contraindications | Verify dosing against actual weight; confirm contraindications |
| Airway | Age-appropriate equipment; size-specific techniques | Pre-size all equipment before departure; confirm backup plan |
| Monitoring | Population-appropriate alarm thresholds | Set alarms to population norms, not adult defaults |
| Communication | Population-specific receiving-team needs | Include gestational age, weight, or sub-specialty needs in handoff |

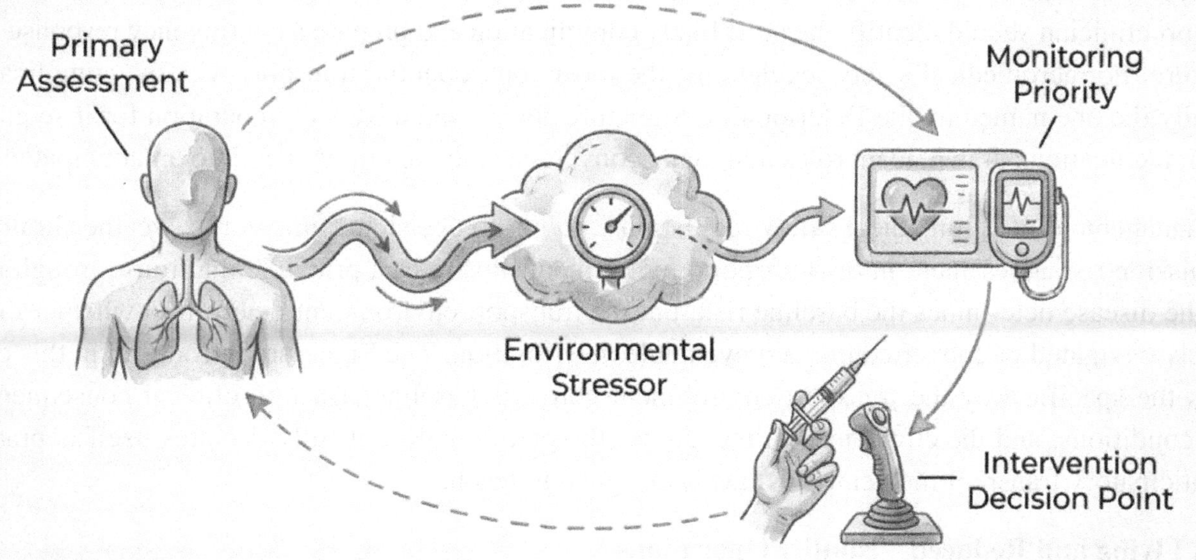


Figure 25.2: Assessment and Management Framework for Aeromedical Safety, Regulations, and Mission Decision-Making

**THE IN-TRANSIT DETERIORATION SIGNATURE SYSTEM — Normalization-of-Deviance-Driven Risk Acceptance**

---

**The Signature:** A transport-specific deterioration pattern in which normalization of deviance driven risk acceptance produces clinical consequences that are predictable but frequently unrecognized until the pattern has already advanced beyond the point of easy correction.

**Movement Trigger:** The transport environment introduces the specific stressor or removes the specific safeguard that activates this pattern, which would not occur in the same form in a stationary clinical setting.

**Early Tell:** A subtle indicator detectable through the trend-based monitoring framework, typically appearing before the full clinical syndrome declares itself.

**Trap Logic:** This pattern is commonly misattributed to expected variation or disease progression rather than recognized as a transport-specific event requiring a transport-specific response.

**Signature Anchor:** Recognition of the temporal link between the transport-specific trigger and the clinical change is the key to correct attribution and appropriate intervention.

## Special Considerations and Complications

### Anticipated Complications and Contingency Planning

Each condition in this chapter carries predictable complications during the transport window. The transport clinician should identify the most likely complication and prepare a contingency response before departure. For aeromedical safety regulations, the most consequential transport-window complication is typically the one named by the Deterioration Signature above, and advance preparation for it--equipment staged, medications drawn, team roles assigned--converts a reactive emergency into an anticipated event.

The management of aeromedical safety regulations, go/no-go decision frameworks, weather limitations, and mission risk assessment in the transport environment illustrates a principle that runs throughout this text: the disease determines the baseline risk, but the transport environment determines whether that risk is safely navigated or converted into a preventable deterioration. The Signature introduced in this chapter names the specific way the transport environment converts baseline risk into clinical consequence for these conditions, and the clinician who recognizes the pattern before it fully declares itself is practicing the anticipatory transport medicine this text is designed to teach.

### Night Flying and Reduced Visibility Operations

Night operations introduce specific risks that are superimposed on all the clinical risks already present during daytime transport: reduced visibility for the pilot increases the risk of spatial disorientation and controlled flight into terrain, reduced lighting in the patient cabin degrades the clinician's ability to assess skin color, perform procedures, and read medication labels, and the circadian performance decrement described in Chapter 1 affects both the pilot's and the clinical crew's cognitive performance. Transport programs should establish specific night-operations protocols that address these risks: enhanced minimum weather requirements for night flights, supplemental cabin lighting for clinical work, and crew alertness verification before accepting night missions during the circadian low point.

### Scene Operations and Landing Zone Safety

When the transport mission involves a scene response rather than an interfacility transfer, the crew faces an additional set of safety considerations at the landing zone or scene: obstacles (power lines, trees, uneven terrain), hazardous materials, bystander safety, and the ongoing threat from the mechanism that caused the patient's injuries (an unstable vehicle, an active fire, a violent perpetrator). The clinical crew should never approach the aircraft while the rotors are turning without specific authorization and escort from the pilot, should maintain awareness of the tail rotor at all times, and should conduct a brief scene safety assessment before committing to patient contact. The patient's clinical urgency, however severe, does not override scene safety: a crew member who is injured or killed at the scene cannot help the patient and creates a second victim that diverts resources from the original mission.

## Post-Accident Incident Plan and Emergency Procedures

Every transport program should maintain and regularly rehearse a post-accident incident plan that addresses the response to a crash or forced landing during a transport mission, including: emergency egress procedures for the clinical crew and patient, fire suppression procedures, communication protocols for activating search and rescue, and clinical management of the patient and crew injuries in a field environment with only the supplies that survived the incident. The plan should be platform-specific (the egress procedure for a rotor-wing aircraft differs fundamentally from a fixed-wing aircraft), should be rehearsed at least annually with the actual flight crew, and should include consideration of the patient's clinical condition in the egress plan, since extracting a ventilated, monitored patient on multiple infusions from a crashed aircraft is a fundamentally different task from extracting an ambulatory passenger.

## Regulatory Framework: CAMTS Accreditation and Its Clinical Implications

The Commission on Accreditation of Medical Transport Systems provides voluntary accreditation for air and ground critical care transport programs based on standards that cover clinical care, safety, training, quality improvement, and operational management. CAMTS accreditation, while voluntary, has become the de facto standard of practice for aeromedical transport programs, and its standards directly affect the transport clinician's practice: minimum training requirements, continuing education mandates, quality review processes, equipment standards, and safety reporting systems are all governed by CAMTS standards in accredited programs. The transport clinician should understand that CAMTS accreditation represents a programmatic commitment to standardized, evidence-based operations that reduces variability and improves safety, and should participate actively in the quality improvement processes that accreditation requires.

## Additional Clinical Considerations for Transport Management

The management of patients in Chapter 25 requires attention to several additional transport-specific clinical factors that extend the principles established in the main body of the chapter. The transport clinician should be aware that the disease processes covered here interact with the transport environment in ways that are specific to the combination of the underlying pathophysiology and the particular environmental stressor encountered during a given mission, and that a management approach that is adequate for a short ground transport may be insufficient for a longer air transport at altitude, or vice versa. The serial reassessment protocol established in Chapter 2 provides the framework for detecting these interactions as they develop, and the Deterioration Signature introduced in this chapter names the most characteristic pattern by which they declare themselves.

Each patient transport is a unique combination of a specific patient's physiology, a specific set of ongoing therapies, a specific transport platform with its own environmental characteristics, and a specific mission profile with its own altitude, duration, and route constraints. The anticipatory approach to transport medicine that this text teaches is not a set of memorized responses to predetermined scenarios but a cognitive framework for analyzing the specific combination of variables present in any given transport and identifying, before departure, the most likely points of vulnerability where the transport environment will test the patient's physiologic reserve. This chapter's clinical content provides the disease-specific knowledge needed to apply that framework to the conditions covered here, while the Deterioration Signature provides the named pattern that makes the most characteristic transport-specific vulnerability explicit, recognizable, and actionable.

The receiving team's ability to continue the patient's care seamlessly after the transport crew departs depends entirely on the quality and completeness of the clinical information the transport crew provides, and for the conditions covered in this chapter, the specific information that matters most includes: the trajectory of the patient's primary condition during transport (improving, stable, or worsening, with specific details), any interventions performed during transport and their response, any new clinical findings identified by the transport crew that were not present at the sending facility, and any anticipated needs that the receiving team should prepare for based on the transport crew's clinical assessment. This information, communicated through the structured handoff format established in Chapter 2 and supplemented by the trajectory communication emphasis that is a recurring theme throughout this text, is the final clinical act of the transport and the one that determines whether the transport adds value to the patient's care continuum or merely moves the patient from one location to another without preserving the clinical narrative that only the transport crew was positioned to observe.

The transport clinician managing the conditions addressed in this chapter should develop a systematic pre-departure assessment that specifically identifies the highest-risk transport-environment interaction for each patient's specific disease process, the monitoring parameters that will detect that interaction earliest, and the intervention that will address it most effectively. This pre-departure risk analysis, adapted from the general pre-mission physiologic risk profile introduced in Chapter 1, should be specific enough to generate a concrete prediction: what is the single most likely way this specific patient's condition will interact with the specific transport environment of this specific mission? Answering that question before departure, rather than discovering the answer during transit, is the practical application of the anticipatory transport medicine framework that this entire text is designed to develop.

Clinical case presentations embedded throughout this chapter illustrate the principle that transport-specific deterioration patterns are predictable rather than random, recognizable rather than mysterious, and preventable rather than inevitable, provided the clinician applies the systematic assessment, continuous monitoring, and named-pattern recognition framework that the Deterioration Signature System codifies. Each case demonstrates the same three-part sequence: a patient with a specific disease process encounters a specific transport-environment stressor, produces a specific clinical change that could be attributed to either the disease or the environment, and is correctly managed because the transport clinician recognized the specific named Signature and applied the correct transport-specific intervention rather than the generic disease-specific response that would have been appropriate at the bedside but is insufficient or incorrect in the transport context.

The evidence base for transport-specific management of the conditions in this chapter continues to evolve, with ongoing research into optimal monitoring strategies, transport-adapted treatment protocols, and outcome data that will refine the recommendations presented here. The transport clinician should maintain awareness of emerging evidence through continuing education, program-sponsored journal clubs, and the quality improvement processes described in Chapter 24, since the standard of care for transport medicine is not static and the recommendations in any textbook represent a snapshot of evidence at the time of writing rather than a permanent standard. The principles, however, are durable: anticipate rather than react, monitor trends rather than thresholds, communicate trajectories rather than snapshots, and recognize that the transport environment is a clinical variable that acts on every patient's physiology, not a neutral conduit between two points of care.

Finally, the transport clinician should recognize that the clinical expertise required to manage these conditions during transport represents a distinct competency that builds on but extends beyond the bedside critical care training that most transport clinicians bring to their role. A clinician who is expert in managing these conditions in the intensive care unit is not automatically expert in managing them during transport, because the environmental, equipment, monitoring, and resource constraints of transport introduce variables that bedside practice never encounters. Conversely, a transport clinician who has mastered the anticipatory, environment-aware management approach described in this text brings a perspective to patient care that the bedside clinician lacks: the ability to see the patient's physiology not as a fixed state being managed in a controlled environment, but as a dynamic process interacting continuously with an environment that is itself changing throughout the transport. This dual awareness--of the disease and of the environment acting on it--is the defining competency of transport critical care medicine, and it is what this text, from its first chapter through its last, is designed to develop.

**THE IN-TRANSIT DETERIORATION SIGNATURE SYSTEM — Normalization-of-Deviance-Driven Risk Acceptance Patterns**

---

**Signature Introduced This Chapter:** Normalization-of-Deviance-Driven Risk Acceptance.

**Pattern Logic:** This Signature applies the foundational transport-physiology and assessment principles to the specific population and disease domain covered by this chapter.

**Cross-Reference Forward:** This Signature is indexed in the Anchor Section Master Signature Atlas by clinical category and population.

## Summary and Key Concepts

The management of aeromedical safety regulations, go/no-go decision frameworks, weather limitations, and mission risk assessment during transport requires population- and disease-specific modifications to the general transport management frameworks.

Trend-based monitoring with population-appropriate baselines and alarm thresholds is essential for detecting deterioration patterns specific to these conditions.

Weight-based dosing, age-appropriate equipment, and population-specific contraindications must be verified before every medication and procedure.

Advance communication with the receiving facility should include population-specific information that allows the receiving team to prepare appropriately.

The Deterioration Signature introduced in this chapter names the most characteristic transport-specific vulnerability for aeromedical safety regulations and provides the anticipatory framework for preventing it.

# CHAPTER 26: PALLIATIVE, ETHICAL, AND END-OF-LIFE CONSIDERATIONS IN CRITICAL CARE TRANSPORT

**Learning Objectives**

1. Apply the principles of goals-of-care discussions, withdrawal of life-sustaining therapy, comfort-focused transport planning, and legal frameworks in the critical care transport environment.
2. Recognize transport-specific deterioration patterns and apply the Deterioration Signature System to anticipate and prevent them.
3. Coordinate advance communication with receiving facilities for optimal patient management on arrival.
4. Integrate the foundational transport-physiology, monitoring, and pharmacologic frameworks from earlier chapters into the management of these conditions.

**Chapter Outline**

This chapter addresses goals-of-care discussions, withdrawal of life-sustaining therapy, comfort-focused transport planning, and legal frameworks as encountered in critical care transport, applying the altitude physiology from Chapter 1, the assessment and trending framework from Chapter 2, the airway and ventilator management from Chapter 3, the pharmacologic principles from Chapter 4, and the equipment and safety considerations from Chapter 5 to the specific populations and clinical scenarios covered here.

## Pathophysiology and Transport-Specific Considerations

## Goals-of-Care Discussions Prior to Transport

### When to Initiate Goals-of-Care Conversations Before Transport

A goals-of-care discussion should occur before any transport of a critically ill patient whose prognosis is uncertain or poor, whose advance directives may limit the interventions available during transport, or whose family has expressed uncertainty about the direction of care. The transport clinician is not typically the physician who initiates these conversations, but they are frequently the clinician who discovers that the conversation has not occurred when they arrive at the sending facility and find that the patient's family has not been told that the prognosis is poor, that the transfer is for a last-resort intervention with a low probability of success, or that the patient has a do-not-resuscitate order that will affect the crew's response to a cardiac arrest during transit.

### Documenting and Communicating Advance Directives During Transport

Advance directives, do-not-resuscitate orders, and physician orders for life-sustaining treatment (POLST or MOLST forms) must be confirmed, documented, and communicated clearly before departure, since a cardiac arrest during transport triggers an automatic resuscitation response unless a valid order to the contrary is immediately available. The transport clinician should confirm the patient's code status verbally with the sending physician, verify that written documentation accompanies the patient, and ensure that every crew member is aware of any limitations on resuscitation before departure. Ambiguity in code status should be resolved before departure, not during a cardiac arrest in a moving aircraft.

## Comfort-Focused Transport Planning

### When the Purpose of Transport Is Comfort, Not Cure

Some interfacility transports are undertaken not for escalation of care but for comfort-focused goals: transfer to a facility closer to the patient's home and family, transfer to a facility with palliative care expertise, or transfer to a hospice facility. The management priorities for these transports differ fundamentally from the clinical optimization framework that governs the rest of this text: the goal is not to prevent physiologic deterioration but to ensure that the patient is comfortable, that symptoms are managed, and that the family's wishes are respected throughout the transport. The transport clinician managing a comfort-focused transport should prioritize analgesia, anxiolysis, and symptom management over hemodynamic optimization, and should resist the impulse to initiate aggressive interventions for changes in vital signs that, in the context of the patient's goals, represent expected and accepted progression toward death rather than a clinical problem requiring correction.

### Symptom Management in the Final Hours

Common symptoms requiring management during comfort-focused transport include pain, dyspnea, anxiety, nausea, and terminal secretions, each of which has a specific pharmacologic approach: opioids for pain and dyspnea, benzodiazepines for anxiety, antiemetics for nausea, and glycopyrrolate or atropine for terminal secretions. The transport clinician should have these medications drawn up and immediately available before departure, and should administer them proactively at the first sign of distress rather than reactively after the patient has been suffering for a prolonged period.

## Legal and Ethical Frameworks for Transport Decision-Making

### EMTALA and the Obligation to Transport

The Emergency Medical Treatment and Labor Act obligates hospitals with emergency departments to provide a medical screening examination and stabilizing treatment for any patient presenting with an emergency medical condition, and to arrange an appropriate transfer when the patient requires a level of care beyond the sending facility's capability. The transport clinician should understand that EMTALA governs the sending facility's obligation to transfer, not the transport crew's obligation to accept, and that the crew retains the right to decline a transport that they judge to be unsafe due to weather, crew fatigue, equipment limitations, or patient instability that exceeds the crew's scope of practice.

### Scope of Practice and Medical Control Authority

Transport clinicians operate under medical control authority that defines their scope of practice, standing orders, and the circumstances under which they must contact medical control for real-time guidance. The transport clinician should know their specific scope of practice, including any transport-specific protocols that differ from their base-hospital protocols, and should contact medical control proactively when a clinical situation exceeds their standing orders or when they face a decision--such as initiating a thrombolytic during transport, performing a surgical airway, or deviating from a standard protocol--that carries sufficient consequence to warrant real-time physician oversight.

## Supporting Family and Crew Through Difficult Transports

### Family Presence and Communication During End-of-Life Transports

Family members accompanying a patient during a comfort-focused or end-of-life transport are themselves in a crisis state, and the transport clinician's communication and emotional support during these transports is as much a part of the clinical care as any medication or intervention. Brief, honest, compassionate communication--explaining what is happening, what the family can expect, and what the crew is doing to keep the patient comfortable--should be offered proactively rather than withheld out of a misplaced concern that discussing death or dying will upset the family. Families consistently report that honest communication, delivered with empathy, is preferable to silence or false reassurance.

### Crew Psychological Support After Difficult Transports

Critical care transport clinicians are exposed to patient death, suffering, and morally distressing situations at rates that exceed most other healthcare roles, and the cumulative psychological burden of this exposure produces burnout, compassion fatigue, and post-traumatic stress symptoms in a significant proportion of transport clinicians. Transport programs should provide structured critical incident stress management resources, peer support programs, and access to mental health professionals for any crew member who requests it, and should establish a culture in which seeking psychological support after a difficult transport is treated as a professional self-care responsibility rather than a sign of inadequacy.

| End-of-Life Transport Consideration | Action | Rationale |
|---|---|---|
| Code status confirmation | Verify and document before departure | Prevents inappropriate resuscitation against patient wishes |
| Symptom management medications | Pre-draw and stage before departure | Enables immediate response to distress |
| Family communication | Proactive, honest, compassionate updates | Reduces family distress and builds trust |
| Crew debrief after transport | Structured debrief with peer support option | Mitigates cumulative psychological burden |

Figure 26.1: Goals-of-Care Documentation Verification for Transport

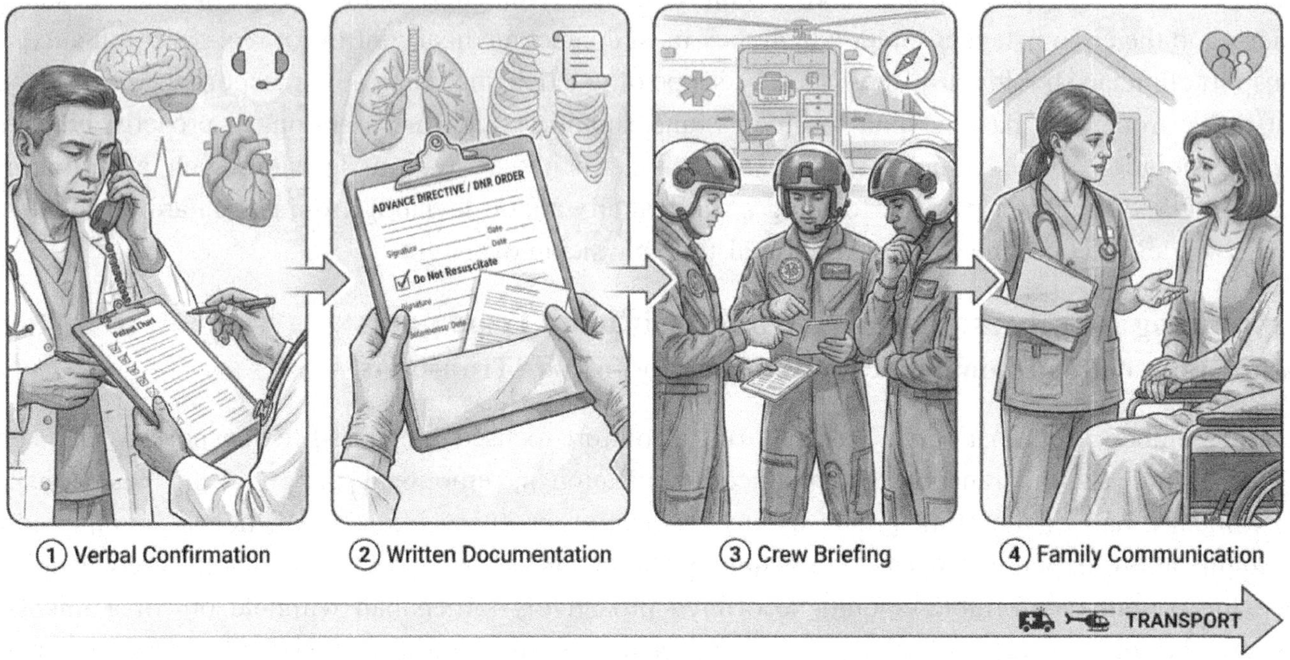


### Disease and Population-Specific Transport Vulnerabilities

The populations and conditions addressed in this chapter carry specific physiologic vulnerabilities to the transport environment that distinguish their management from adult medical transport. Goals-of-care discussions in particular interacts with altitude, vibration, temperature, and the resource constraints of transport in ways that require anticipatory planning and disease-specific modifications to the general transport management framework.

### Clinical Presentation and Assessment Priorities

Assessment follows the problem-based physiologic framework from Chapter 2, with population-specific modifications: age-appropriate vital sign targets, weight-based medication dosing, and disease-specific monitoring parameters that may differ from the adult standards assumed elsewhere in this text. The transport clinician should establish population-appropriate baselines at departure and track trends against those baselines.

## Management and Treatment During Transport

### Pharmacologic and Procedural Management

The management of goals-of-care discussions, withdrawal of life-sustaining therapy, comfort-focused transport planning, and legal frameworks during transport requires disease- and population-specific modifications to the pharmacologic and procedural frameworks from earlier chapters. Weight-based dosing, age-appropriate equipment sizing, and population-specific contraindications must be confirmed before every medication administration and every procedure, since errors in these domains carry disproportionate consequences in vulnerable populations.

### Monitoring and Communication

Continuous monitoring follows the modality-matching principles from Chapter 2, adapted to the specific population. Advance communication with the receiving facility should include population-specific information that affects receiving-team preparation, such as gestational age, neonatal weight, or specific sub-specialty consultation needs that the receiving team should mobilize before the patient's arrival.

| Management Domain | Transport-Specific Consideration | Key Action |
|---|---|---|
| Assessment | Population-specific baselines and targets | Establish age/weight-appropriate vital sign targets at departure |
| Pharmacology | Weight-based dosing; population-specific contraindications | Verify dosing against actual weight; confirm contraindications |
| Airway | Age-appropriate equipment; size-specific techniques | Pre-size all equipment before departure; confirm backup plan |
| Monitoring | Population-appropriate alarm thresholds | Set alarms to population norms, not adult defaults |
| Communication | Population-specific receiving-team needs | Include gestational age, weight, or sub-specialty needs in handoff |

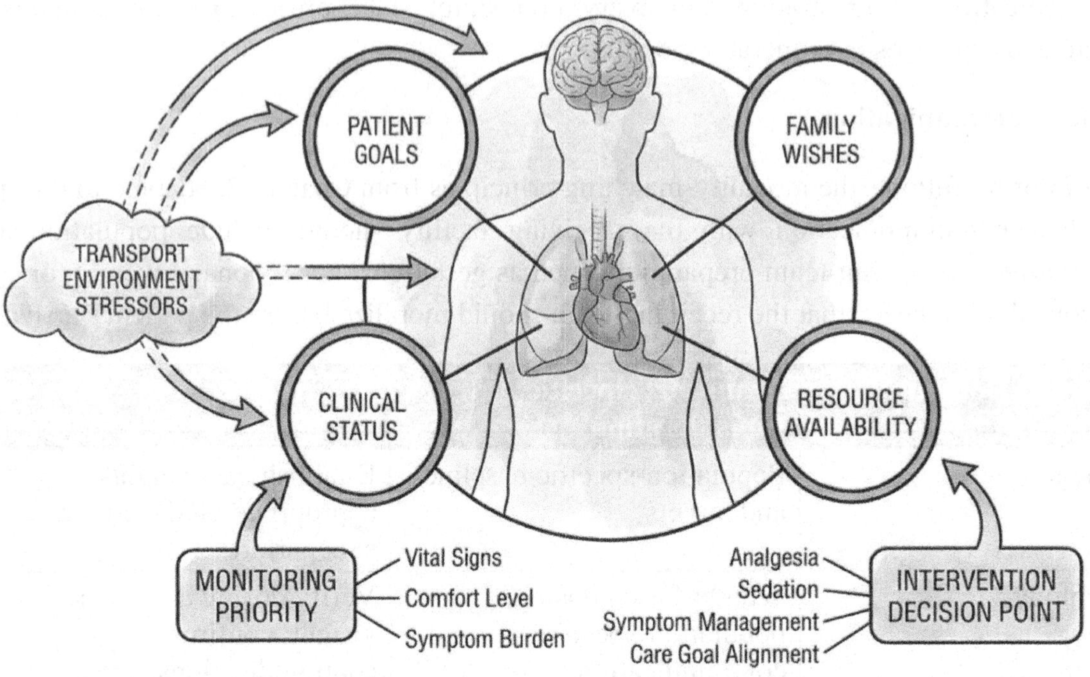


**Figure 26.2**: Assessment and Management Framework for Palliative, Ethical, and End-of-Life Considerations in Critical Care Transport.

**THE IN-TRANSIT DETERIORATION SIGNATURE SYSTEM — Unrecognized Goals-Mismatch Between Transport Indication and Patient Wishes**

**The Signature:** A transport-specific deterioration pattern in which unrecognized goals mismatch between transport indication and patient wishes produces clinical consequences that are predictable but frequently unrecognized until the pattern has already advanced beyond the point of easy correction.

**Movement Trigger:** The transport environment introduces the specific stressor or removes the specific safeguard that activates this pattern, which would not occur in the same form in a stationary clinical setting.

**Early Tell:** A subtle indicator detectable through the trend-based monitoring framework, typically appearing before the full clinical syndrome declares itself.

**Trap Logic:** This pattern is commonly misattributed to expected variation or disease progression rather than recognized as a transport-specific event requiring a transport-specific response.

**Signature Anchor:** Recognition of the temporal link between the transport-specific trigger and the clinical change is the key to correct attribution and appropriate intervention.

## Special Considerations and Complications

### Anticipated Complications and Contingency Planning

Each condition in this chapter carries predictable complications during the transport window. The transport clinician should identify the most likely complication and prepare a contingency response before departure. For goals-of-care discussions, the most consequential transport-window complication is typically the one named by the Deterioration Signature above, and advance preparation for it--equipment staged, medications drawn, team roles assigned--converts a reactive emergency into an anticipated event.

The management of goals-of-care discussions, withdrawal of life-sustaining therapy, comfort-focused transport planning, and legal frameworks in the transport environment illustrates a principle that runs throughout this text: the disease determines the baseline risk, but the transport environment determines whether that risk is safely navigated or converted into a preventable deterioration. The Signature introduced in this chapter names the specific way the transport environment converts baseline risk into clinical consequence for these conditions, and the clinician who recognizes the pattern before it fully declares itself is practicing the anticipatory transport medicine this text is designed to teach.

### Moral Distress in Transport Medicine

Moral distress--the psychological distress experienced when a clinician knows the ethically appropriate action but is constrained from taking it--is a common experience in transport medicine, arising from situations where the transport clinician perceives that the transfer is not in the patient's best interest (a futile transfer for aggressive intervention when the patient's goals favor comfort), where the system requires actions that conflict with the clinician's clinical judgment (transporting a patient who is too unstable to move safely), or where the clinician is unable to provide adequate care due to resource limitations (a patient who needs an intervention beyond the crew's scope or equipment). Programs should acknowledge moral distress as a legitimate occupational hazard of transport medicine, provide structured support for clinicians experiencing it, and create channels for clinicians to raise system-level concerns about recurring sources of moral distress without fear of professional consequence.

### Organ Donation and the Transport Clinician's Role

Transport clinicians occasionally participate in the transport of patients who have been declared brain dead and are being maintained on organ-support measures for the purpose of organ procurement, a clinical scenario that requires specific management: the goal is to maintain adequate organ perfusion and function rather than to treat the underlying condition, and the hemodynamic targets, ventilator settings, and fluid management are all directed toward preserving organ viability for the recipients rather than toward any benefit for the patient. The transport clinician managing an organ-preservation transport should understand the specific organ-directed management protocols provided by the organ procurement organization, should maintain meticulous hemodynamic and ventilatory management to protect donor organ function, and should approach the mission with the same professionalism and clinical rigor applied to any other transport, recognizing that the quality of organ preservation during transport directly affects the outcomes of the transplant recipients who will receive those organs.

### Cultural Sensitivity in End-of-Life Transport

Death and dying are experienced differently across cultures, religions, and individual belief systems, and the transport clinician managing a comfort-focused or end-of-life transport should approach the patient and family with cultural humility--the recognition that the clinician's own cultural framework for understanding death may differ from the patient's and family's, and that the family's needs, rituals, and communication preferences should guide the transport experience to the extent that patient safety and clinical management allow. Specific cultural considerations may include the presence of religious objects or texts, the involvement of religious or spiritual leaders in decision-making, specific beliefs about the moment of death and the handling of the body, and the family's communication preferences regarding prognostic information (some cultures prefer indirect communication about death, while others prefer direct disclosure). The transport clinician need not be an expert in every cultural tradition but should be willing to ask, to listen, and to accommodate requests that do not compromise patient safety.

### Documentation of End-of-Life Decisions and Their Legal Protection

The documentation of goals-of-care decisions, do-not-resuscitate orders, and the clinical rationale for comfort-focused management during transport serves a dual purpose: it communicates the patient's wishes and the clinical plan to the receiving team, and it provides legal protection for the transport clinician who honors a valid DNR order by not initiating resuscitation during a cardiac arrest in transit. The documentation should include: the specific advance directive or POLST/MOLST form accompanying the patient, the verbal confirmation of code status obtained from the sending physician, the names and relationship of any family members who participated in goals-of-care discussions, and the specific comfort-focused interventions administered during transport with their timing and the patient's response. This documentation should be contemporaneous (written at the time of the events rather than reconstructed later) and should clearly distinguish between the patient's stated wishes, the sending physician's medical orders, and the transport clinician's clinical actions, so that any subsequent review can reconstruct the decision chain without ambiguity.

### Additional Clinical Considerations for Transport Management

The management of patients in Chapter 26 requires attention to several additional transport-specific clinical factors that extend the principles established in the main body of the chapter. The transport clinician should be aware that the disease processes covered here interact with the transport environment in ways that are specific to the combination of the underlying pathophysiology and the particular environmental stressor encountered during a given mission, and that a management approach that is adequate for a short ground transport may be insufficient for a longer air transport at altitude, or vice versa. The serial reassessment protocol established in Chapter 2 provides the framework for detecting these interactions as they develop, and the Deterioration Signature introduced in this chapter names the most characteristic pattern by which they declare themselves.

Each patient transport is a unique combination of a specific patient's physiology, a specific set of ongoing therapies, a specific transport platform with its own environmental characteristics, and a specific mission profile with its own altitude, duration, and route constraints. The anticipatory approach to transport medicine that this text teaches is not a set of memorized responses to predetermined scenarios but a cognitive framework for analyzing the specific combination of variables present in any given transport and identifying, before departure, the most likely points of vulnerability where the transport environment will test the patient's physiologic reserve. This chapter's clinical content provides the disease-specific knowledge needed to apply that framework to the conditions covered here, while the Deterioration Signature provides the named pattern that makes the most characteristic transport-specific vulnerability explicit, recognizable, and actionable.

The receiving team's ability to continue the patient's care seamlessly after the transport crew departs depends entirely on the quality and completeness of the clinical information the transport crew provides, and for the conditions covered in this chapter, the specific information that matters most includes: the trajectory of the patient's primary condition during transport (improving, stable, or worsening, with specific details), any interventions performed during transport and their response, any new clinical findings identified by the transport crew that were not present at the sending facility, and any anticipated needs that the receiving team should prepare for based on the transport crew's clinical assessment. This information, communicated through the structured handoff format established in Chapter 2 and supplemented by the trajectory communication emphasis that is a recurring theme throughout this text, is the final clinical act of the transport and the one that determines whether the transport adds value to the patient's care continuum or merely moves the patient from one location to another without preserving the clinical narrative that only the transport crew was positioned to observe.

The transport clinician managing the conditions addressed in this chapter should develop a systematic pre-departure assessment that specifically identifies the highest-risk transport-environment interaction for each patient's specific disease process, the monitoring parameters that will detect that interaction earliest, and the intervention that will address it most effectively. This pre-departure risk analysis, adapted from the general pre-mission physiologic risk profile introduced in Chapter 1, should be specific enough to generate a concrete prediction: what is the single most likely way this specific patient's condition will interact with the specific transport environment of this specific mission? Answering that question before departure, rather than discovering the answer during transit, is the practical application of the anticipatory transport medicine framework that this entire text is designed to develop.

Clinical case presentations embedded throughout this chapter illustrate the principle that transport-specific deterioration patterns are predictable rather than random, recognizable rather than mysterious, and preventable rather than inevitable, provided the clinician applies the systematic assessment, continuous monitoring, and named-pattern recognition framework that the Deterioration Signature System codifies. Each case demonstrates the same three-part sequence: a patient with a specific disease process encounters a specific transport-environment stressor, produces a specific clinical change that could be attributed to either the disease or the environment, and is correctly managed because the transport clinician recognized the specific named Signature and applied the correct transport-specific intervention rather than the generic disease-specific response that would have been appropriate at the bedside but is insufficient or incorrect in the transport context.

The evidence base for transport-specific management of the conditions in this chapter continues to evolve, with ongoing research into optimal monitoring strategies, transport-adapted treatment protocols, and outcome data that will refine the recommendations presented here. The transport clinician should maintain awareness of emerging evidence through continuing education, program-sponsored journal clubs, and the quality improvement processes described in Chapter 24, since the standard of care for transport medicine is not static and the recommendations in any textbook represent a snapshot of evidence at the time of writing rather than a permanent standard. The principles, however, are durable: anticipate rather than react, monitor trends rather than thresholds, communicate trajectories rather than snapshots, and recognize that the transport environment is a clinical variable that acts on every patient's physiology, not a neutral conduit between two points of care.

Finally, the transport clinician should recognize that the clinical expertise required to manage these conditions during transport represents a distinct competency that builds on but extends beyond the bedside critical care training that most transport clinicians bring to their role. A clinician who is expert in managing these conditions in the intensive care unit is not automatically expert in managing them during transport, because the environmental, equipment, monitoring, and resource constraints of transport introduce variables that bedside practice never encounters. Conversely, a transport clinician who has mastered the anticipatory, environment-aware management approach described in this text brings a perspective to patient care that the bedside clinician lacks: the ability to see the patient's physiology not as a fixed state being managed in a controlled environment, but as a dynamic process interacting continuously with an environment that is itself changing throughout the transport. This dual awareness--of the disease and of the environment acting on it--is the defining competency of transport critical care medicine, and it is what this text, from its first chapter through its last, is designed to develop.

**THE IN-TRANSIT DETERIORATION SIGNATURE SYSTEM — Unrecognized Goals-Mismatch Between Transport Indication and Patient Wishes Patterns**

---

**Signature Introduced This Chapter:** Unrecognized Goals-Mismatch Between Transport Indication and Patient Wishes.

**Pattern Logic:** This Signature applies the foundational transport-physiology and assessment principles to the specific population and disease domain covered by this chapter.

**Cross-Reference Forward:** This Signature is indexed in the Anchor Section Master Signature Atlas by clinical category and population.

## Summary and Key Concepts

The management of goals-of-care discussions, withdrawal of life-sustaining therapy, comfort-focused transport planning, and legal frameworks during transport requires population- and disease-specific modifications to the general transport management frameworks.

Trend-based monitoring with population-appropriate baselines and alarm thresholds is essential for detecting deterioration patterns specific to these conditions.

Weight-based dosing, age-appropriate equipment, and population-specific contraindications must be verified before every medication and procedure.

Advance communication with the receiving facility should include population-specific information that allows the receiving team to prepare appropriately.

The Deterioration Signature introduced in this chapter names the most characteristic transport-specific vulnerability for goals-of-care discussions and provides the anticipatory framework for preventing it.

# THE IN-TRANSIT DETERIORATION MASTER SIGNATURE ATLAS

This atlas consolidates every Deterioration Signature introduced across the twenty-six chapters of this text into a single, indexed reference organized by clinical category and cross-referenced to the chapter of origin. It is built to be scanned in the seconds before wheels-up, during a midpoint reassessment, or at any moment when a clinician recognizes a developing pattern and needs to confirm the named Signature, its movement trigger, and its correct first response. Each entry carries the Signature name, the movement trigger, the early tell, the trap logic, and the signature anchor from the chapter in which it was introduced. No entry contains practice questions, drills, or answer choices of any kind.

## Foundational and Equipment Signatures

**Ascent-Triggered Device Flow Compromise (Chapter 1)**

Progressive fall in VAD flow or cardiac output monitor readings beginning within minutes of takeoff or climb. Movement trigger: altitude-related preload reduction via gravitational venous pooling. Early tell: ten to fifteen percent flow decrement in the first five minutes of climb. Trap logic: frequently misread as device malfunction or thrombus; timing with ascent is the discriminator. Anchor: confirm euvolemia, elevate legs, treat as preload event before device-focused troubleshooting.

**Occult Pneumothorax Expansion at Altitude (Chapter 1)**

Progressive desaturation, rising peak airway pressures, and new hemodynamic instability during or shortly after ascent. Movement trigger: Boyle's law expansion of trapped pleural air. Early tell: subtle, sustained rise in peak inspiratory pressure or fall in dynamic compliance in the first ten to fifteen minutes of climb. Trap logic: easily mistaken for tube migration, mucus plugging, or bronchospasm. Anchor: treat new pressure or saturation change during ascent as pleural in origin until excluded; proceed to decompression without delay if tension physiology develops.

**Undisclosed Trajectory Mismatch (Chapter 2)**

A patient who appears stable at departure but whose sending-facility trend data shows a worsening trajectory not verbally emphasized during handoff. Movement trigger: the handoff moment itself. Early tell: escalating vasopressor or ventilator support over the preceding one to two hours. Trap logic: the most recent single vital sign may still look acceptable. Anchor: explicitly request trend of support requirements over the preceding two hours before every departure.

**Silent Lung-Protection Lapse at Equipment Transition (Chapter 3)**

Inadvertent ventilation with higher tidal volume or plateau pressure after switching to the transport ventilator. Movement trigger: the equipment transition itself. Early tell: delivered tidal volume exceeds lung-protective target when recalculated against predicted body weight. Trap logic: no ventilator alarm because the device is functioning as set. Anchor: explicitly recalculate tidal volume against predicted body weight at every ventilator transition.

### Masked Hemodynamic Collapse Under Deep Sedation (Chapter 4)

Insidious blood pressure decline without compensatory tachycardia in a deeply sedated or paralyzed patient. Movement trigger: deep sedation suppresses compensatory sympathetic responses while transport stressors produce cumulative hemodynamic burden. Early tell: narrowing pulse pressure or downward MAP drift without tachycardic response. Trap logic: attributed to expected sedation effect. Anchor: treat sustained downward pressure trend beyond the expected bolus effect as a hemodynamic event requiring volume assessment and vasopressor readiness.

### Equipment-Masked Physiologic Deterioration (Chapter 5)

A genuine patient-level event dismissed as equipment artifact. Movement trigger: high background rate of transport-related artifact conditions the crew to default to equipment explanations. Early tell: parameter change persists beyond typical artifact duration or is accompanied by concordant change in a second modality. Trap logic: crew dismisses alarm as noise. Anchor: check concordance across at least one additional independent monitoring modality before attributing any change to equipment artifact.

## Cardiovascular Signatures

### Altitude-Exacerbated Myocardial Ischemia (Chapter 6)

New or worsening ECG ischemic changes, chest pain, or hemodynamic instability developing during ascent or at altitude in an ACS patient. Movement trigger: reduced alveolar oxygen tension tips the myocardial supply-demand balance. Early tell: new ST-segment changes temporally linked to climb. Trap logic: attributed to disease progression. Anchor: optimize oxygen, request lower cabin altitude, and treat as supply-demand mismatch.

### Deceleration-Triggered Pulmonary Edema (Chapter 7)

Acute worsening of respiratory distress during descent or deceleration in a heart failure patient. Movement trigger: transient preload surge from deceleration. Early tell: subtle rise in oxygen requirement beginning during descent. Trap logic: attributed to general disease progression. Anchor: have vasodilator and diuretic ready for the descent phase.

### Vibration-Obscured Rhythm Deterioration (Chapter 8)

Progressive rhythm deterioration masked by vibration-induced monitor artifact. Movement trigger: continuous vibration degrades cardiac monitor signal-to-noise ratio. Early tell: persistent alarm combined with concordant hemodynamic change. Trap logic: crew dismisses alarm as vibration artifact. Anchor: check arterial waveform or manual pulse before dismissing any persistent cardiac alarm.

### Suction-Event Cascade at Altitude (Chapter 9)

Escalating VAD flow alarms with oscillating power consumption during ascent, progressing toward ventricular collapse. Movement trigger: altitude-related preload reduction empties the ventricle around the inflow cannula. Early tell: intermittent, self-resolving flow dips coinciding with respiratory cycle. Trap logic: attributed to pump thrombus. Anchor: reduce pump speed, elevate legs, assess volume before pursuing thrombus workup.

## Neurologic Signatures

### Altitude-Potentiated Intracranial Pressure Elevation (Chapter 10)

New or worsening signs of elevated ICP during ascent in a patient with acute intracranial pathology. Movement trigger: gas-law expansion of intracranial air and altered transmural venous pressures. Early tell: subtle GCS decline or new headache worsening linked to ascent. Trap logic: attributed to disease progression. Anchor: request lower cabin altitude, confirm head positioning, ready hyperosmolar therapy.

### Position-Triggered Herniation Progression (Chapter 11)

Acute neurologic deterioration linked to a positional change in a TBI patient with marginal compensatory reserve. Movement trigger: head-down tilt, lateral head rotation, or acceleration-related cerebral perfusion pressure drop. Early tell: subtle pupillary change or one-to-two-point GCS motor decline linked to a specific positional event. Trap logic: attributed to disease progression. Anchor: immediately reverse position, confirm head elevation and midline, deploy hyperosmolar therapy.

### Sedation-Masked Seizure Recurrence (Chapter 12)

Seizure recurrence beneath pharmacologic suppression, detectable only through indirect signs. Movement trigger: anticonvulsant infusion becomes subtherapeutic from pump interruption or flow irregularity. Early tell: unexplained concordant rise in heart rate, blood pressure, and ETCO2. Trap logic: attributed to inadequate sedation or primary hemodynamic event. Anchor: verify anticonvulsant infusion, administer benzodiazepine bolus, communicate for urgent EEG on arrival.

## Respiratory and Thoracic Signatures

### Altitude-Driven ARDS Oxygenation Collapse (Chapter 13)

Progressive oxygenation decline exceeding predicted altitude effect in an ARDS patient. Movement trigger: reduced ambient pressure promotes alveolar de-recruitment superimposed on altitude hypoxemia. Early tell: oxygenation continues to worsen after reaching cruise rather than stabilizing. Trap logic: initial decline correctly attributed to altitude, but continued worsening missed as de-recruitment. Anchor: increase PEEP, consider recruitment maneuver, request lower cabin altitude.

### Chest Tube Obstruction Masquerading as Primary Pulmonary Deterioration (Chapter 14)

Respiratory distress from recurrent pneumothorax or hemothorax due to mechanically obstructed chest tube. Movement trigger: transport-related tube kinking, displacement, or connection disconnection. Early tell: cessation of drainage output, loss of respiratory swing. Trap logic: chest tube presence creates false security. Anchor: inspect tube and drainage system for patency before treating as primary pulmonary process.

## Trauma Signatures

### Rebleeding After Position-Disrupted Tamponade (Chapter 15)

Sudden hemodynamic deterioration from re-initiated hemorrhage during or after a positional change. Movement trigger: loading tilt, acceleration, or repositioning disrupts a tamponaded hemorrhage source. Early tell: abrupt, disproportionate heart rate rise and blood pressure fall linked to a movement event. Trap logic: attributed to expected preload shift. Anchor: treat as possible rebleeding, initiate resuscitation, verify hemorrhage control measures.

### Inhalation-Masked Airway Compromise (Chapter 16)

Progressive upper airway edema from thermal or chemical inhalation that develops insidiously during transport. Movement trigger: the time-dependent progression of inhalation injury coincides with the transport window. Early tell: progressive voice change, stridor, or increased secretions. Anchor: secure the airway early and definitively when inhalation injury is suspected; do not wait for overt obstruction.

## Systemic and Special Population Signatures

### Cryptic Hypoperfusion Behind Normalizing Vitals (Chapter 17)

Improving vital signs masking worsening tissue perfusion in sepsis. Early tell: discordance between normalizing blood pressure and worsening lactate, capillary refill, or mottling. Anchor: assess perfusion markers, not just vital signs.

### Insulin-Infusion-Interrupted Metabolic Rebound (Chapter 18)

Rising anion gap and worsening acidosis from interrupted insulin infusion. Early tell: rising point-of-care glucose or worsening acidosis despite unchanged clinical picture. Anchor: verify insulin infusion continuity at every reassessment.

### Temperature-Shifted Electrolyte Toxicity (Chapter 19)

Electrolyte-driven cardiac or neuromuscular event during temperature shifts. Early tell: new ECG changes during rewarming or cooling. Anchor: recheck electrolytes during any temperature management intervention.

**Delayed Toxidrome Declaration During Extended Transport (Chapter 20)**

Toxic syndrome declaring itself during transport because of delayed absorption or peak effect. Early tell: new symptom pattern developing mid-transport inconsistent with the initial clinical picture. Anchor: reassess for evolving toxidrome at each interval; do not assume the pre-departure assessment captured the full syndrome.

**Aortocaval Compression-Triggered Maternal Deterioration (Chapter 21)**

Hemodynamic compromise in a pregnant patient from supine positioning. Anchor: maintain left lateral uterine displacement throughout transport.

**Thermoregulatory Failure Cascade in the Transported Neonate (Chapter 22)**

Progressive hypothermia driving metabolic acidosis and hypoglycemia in a neonate during transport. Anchor: continuous temperature monitoring with active warming from the moment of departure.

**Weight-Estimation-Driven Dosing Error in the Transported Child (Chapter 23)**

Medication dosing error from inaccurate weight estimation. Anchor: measure or weigh the child directly whenever feasible; use length-based estimation only as a backup.

**Fixation-Driven Diagnostic Anchoring Under Workload Pressure (Chapter 24)**

Cognitive fixation on an initial diagnosis preventing recognition of a new or different process. Anchor: deliberately verbalize the working diagnosis and its alternatives at each reassessment interval.

**Normalization-of-Deviance-Driven Risk Acceptance (Chapter 25)**

Incremental acceptance of escalating mission risk because each individual deviation seems small. Anchor: apply the go/no-go framework at each decision point, not only at the initial mission acceptance.

**Unrecognized Goals-Mismatch Between Transport Indication and Patient Wishes (Chapter 26)**

A transport initiated for aggressive intervention when the patient's actual goals of care favor comfort. Anchor: confirm goals of care with the patient or surrogate before departure; document and communicate any advance directive or limitation.

## Quick-Lookup Signature Index

| Signature Name | Chapter | Primary Trigger Category |
|---|---|---|
| Ascent-Triggered Device Flow Compromise | 1 | Altitude / Preload |
| Occult Pneumothorax Expansion at Altitude | 1 | Altitude / Gas Expansion |

| | | |
|---|---|---|
| Undisclosed Trajectory Mismatch | 2 | Handoff / Data |
| Silent Lung-Protection Lapse at Equipment Transition | 3 | Equipment Transition |
| Masked Hemodynamic Collapse Under Deep Sedation | 4 | Pharmacologic |
| Equipment-Masked Physiologic Deterioration | 5 | Equipment / Artifact |
| Altitude-Exacerbated Myocardial Ischemia | 6 | Altitude / Oxygenation |
| Deceleration-Triggered Pulmonary Edema | 7 | Deceleration / Preload |
| Vibration-Obscured Rhythm Deterioration | 8 | Vibration / Monitoring |
| Suction-Event Cascade at Altitude | 9 | Altitude / Preload |
| Altitude-Potentiated ICP Elevation | 10 | Altitude / Gas Expansion |
| Position-Triggered Herniation Progression | 11 | Position / Perfusion |
| Sedation-Masked Seizure Recurrence | 12 | Pharmacologic / Infusion |
| Altitude-Driven ARDS Oxygenation Collapse | 13 | Altitude / De-recruitment |
| Chest Tube Obstruction Masquerading as Pulmonary Deterioration | 14 | Equipment / Mechanical |
| Rebleeding After Position-Disrupted Tamponade | 15 | Position / Hemorrhage |
| Inhalation-Masked Airway Compromise | 16 | Time-Dependent |
| Cryptic Hypoperfusion Behind Normalizing Vitals | 17 | Monitoring / Discordance |
| Insulin-Infusion-Interrupted Metabolic Rebound | 18 | Infusion / Interruption |
| Temperature-Shifted Electrolyte Toxicity | 19 | Temperature / Electrolyte |
| Delayed Toxidrome Declaration | 20 | Time-Dependent / Absorption |

| | | |
|---|---|---|
| Aortocaval Compression-Triggered Maternal Deterioration | 21 | Position / Compression |
| Thermoregulatory Failure Cascade in the Neonate | 22 | Temperature / Metabolic |
| Weight-Estimation-Driven Dosing Error | 23 | Pharmacologic / Dosing |
| Fixation-Driven Diagnostic Anchoring | 24 | Cognitive / Human Factors |
| Normalization-of-Deviance-Driven Risk Acceptance | 25 | Cognitive / Safety Culture |
| Unrecognized Goals-Mismatch | 26 | Communication / Ethics |

# CONCLUSION

This text began with a simple premise: the transport environment is not a neutral conduit between two points of care but an active physiologic variable that acts on every critically ill patient who passes through it. Twenty-six chapters later, that premise has been tested against every major disease domain encountered in critical care transport--cardiovascular, neurologic, respiratory, traumatic, metabolic, toxicologic, obstetric, neonatal, and pediatric--and in every domain, the same pattern holds. The disease determines the patient's baseline vulnerability. The transport environment determines whether that vulnerability is safely navigated or converted into a preventable deterioration. And the transport clinician's anticipatory recognition of the specific interaction between the two is the skill that separates a transport that adds clinical value from one that merely moves a patient from one building to another.

The In-Transit Deterioration Signature System, introduced in the preface and built into every chapter, is the structural expression of that premise. Its twenty-six named Signatures are not an exhaustive catalog of everything that can go wrong during transport; they are the most characteristic, most predictable, and most preventable patterns by which the transport environment converts a stable-appearing patient into a deteriorating one. Each Signature names a specific pattern, identifies the movement trigger that provokes it, describes the earliest detectable sign that it is developing, explains the trap logic that leads clinicians to misattribute it to something else, and closes with the decisive intervention--the Signature Anchor--that resolves the clinical question. These Signatures are designed to be recalled in seconds, not studied at leisure, because the clinical value of recognizing a pattern exists only if the recognition occurs before the pattern has progressed beyond the point of easy correction.

The Master Signature Atlas that immediately precedes this conclusion consolidates every Signature into a single indexed reference, organized by clinical category and cross-referenced to the chapter of origin. It is built for the moments when the clinician has seconds rather than minutes: the pre-departure scan, the midpoint reassessment, the moment when a monitor change triggers a flash of recognition that something they have read about is happening right now. If this text has succeeded in its purpose, the clinician who reaches for the Atlas during a transport will find a named pattern that matches their clinical observation, a movement trigger that explains why it is happening at this specific moment, and an anchor intervention that tells them what to do about it--all within the time it takes to read a single indexed entry.

But the Signatures are only the most visible layer of a deeper clinical framework that runs through the entire text. Beneath the named patterns lies the assessment architecture from Chapter 2: the problem-based physiologic framework, the patient-specific baseline, the trend-based monitoring discipline, and the trajectory communication that preserves the clinical narrative for the receiving team. Beneath that lies the transport physiology from Chapter 1: the gas laws, the hemodynamic effects of acceleration and vibration, the thermoregulatory and humidity challenges, and the altitude-mediated changes in oxygenation, drug metabolism, and device behavior that make the transport environment physiologically distinct from the bedside. And beneath all of it lies the pharmacologic, equipment, and human-factors infrastructure from Chapters 4, 5, and 24: the infusion logistics, the power management, the crew communication practices, and the cognitive discipline that allow the clinical framework to function reliably under the workload, noise, confined space, and time pressure of a moving vehicle or aircraft.

These layers are not separable. A clinician who knows the Signatures but does not understand the transport physiology that drives them will recognize patterns without understanding why they occur, which limits their ability to anticipate patterns in novel clinical situations that no named Signature covers. A clinician who understands the physiology but does not apply the structured assessment and trending framework will have the knowledge to predict deterioration but not the monitoring discipline to detect it. And a clinician who has both the knowledge and the monitoring discipline but operates with inadequate equipment, interrupted infusions, or unchecked cognitive biases will be undermined by system-level failures that no amount of individual clinical expertise can overcome. Transport critical care medicine is the integration of all these layers, and the competency it demands is not mastery of any single layer but the ability to operate all of them simultaneously, continuously, under the specific constraints that the transport environment imposes.

The evidence base for transport medicine continues to evolve. The specific drug doses, ventilator targets, blood pressure thresholds, and procedural techniques described in this text reflect the best available evidence at the time of writing, and some of them will be revised as new evidence emerges. The principles, however, are more durable than the specifics. Anticipate rather than react. Monitor trends rather than thresholds. Communicate trajectories rather than snapshots. Treat the transport environment as a clinical variable, not a logistic inconvenience. Prepare for the most likely deterioration before departure rather than discovering it during transit. These principles will remain valid regardless of which specific drug or ventilator mode is in favor in any given year, because they describe how to think about transport medicine rather than what to do in any single clinical scenario.

The patients who benefit most from the approach this text teaches will never know that they benefited. The deterioration that was anticipated and prevented, the hemodynamic shift that was detected one reassessment interval before it would have become a crisis, the altitude-mediated device alarm that was correctly attributed to a preload phenomenon and resolved with positioning rather than escalated into an unnecessary and counterproductive troubleshooting sequence--these are events that, precisely because they were managed well, produced no drama, no emergency, and no story to tell afterward. The transport clinician who applies this framework consistently will have many quiet, uneventful transports in which nothing appeared to go wrong, and the quiet itself is the evidence that everything went right: the patient arrived at the receiving facility in the same condition or better than they left the sending facility, the trajectory was preserved and communicated, and the receiving team began their care with the clinical narrative intact. That quiet transport, invisible to everyone except the clinician who made it possible, is the measure of success in transport critical care medicine.

Finally, a word about the clinicians who do this work. Critical care transport demands a combination of clinical expertise, environmental adaptability, physical endurance, and psychological resilience that few other roles in medicine require, and it demands them simultaneously, in a confined space, under time pressure, often during the hours when the rest of the healthcare system is asleep. The transport nurse who manages a cardiogenic shock patient through a turbulent night flight, the flight paramedic who recognizes a suction event at altitude and corrects it before the alarm escalates, the transport physician who communicates a trajectory change that allows the receiving team to mobilize resources ten minutes earlier--these clinicians are practicing a form of medicine that is as demanding and as consequential as any subspecialty in the hospital, and they deserve a clinical reference that takes their work as seriously as they do. This text was written to be that reference.

Made in the USA
Monee, IL
05 November 2026

67806917R00188